MRI-Guided Focused Ultrasound Surgery

MRI-Guided Focused Ultrasound Surgery

Edited by
Ferenc A. Jolesz
Brigham and Women's Hospital
Harvard Medical School
Boston, Massachusetts, USA
Kullervo H. Hynynen
University of Toronto
Toronto, Ontario, Canada

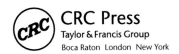

CRC Press
Taylor & Francis Group
Boca Raton London New York

CRC Press is an imprint of the
Taylor & Francis Group, an **informa** business

CRC Press
Taylor & Francis Group
6000 Broken Sound Parkway NW, Suite 300
Boca Raton, FL 33487-2742

First issued in paperback 2019

© 2008 by Taylor & Francis Group, LLC
CRC Press is an imprint of Taylor & Francis Group, an Informa business

No claim to original U.S. Government works

ISBN-13: 978-0-8493-7370-1 (hbk)
ISBN-13: 978-0-367-38856-0 (pbk)

This book contains information obtained from authentic and highly regarded sources. While all reasonable efforts have been made to publish reliable data and information, neither the author[s] nor the publisher can accept any legal responsibility or liability for any errors or omissions that may be made. The publishers wish to make clear that any views or opinions expressed in this book by individual editors, authors or contributors are personal to them and do not necessarily reflect the views/opinions of the publishers. The information or guidance contained in this book is intended for use by medical, scientific or health-care professionals and is provided strictly as a supplement to the medical or other professional's own judgement, their knowledge of the patient's medical history, relevant manufacturer's instructions and the appropriate best practice guidelines. Because of the rapid advances in medical science, any information or advice on dosages, procedures or diagnoses should be independently verified. The reader is strongly urged to consult the relevant national drug formulary and the drug companies' and device or material manufacturers' printed instructions, and their websites, before administering or utilizing any of the drugs, devices or materials mentioned in this book. This book does not indicate whether a particular treatment is appropriate or suitable for a particular individual. Ultimately it is the sole responsibility of the medical professional to make his or her own professional judgements, so as to advise and treat patients appropriately. The authors and publishers have also attempted to trace the copyright holders of all material reproduced in this publication and apologize to copyright holders if permission to publish in this form has not been obtained. If any copyright material has not been acknowledged please write and let us know so we may rectify in any future reprint.

Library of Congress Cataloging-in-Publication Data

MRI-guided focused ultrasound surgery / edited by Ferenc A. Jolesz, Kullervo H. Hynynen.
    p. ; cm.
    Includes bibliographical references and index.
    ISBN-13: 978-0-8493-7370-1 (hardcover : alk. paper)
    ISBN-10: 0-8493-7370-0 (hardcover : alk. paper) 1. Operative ultrasonography.
  2. Magnetic resonance imaging. I. Jolesz, Ference A. II. Hynynen, Kullervo.
    [DNLM: 1. Magnetic Resonance Imaging–methods. 2. Neoplasms–surgery.
  3. Ultrasonic Therapy–methods. WN 185 M9387 2007]
    RD33.7.M75 2007
    617'.07543–dc22   2007020668

Visit the Informa web site at
www.informa.com

and the Informa Healthcare Web site at
www.informahealthcare.com

Preface

The use of acoustic energy for thermal ablation is a relatively old idea. Despite serious attempts by several investigators to develop focused ultrasound surgery into an effective ablative therapy, it has been in the incubation stage as a noninvasive surgical method for a long time. In the last decade, however, since the introduction of monitoring and control by magnetic resonance imaging, remarkable progress has taken place in focused ultrasound surgery.

The goal of this book is to survey this method's extraordinary improvement and advancement when it is integrated with the best diagnostic imaging technique available. Anatomic and functional imaging with magnetic resonance imaging can optimally localize and define targets since magnetic resonance imaging–based thermometry accurately controls energy deposition. The resulting therapy delivery system with closed-loop control—first produced as a commercial product by InSightec, Ltd. (Dallas, Texas, U.S.A.)—is one of the most complex medical devices of our times.

Though we have tried to introduce and present the technique and its applications as completely as possible, a single book on magnetic resonance imaging–guided focused ultrasound surgery cannot adequately cover all recent advances. With that admission, we did detail the technical and physical principles behind the method, explain the biological effects caused by thermal and non-thermal interactions with tissue, and devote a substantial portion of the book to already proven applications, including treatment of uterine fibroids and breast cancer. In addition, we tried to demonstrate the enormous potential of this method for the noninvasive treatment of several malignancies, such as prostate and liver cancer or bone metastasis. Since the most challenging clinical application of focused ultrasound is the ablation of brain tumors, we went into considerable detail in describing this treatment method. Finally, the book discusses such exciting non-thermal applications of magnetic resonance imaging–guided focused ultrasound surgery as targeted drug delivery and gene therapy. We believe that these innovative uses of the technique will have significant clinical impact in the near future.

Targeted delivery of larger molecules into the brain through the transiently opened blood- brain barrier is considered the most promising therapeutic use of magnetic resonance imaging–guided focused ultrasound surgery. This application alone has the potential to drastically change the entire field of clinical neuroscience and neuropharmacology.

Even before this, however, magnetic resonance imaging–guided focused ultrasound surgery will have significant impact on surgery and radiation oncology. It can be characterized as a "disruptive technology" that will radically change existing medical disciplines. Our vision is that this noninvasive surgical method will eventually replace several invasive surgical procedures and, in some cases, eliminate the need for ionizing radiation.

We believe that this image-guided and controlled technique is safer and more efficient than most of those for open surgery and radiation therapy procedures. However, there is no doubt about the need to further improve the technology in order to advance clinical knowledge and experience.

Although the development of this method originated in academic institutions, it is a very complex technology that must be built with industry involvement. The device, the best example of an advanced image-guided therapy delivery system, requires magnetic resonance imaging to integrate fully with acoustic technology. To accomplish this integration, contributions from General Electric Corporation and InSightec, Ltd. have been critical.

They are not alone. Other medical companies have also become interested in advancing magnetic resonance imaging–guided focused ultrasound surgery.

In the future, specific applications and their clinical success will define the direction of magnetic resonance imaging–guided focused ultrasound surgery. It may consist of the use of high-field magnets with large phased arrays, or it may apply local focused ultrasound surgery probes or applicators. In either case, we believe that magnetic resonance imaging is essential for the technique, not only for providing thermal images but also for accurate targeting and localization. We hope the book elucidates the advantages of magnetic resonance imaging for monitoring and controlling focused ultrasound surgery therapy.

We, the editors, extend our gratitude to the publisher for devoting an entire book to magnetic resonance imaging–guided focused ultrasound surgery—a literary first. To this point, we are very thankful for the opportunity to introduce this exciting technology to a larger audience. We also wish to thank our colleagues who contributed to this book and provided early insight into the development and clinical use of this method. We hope that our collective vision of this technology is correct, and that this initial publication will be followed by several others, each elaborating on magnetic resonance imaging–guided focused ultrasound surgery's full potential.

Ferenc A. Jolesz
Kullervo H. Hynynen

Contents

Preface   iii
Contributors   vii

1. Introduction   *1*
   Ferenc A. Jolesz and Kullervo H. Hynynen

2. Fundamental Principles of Therapeutic Ultrasound   *5*
   Kullervo H. Hynynen

3. Fundamental Principles of Magnetic Resonance Temperature Imaging   *25*
   R. Jason Stafford and John D. Hazle

4. Experimental Uses of Magnetic Resonance Imaging–Guided Focused
   Ultrasound Surgery   *43*
   Nathan McDannold

5. Integrated Therapy Delivery Systems   *55*
   Kullervo H. Hynynen and Nathan McDannold

6. Treatment Planning   *69*
   Gregory T. Clement

7. Current and Future Clinical Applications of Magnetic Resonance
   Imaging–Guided Focused Ultrasound Surgery   *81*
   Ferenc A. Jolesz and Clare M.C. Tempany

8. Magnetic Resonance Imaging–Guided Breast Focused Ultrasound Surgery   *101*
   Eva C. Gombos and Daniel F. Kacher

9. Uterine Fibroids and MRI-Guided Focused Ultrasound Surgery   *111*
   Miriam M.F. Hanstede, Elizabeth A. Stewart, and Clare M.C. Tempany

10. MRI-Guided Focused Ultrasound Treatment of the Brain   *129*
    Kullervo H. Hynynen and Ferenc A. Jolesz

11. New Clinical Applications of Magnetic Resonance–Guided
    Focused Ultrasound   *137*
    Wladyslaw M.W. Gedroyc

12. Targeted Drug Delivery   *147*
    Manabu Kinoshita

13. Blood-Brain Barrier Opening   *161*
    Nathan McDannold and Kullervo H. Hynynen

14. Ultrasound-Induced Expression of a Heat Shock Promoter-Driven Transgene
Delivered in the Kidney by Genetically Modified Mesenchymal Stem Cells:
A Feasibility Study   *171*
*Béatrice Letavernier, Rares Salomir, Yahsou Delmas, Claire Rome,
Franck Couillaud, Alexis Desmoulière, Isabelle Dubus, François Moreau-Gaudry,
Christophe Grosset, Olivier Hauger, Jean Rosenbaum, Nicolas Grenier,
Christian Combe, Jean Ripoche, and Chrit Moonen*

15. Ultrasound-Induced Apoptosis   *181*
Natalia Vykhodtseva and Manabu Kinoshita

Index   195

Contributors

Gregory T. Clement Department of Radiology, Brigham and Women's Hospital and Harvard Medical School, Boston, Massachusetts, U.S.A.

Christian Combe INSERM, E362, Université Victor Segalen Bordeaux 2, CHRU Bordeaux and Département de Néphrologie, Hôpital Bordeaux, Bordeaux, France

Franck Couillaud CNRS, ERT Imagerie Moléculaire et Fonctionnelle and Université Victor Segalen Bordeaux 2, Bordeaux, France

Yahsou Delmas INSERM, E362 and Université Victor Segalen Bordeaux 2 and Département de Néphrologie, Hôpital Bordeaux, Bordeaux, France

Alexis Desmoulière INSERM, E362 and Université Victor Segalen Bordeaux 2, Bordeaux, France

Isabelle Dubus INSERM, E362 and Université Victor Segalen Bordeaux 2, Bordeaux, France

Wladyslaw M.W. Gedroyc St. Mary's Hospital, Imperial College London, London, U.K.

Eva C. Gombos Department of Radiology, Brigham and Women's Hospital and Harvard Medical School, Boston, Massachusetts, U.S.A.

Nicolas Grenier CNRS, UMR5231 Imagerie Moléculaire et Fonctionnelle, Université Victor Segalen Bordeaux 2, CHRU Bordeaux and Département de Radiologie, Hôpital Bordeaux, Bordeaux, France

Christophe Grosset INSERM, E362 and Université Victor Segalen Bordeaux 2, Bordeaux, France

Miriam M.F. Hanstede Departments of Obstetrics, Gynecology, and Reproductive Biology and Radiology, Brigham and Women's Hospital and Harvard Medical School, Boston, Massachusetts, and Mayo Clinic, Rochester, Minnesota, U.S.A.

Olivier Hauger CNRS, UMR5231 Imagerie Moléculaire et Fonctionnelle, Université Victor Segalen Bordeaux 2, CHRU Bordeaux and Département de Radiologie, Hôpital Bordeaux, Bordeaux, France

John D. Hazle Department of Imaging Physics, The University of Texas M. D. Anderson Cancer Center, Houston, Texas, U.S.A.

Kullervo H. H. Hynynen Department of Medical Biophysics, University of Toronto and Department of Imaging Research, Sunnybrook Health Sciences Centre, Toronto, Ontario, Canada

Ferenc A. Jolesz   Department of Radiology, Brigham and Women's Hospital and Harvard Medical School, Boston, Massachusetts, U.S.A.

Daniel F. Kacher   Department of Radiology, Brigham and Women's Hospital and Harvard Medical School, Boston, Massachusetts, U.S.A.

Manabu Kinoshita   Department of Radiology, Brigham and Women's Hospital and Harvard Medical School, Boston, Massachusetts, U.S.A.

Béatrice Letavernier   INSERM, E362 and Université Victor Segalen Bordeaux 2, Bordeaux, France

Nathan McDannold   Department of Radiology, Brigham and Women's Hospital and Harvard Medical School, Boston, Massachusetts, U.S.A.

Chrit Moonen   CNRS, UMR5231 Imagerie Moléculaire et Fonctionnelle and Université Victor Segalen Bordeaux 2, Bordeaux, France

François Moreau-Gaudry   INSERM, E217 and Université Victor Segalen Bordeaux 2, Bordeaux, France

Jean Ripoche   INSERM, E362 and Université Victor Segalen Bordeaux 2, Bordeaux, France

Claire Rome   CNRS, ERT Imagerie Moléculaire et Fonctionnelle and Université Victor Segalen Bordeaux 2, Bordeaux, France

Jean Rosenbaum   INSERM, E362 and Université Victor Segalen Bordeaux 2, Bordeaux, France

Rares Salomir   INSERM, U 386, Lyon, France

R. Jason Stafford   Department of Imaging Physics, The University of Texas M. D. Anderson Cancer Center, Houston, Texas, U.S.A.

Elizabeth A. Stewart   Department of Obstetrics and Gynecology, Mayo Clinic, Rochester, Minnesota, U.S.A.

Clare M.C. Tempany   Division of MRI, Department of Radiology, Brigham and Women's Hospital and Harvard Medical School, Boston, Massachusetts, U.S.A.

Natalia Vykhodtseva   Department of Radiology, Brigham and Women's Hospital and Harvard Medical School, Boston, Massachusetts, U.S.A.

1
Introduction

Ferenc A. Jolesz
Department of Radiology, Brigham and Women's Hospital and Harvard Medical School, Boston, Massachusetts, U.S.A.

Kullervo H. Hynynen
Department of Medical Biophysics, University of Toronto and
Department of Imaging Research, Sunnybrook Health Sciences Centre, Toronto, Ontario, Canada

The concept of "ideal" tumor surgery is to excise or remove the neoplastic tissue without damaging adjacent normal structures. This concept requires a noninvasive nonincisional surgical approach, which limits the tissue destruction to the targeted tumor. Noninvasive surgery would lead to even shorter recovery time and result in even less complications than minimally invasive techniques. Implementing such noninvasive surgical procedures will transform current medical specialties, change existing clinical practices, and could therefore be an important tool in reducing the cost of patient care. It is obvious that the introduction of a noninvasive tumor destruction method will disrupt the current way of patient management and require changes in the related infrastructures too. In the surgical specialty, emphasis on manual skills and practical training will be replaced by a mostly technical knowledge base. Sterile operating rooms, anesthesiology, and postoperative intensive care units will not be required, and their relatively outdated equipment will be replaced by a more advanced technology. Patients will return home and to work much faster without any significant reduction in quality-of-life caused by the procedure. Therefore any noninvasive surgical technology, when it is established and introduced in practice, will be a disruptive technology.

We think magnetic resonance imaging (MRI)–guided focused ultrasound (MRIgFUS) is such a disruptive technology. Unlike invasive surgery, it requires no incision, and the acoustic energy penetrates through the intact skin and through the tissues surrounding the tumor, without causing any significant bioeffects. Energy deposition takes place mainly at the focal spot where heat-induced thermal coagulation of the targeted tissue is accomplished. As in ionizing radiation-based therapy, the localization of the target volume requires image guidance. Using intraprocedural MRI, this technique provides the best possible tumor margin definition and with real-time MRI thermometry, the closed-loop feedback control of energy deposition is also accomplished. This real-time targeting and control makes MRIgFUS superior to radiation surgery. In addition, because of the lack of any tissue toxicity, focused ultrasound surgery (FUS), unlike radiosurgery, can be repeated multiple times if necessary.

The idea of using focused acoustic energy for thermal coagulation deep within the tissue as a noninvasive surgical method is not new. It was first proposed over 60 years ago for the destruction of central nervous system tissue (1). In the 1950s, a complex sonication system that used X rays to determine the target location with respect to skull bones was developed by William and Francis Fry at the University of Illinois (2–4). The system was clinically tested for the treatment of Parkinson's disease with success, but was not used outside the research setting (5). The primary difficulty with the treatment was the localization of target tissues and the complexity of the procedure. There were also several other researchers exploring the feasibility of using FUS for noninvasive surgery in animals and a limited number of patients [see review by Kremkau (6)]. More recently, FUS surgery systems were combined with diagnostic ultrasound (US) imaging (7) to make soft tissue tumor targeting and sonication possible. Several clinical trials for the treatment of the eye (8), prostate (9,10), bladder (11), kidney (11,12), liver (11,13,14), breast (15), bone, and other cancers (16,17) have been conducted with these devices.

Currently, two transrectal US surgery devices for prostate cancer are in clinical use in Europe and several other countries. Furthermore, external US-guided devices are in clinical use in China, where tens of thousands of patients have been treated so far. Although targeting using diagnostic US works well in some cases, the treatment is still relying on open-loop, uncontrolled energy delivery. This means that the power settings for the exposures are based on experimental and theoretical models and clinical experience, and no online monitoring of the location or the magnitude of the temperature elevation is used. This makes the treatment sensitive to patient-to-patient variations. Just the propagation of the wave through the overlying tissue layers can significantly distort the power deposition pattern at the focus (18). To eliminate these variations, the energy delivery and its biological effects should be monitored online, and exposure variations should be adjusted to give comparable thermal exposure to all patients while avoiding overexposing tissues outside of the target volume.

By using the temperature sensitivity of MRI, the monitoring of thermal ablations became possible (19). It was a logical step to introduce MRI-based thermometry for the control of FUS procedures (20,21). To do this, researchers at the Brigham and Women's Hospital and Harvard Medical School have worked with engineers and scientists, first from General Electric Medical Systems and later from InSightec, Inc., to develop US surgery systems combined with MRI. This makes online temperature information available for monitoring and controlling the energy delivery. In addition, and maybe more importantly, MRI gives more accurate definition of the targeted tumor volume than surgical inspection with eye. MRI is also superior to other imaging techniques such as the US and computed tomography in tumor localization.

The successful testing and early development or the MRIgFUS technique at the Brigham and the confirmation of their results from many research groups have resulted in the development of a commercial device that is in routine clinical use in many medical centers around the world. The device has been approved in many countries, most notably in the United States by the Food and Drug Administration for the treatment of uterine fibroids. Currently, its use is being further investigated for several other clinical applications. If our vision is correct, the future of MRIgFUS is extremely promising as a replacement for invasive tumor surgery at multiple organs and anatomic sites. Currently the usage of the InSightec system clinical trials has begun in prostate, breast, and brain tumor treatment, and there are extremely encouraging early results in palliative pain treatment of bone tumors. At the same time, there is significant research effort concerning the nonablative use of MRIgFUS for targeted drug delivery (22), focal blood-brain barrier disruption (23), and gene therapy (24–26). There is also significant progress in developing more efficient phased array transducers that can apply the treatment within shorter time and can sonicate targets within moving organs or in locations where acoustic windows are limited.

Although there is only one commercial device currently on the market, other manufacturers appear to be working toward developing their own MRIgFUS devices (27). Therefore, the editors believe that it is the best time to provide a book with an up-to-date review of MRI-guided and controlled therapeutic US for the scientists, clinicians, and trainees who are entering this rapidly growing and exciting field.

REFERENCES

1. Lynn JG, Zwemer RL, Chick AJ, Miller AE. A new method for the generation and use of focused ultrasound in experimental biology. J Gen Physiol 1942; 26:179–193.
2. Fry WJ. Brain surgery by sound. US Office Naval Res 1953:23–26.
3. Fry WJ, Barnard JW, Fry FJ, Krumins RF, Brennan JF. Ultrasonic lesions in the mammalian central nervous system. Science 1955; 122:517–518.
4. Fry WJ, Barnard JW, Fry FJ. Ultrasonically produced localized selective lesions in the central nervous system. Am J Phys Med 1955; 34:413–423.
5. Fry WJ, Fry FJ. Fundamental neurological research and human neurosurgery using intense ultrasound. IRE Trans Med Electron 1960; ME-7:166–181.
6. KremKau FW. Cancer therapy with ultrasound: a historical review. J Clin Ultrasound 1979; 7(4):287–300.
7. Fry WJ. Intracranial anatomy and ultrasonic lesions visualized by ultrasound. In: Bock J, Ossoinig K, eds. Ultrasonographia Medica. Vienna: Verlag der Wiener Medizinischen Akademie, 1971.
8. Coleman DJ, Lizzi FL, Driller J, et al. Therapeutic ultrasound in the treatment of glaucoma. Ophthalmology 1985; 92:339–346.
9. Bihrle R, Foster RS, Sanghvi NT, Fry FJ, Donohue JP. High-intensity focused ultrasound in the treatment of prostate tissue. Suppl Urol 1994; 43(2):21–26.
10. Chapelon JY, Ribault M, Vernier F, Souchon R, Gelet A. Treatment of localised prostate cancer with transrectal high intensity focused ultrasound. Eur J Ultrasound 1999; 9(1):31–38.
11. Vallancien G, Harouni M, Veillon B, et al. Focused extracorporeal pyrotherapy: feasibility study in man. J Endourol 1992; 6:173–180.
12. Kohrmann KU, Michel MS, Gaa J, Marlinghaus E, Alken P. High intensity focused ultrasound as noninvasive therapy for multilocal renal cell carcinoma: case study and review of the literature. J Urol 2002; 167(6):2397–2403.
13. Wu F, Wang ZB, Chen WZ, et al. Extracorporeal high intensity focused ultrasound ablation in the treatment of patients with large hepatocellular carcinoma. Ann Surg Oncol 2004; 11(12): 1061–1069.
14. Kennedy JE, Wu F, ter Haar GR, et al. High-intensity focused ultrasound for the treatment of liver tumours. Ultrasonics 2004; 42(1–9):931–935.
15. Wu F, Wang ZB, Zhu H, et al. Extracorporeal high intensity focused ultrasound treatment for patients with breast cancer. Breast Cancer Res Treat 2005; 92(1):51–60.
16. Wu F, Chen WZ, Bai J, et al. Pathological changes in human malignant carcinoma treated with high-intensity focused ultrasound. Ultrasound Med Biol 2001; 27(8):1099–1106.
17. Wu F. Extracorporeal high intensity focused ultrasound in the treatment of patients with solid malignancy. Minim Invasive Ther Allied Technol 2006; 15(1):26–35.
18. Liu H-L, McDannold N, Hynynen K. Focal beam distortion and treatment planning in abdominal focused ultrasound surgery. Med Phys 2005; 32(5):1270–80.
19. Jolesz FA, Bleier AR, Jakab P, Ruenzel PW, Huttl K, Jako GJ. MRI imaging of laser tissue interactions. Radiology 1988; 168:249–253.
20. Hynynen K, Darkazanli A, Unger E, Schenck JF. MRI-guided noninvasive ultrasound surgery. Med Phys 1993; 20:107–115.

21. Darkazanli A, Hynynen K, Unger E, Schenck JF. On-line monitoring of ultrasound surgery with MRI. J Mag Res Imag 1993; 3:509–514.

22. Bednarski MD, Lee JW, Callstrom MR, King CP. In vivo target-specific delivery of macromolecular agents with MR-guided focused ultrasound. Radiology 1997; 204:263–268.

23. Hynynen K, McDannold N, Vykhodtseva N, Jolesz FA. Noninvasive MR imaging-guided focal opening of the blood-brain barrier in rabbits. Radiology 2001; 220(3):640–646.

24. Bednarski MD, Lee JW, Yuh EL, Li KCP. In vivo target-specific delivery of genetic materials with MR-guided focused ultrasound. Ultrasonics 1998; 30(5):325–330.

25. Moonen C, Madio D, de Zwart J, et al. MRI-guided focused ultrasound as a potential tool for control of gene therapy. Eur Radiol 1997; 7:1165.

26. Silcox CE, Smith RC, King R, et al. MRI-guided ultrasonic heating allows spatial control of exogenous luciferase in canine prostate. Ultrasound Med Biol 2005; 31(7):965–970.

27. Huber PE, Jenne JW, Rastert R, et al. A new noninvasive approach in breast cancer therapy using magnetic resonance imaging-guided focused ultrasound surgery. Cancer Res 2001; 61(23): 8441–8447.

2

Fundamental Principles of Therapeutic Ultrasound

Kullervo H. Hynynen

Department of Medical Biophysics, University of Toronto and Department of Imaging Research, Sunnybrook Health Sciences Centre, Toronto, Ontario, Canada

INTRODUCTION

Ultrasound is a pressure wave with a frequency above the audible range of a human ear (18–20 kHz); it is generated by a mechanical motion that induces the molecules in a medium to oscillate around their rest positions. Due to the bonding between the molecules, the disturbance is transmitted to neighboring molecules. The motion causes compressions and rarefactions of the medium and thus a pressure wave travels with the mechanical disturbance (Figs. 1 and 2).

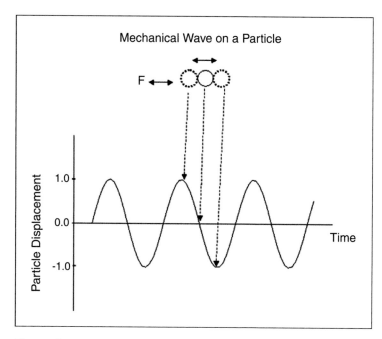

Figure 1 A diagram showing the particle motion induced by an ultrasound wave as a function of time.

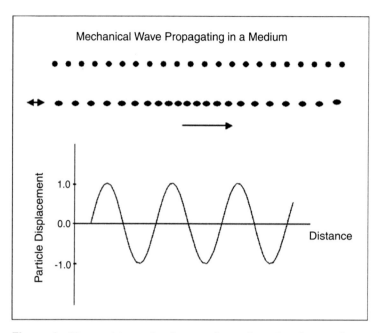

Figure 2 The particle motion in a medium where the ultrasound wave is propagating as a function of location.

As a result, an ultrasound wave requires a medium for propagation. In most cases, the molecules vibrate along the direction of the propagation (longitudinal wave), but in some instances, the molecular motion is across the direction of the wave propagation (shear wave). Shear waves propagate in solids such as bone but are quickly attenuated in soft tissues. Therefore, most current medical ultrasound methods utilize longitudinal waves (1–4).

GENERATION OF ULTRASOUND

Ultrasound Transducers

Ultrasound is generated by applying radiofrequency (RF) voltage across a material that is piezoelectric, i.e., it expands and contracts in proportion to the applied voltage. This phenomenon is the inverse of the piezoelectric effect, which was discovered by Jacques and Pierre Curie in natural quartz crystals in 1880. Since then, many piezoelectric materials have been discovered and developed. From these materials, a group of artificial piezoelectric materials known as polarized polycrystalline ferroelectrics (for example, lead zirconate titanate or PZT) is used for medical ultrasound applications. The piezoelectric property is lost above a material-specific temperature—the Curie point (for example, 328°C for PZT-4). Also, piezoelectric material rods or grains can be placed into a polymer matrix to have more control over the acoustic and electrical properties of the material. These so-called piezo composite materials are used especially in phased array transducers.

For many applications of ultrasound therapy, transducers capable of producing high-power, single-frequency, continuous waves are needed. In Figure 3, a simplified version of a high-powered transducer is shown.

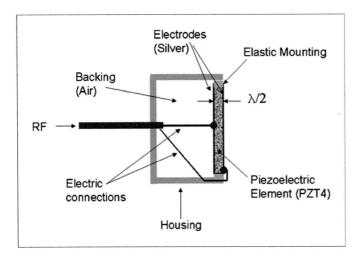

Figure 3   A diagram of an ultrasound therapy transducer. *Abbreviation*: PZT, lead zirconate titanate.

The ultrasound wave is generated by a piezoelectric plate of uniform thickness that has electrodes on its front and back surfaces. The electrodes are connected to the driving RF-line. Maximum power from a transducer can be delivered when it is operated close to its resonant frequency, which is achieved when the thickness of the plate is equal to the wavelength/2. However, a range of frequencies can be used with piezo composite materials. The frequency, which corresponds to the half-wavelength thickness, is called the fundamental resonant frequency of the transducer and it gives the maximum displacement amplitude at the transducer faces. The transducer can be driven at a frequency which is three, five, or so on, times its fundamental frequency. The conversion efficiency is, however, reduced when compared with the fundamental frequency operation. At a frequency of 1 MHz, the half-wavelength thickness is approximately 2 mm in PZT-4, thus high-frequency transducers are thin and more difficult to manufacture.

In order to maximize energy output, all of the acoustic energy should be radiated through the face of the transducer. This can be achieved by selecting a backing material so that the acoustic impedance of the transducer is much larger than the acoustic impedance of the backing. In practice, air-backing gives almost complete energy transmission through the front of the transducer.

Ultrasound transducers can be manufactured in practically any desired shape and size. Spherically curved focused transducers of various sizes up to 30 cm diameter hemispherical transducer arrays have been manufactured (5–7). Both nonfocused and focused, single and multielement transducers and arrays have been manufactured for endocavity use (8–14). Interstitial applicators inserted directly into the tissue via catheter have been constructed down to the size of 1 mm in diameter (15,16). Catheter-based applicators, inserted via the vascular route into the heart, have been developed for ablating cardiac tissue (17,18). Special care in the selection of transducer materials has to be taken when applicators for use in magnetic resonance imaging (MRI)-guided interventions are developed. For a detailed example of the material description see Ref. (19).

Basic Ultrasound Driving System

The generation of RF signals for conversion into mechanical motion is in principle similar in all systems. A typical system diagram is presented in Figure 4.

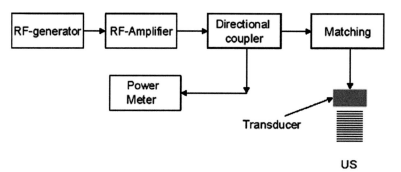

Figure 4 A block diagram of basic components of an ultrasound therapy system. *Abbreviations*: US, ultrasound; RF, radiofrequency.

The RF-signal is generated by a signal generator (analog or digital) or an oscillator and is amplified by an RF-amplifier. Commercial amplifiers and frequency generators are used in many lab systems. The forward and reflected electric power are measured after amplification in order to obtain the total RF-power that is proportional to the acoustic power output (the system must be calibrated to give acoustic power as a function of net electric power). Before the signal enters into the transducer element, it passes through a matching and tuning network that couples the electric impedance of the transducer to the output impedance of the power amplifier. The power output can be controlled either by using a fixed gain amplifier and controlling the level and/or duty cycle of the input signal from the frequency generator or by controlling the gain of the amplifier. For phased array transducers, this driving line is required for each transducer element. This has become possible with the development of low-cost drivers.

ULTRASOUND FIELDS

The ultrasound field generated by a transducer depends on the size, shape, and vibration frequency of the source. Only continuous wave fields from ideal, uniformly vibrating sources will be discussed in order to provide a simple illustration of the main character-istics of ultrasound fields.

Ultrasonic Fields from a Planar Transducer

The acoustical pressure amplitude distribution emitted by a planar, circular transducer, oscillating as a piston (radius $= a$) in simple harmonic motion, is dependent on the ratio between the diameter and the wavelength. In the case where the diameter of the transducer is equal to or smaller than half of the wavelength, a hemispherical wave is launched. When the diameter of the transducer increases, the field becomes more and more directed with a complex pressure-amplitude pattern located close to the transducer (the near field or Fresnel zone) transitioning to a smoothly decaying field past the last axial maximum that is located approximately at a distance of a^2/λ from the transducer face (Fig. 5).

The ultrasonic field beyond the last axial maximum (the far field or Fraunhofer zone) is diverging and the pressure amplitude follows the inverse law and is proportional to 1/distance. The beam also narrows toward the last axial maximum, being about 1/4 of the diameter of the transducer (-3 dB beam diameter of the intensity) at the last axial maximum.

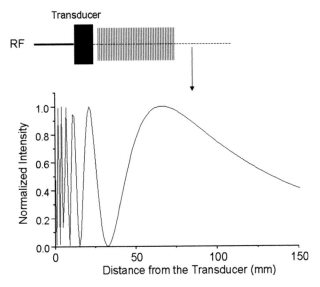

Figure 5 An axial ultrasound intensity distribution from a planar transducer (frequency, 1 MHz; diameter, 20 mm). *Abbreviation*: RF, radiofrequency.

Focused Ultrasonic Fields

If the diameter of an ultrasound source is much larger than the wavelength in the medium, then the ultrasonic wave can be focused by lenses or reflectors, or by making the transducer self-focusing (Fig. 6).

Focusing can be achieved by using arrays of small transducers that are driven with signals having suitable phase delays to obtain a common focal point (electrical focusing). The wavelength imposes a limitation on the size of the focal region and the sharpness of the focus is determined by the ratio of the aperture of the radiator to the wavelength, and the distance of the focus from the transducer.

Spherically Curved Transducers

The theory of spherically curved transducers vibrating with uniform normal surface velocity was developed by O'Neil (20). Theoretical axial intensity distributions from spherically focused transducers are shown in Figure 6. It is possible to focus energy in the near field of an equivalent diameter planar transducer, due to the finite size of the wavelength. The ultrasound field between the acoustical focus and the transducer resembles the near field of a planar transducer. Beyond the focus, the field follows the geometrical divergence angle of the transducer. The shape of the focus is a long narrow ellipsoid with dimensions dependent on the transducer diameter, radius of curvature, and frequency. The geometrical focusing of a transducer is often described by an F-number, which is the ratio between the radius of curvature and the diameter of the transducer (F-number $= R/d$). By increasing the radius of curvature (R), the maximum intensity can be pushed deeper into the tissue but at the cost of the focal region becoming longer and the peak intensity lower. This is due to the reduced focusing effect of the transducer and the attenuation within the tissue. It is possible to induce an intensity maximum at any practical depth in a human body with a suitable choice of transducer parameters, as long as the beam entry is not restricted by gas or bone (21).

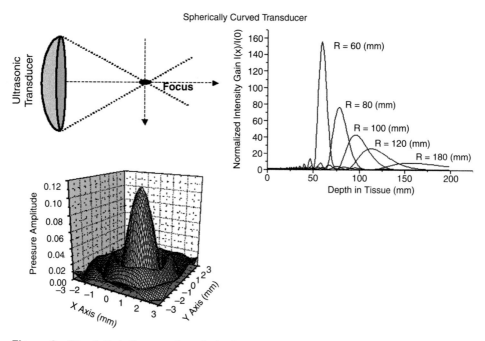

Figure 6 (*Top left*) A diagram of a spherically curved ultrasound transducer and (*top right*) the simulated axial intensity distributions in soft tissue of transducers with different radius of curvature (diameter, 60 mm; frequency, 1 MHz). (*Bottom*) A measured pressure amplitude distribution across the focus of a transducer (frequency, 1.1 MHz; F-number, 0.8).

Ultrasonic Lenses

Acoustic lenses are made of materials in which the speed of sound (V_L) is different from that in the coupling medium (V_m), causing the ultrasound beam to focus if the lens shape is appropriate. Lenses made of solids, e.g., plastics, metals, where the speed of sound is higher than in water, or liquids where the speed is lower than in water, have been used. The ideal shape of a lens is planoconcave, with $V_L > V_m$, where the generating curve of the concave surface is elliptic. By using a liquid lens with suitable mechanical structures, a single lens can offer a wide variety of different focal distances (22). Lenses have also been used to produce multiple foci in order to increase the size of the exposed tissue volume (23,24). It is possible to design low-profile lenses that can be made thinner than curved transducers (25).

Reflectors

The absorption losses caused by lenses can be avoided by using acoustical reflectors. However, the manufacturing of reflectors requires great care and is expensive. Thus, reflectors are used only in special applicator designs (26).

Electrical Focusing

Ultrasonic beams can be focused by using one- or two-dimensional arrays of transducers, with each element driven by RF-signals of a specified phase and amplitude, so that the waves emitted by all of the elements are in phase at the desired focal point. The element size will determine the volume within which the focus can be moved because the focus has to be within the volume where all of the beams generated by the elements are overlapping. Focusing to a location outside this volume will result in secondary focal spots. An ultrasound beam can be focused anywhere in front of the array when the element center-to-center spacing is wavelength/2 or smaller (Fig. 7).

So far, all of the phased array systems developed for ultrasound treatments have had a limited focal range because the large size of the arrays needed results in thousands of elements. However, it has been demonstrated that adequate power outputs can be achieved with wavelength/2 test arrays (27) and thus there is no technology barrier to constructing such arrays.

Although electric focusing and beam steering has been used extensively in diagnostic ultrasound (28), its adoption in the therapy systems has been much slower. The first attempt to utilize electrical focusing in ultrasound therapy was done by Do-Huu and Hartemann (29). They constructed a concentric ring transducer that allowed the focus to be moved along the axis but not in any other direction. Full range of axial focal spot movement can be achieved with ring center spacing of one wavelength (30). Large spacing can be used if the array is spherically curved and the focal range is limited (31,32). A similar approach can be used for achieving a limited range, three-dimensional motion with phased arrays with large element sizes (5).

There has been a lot of progress in using phased arrays for ultrasound surgery and especially for MRI-guided ultrasound surgery (32–34). Today, phased arrays are the method of choice for clinical devices, with the concentric ring design providing control over the depth of focus with added sectors to provide limited beam steering to make the focus larger (35). Phased arrays have also made it possible to compensate for wave distortion induced by overlying tissues such as skull (6). Similarly, phased arrays offer significant advantages for applicators that deliver the ultrasound energy via body cavities (36,37).

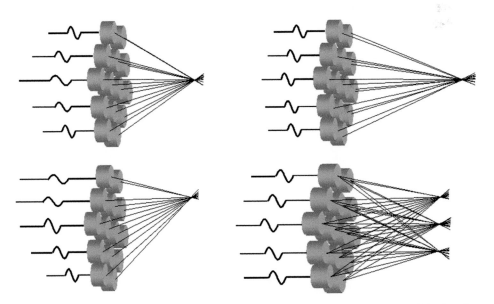

Figure 7 A diagram of a phased array focusing demonstrating the ability to control the location of the focus by the phase and amplitude of the RF-signals driving each element. *Abbreviation*: RF, radiofrequency.

ULTRASOUND PROPAGATION THROUGH TISSUE

In order to be able to use ultrasound for therapy, it is essential to know the ultrasonic properties of tissues. For instance, the ultrasonic velocity that determines the field shape and the amount of reflected energy at tissue interfaces is dependent on the acoustical impedance (=speed of sound × tissue density) differences between two neighboring tissues. The temperature elevation induced at the focus is partially dependent on the ultrasound attenuation, while the beam propagates through the overlying tissues, and the tissue absorption coefficient at the target site. The ultrasound properties have been compiled by several papers (38–40), and they have been used as the main sources for the values presented in the following sections.

Speed of Sound

The speed of ultrasound is not frequency-dependent and has a similar average magnitude of 1550 m/sec in all soft tissues (excluding lung). The velocity in fatty tissues is less than that in other soft tissues, being about 1480 m/sec while in the lungs the air spaces reduce the velocity to about 600 m/sec. The highest values have been measured in bones, between 1800 and 3700 m/sec depending on the density, structure, and frequency of the wave. In various soft tissues, the speed of ultrasound increases gradually as a function of temperature, with the slope between 0.04 and $0.08°\%K^{-1}$. In fatty tissues, the speed of ultrasound decreases as the temperature increases (41). The effect of the temperature-dependent sound speed is small on the field shape and can be ignored when sharply focused fields are used (42–44).

Absorption and Attenuation

Ultrasonic attenuation in tissues is a sum of the losses due to absorption and scattering, and it determines the penetration of the beam into the tissue (Fig. 8).

In experimental studies, attenuation has been found to be dominated by absorption (45) and thus follows a frequency dependence similar to that of absorption. Therefore, the amount of scattered energy is small and it will also be absorbed by the tissue although it may broaden the energy distribution beyond what is expected from free field measurements (46).

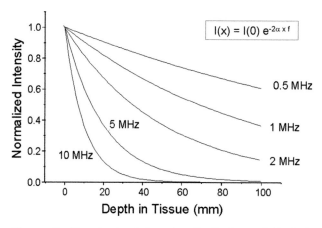

Figure 8 The simulated intensity distributions of ideal plane wave ultrasound fields, with different frequencies as a function of depth, in soft tissues (amplitude attenuation coefficient 4 Np/m/MHz).

Ultrasound absorption in a viscous medium is well understood and is a result of viscous forces between the moving particles that cause a lag between the particle pressure and velocity (or change in density). Therefore, an energy loss during each cycle will result. However, the tissue viscosity can explain only part of the energy loss experienced by ultrasound while propagating through soft tissues. In tissues there is energy absorption due to a relaxation mechanism that can be briefly described as follows. During the compressive part of the cycle, energy is stored in the medium in a number of forms, such as lattice vibrational energy, molecular vibrational energy, translational energy, etc. During the expansion part of the ultrasound wave cycle, this stored energy is returned to the wave and the temperature of the medium returns to the original level. In tissue, the increased kinetic energy of the molecules is not in balance with the environment and the system tries to redistribute the energy. This transfer of energy takes time and thus, during the decompression cycle, kinetic energy will return out of phase to the wave and absorption results. The ultrasonic absorption mechanism in tissues has been reviewed in detail by Wells (1) and Mortimer (47).

The measured absorption coefficients of tissue increase as a function of frequency according to the following relations:

$$a = a_o(f)^m$$

where a_o is the absorption coefficient/MHz and f is the frequency in MHz; a_o and m are dependent on the tissue type and m has been found experimentally to be between 1 and 1.2 (45). The measured absorption coefficients for various tissues in cat, mouse, pig, and cow are similar, with little difference among the species studied (45). However, there are more variations among the absorption coefficients of the different tissues. Generally, the absorption coefficient in soft tissues is on average approximately 3 to $5 \, m^{-1} \, MHz^{-1}$, excluding tendon and testis, which have absorption coefficients 14 and $1.5 \, m^{-1} \, MHz^{-1}$, respectively. Ultrasound absorption/attenuation has been found to be a nonlinear function of bone density and frequency with a minimum attenuation at a frequency-dependent density (48).

Characteristic Acoustic Impedance

The acoustic impedance of a tissue is the product of the speed of sound and the density of the medium. Generally, most soft tissues have an impedance roughly equal to that of water, having a density around $1000 \, kg/m^3$ and an acoustical impedance $1.6 \times 10^6 \, kgm^{-2} \, s^{-1}$. Fat has a slightly lower impedance value of $1.35 \times 10^6 \, kgm^{-2} \, s^{-1}$ due to its lower density and lower speed of sound. Bone and lung have impedances significantly higher and lower, respectively. In practice, these impedance differences mean that an ultrasound beam suffers little reflection loss while penetrating from one soft tissue to another, unless the angle of incidence is large. This may become an issue in strongly curved tissues such as breast (49). Soft tissue–bone is an exception with 30% to 40% reflection at the normal incidence of the wave, and total reflection of the longitudinal wave at angles larger than 25° to 30°. At a tissue-gas interface, all the energy is reflected back into the tissue.

Shear Wave Properties

At interfaces between different tissues, longitudinal ultrasonic waves may be converted into shear waves when the wave incidence is not normal to the interface. The attenuation of shear waves is higher than for longitudinal ones, being about $15 \times 10^3/m$ at 1 MHz in soft tissues (50,51). This mode conversion is important at the interfaces between soft tissues and bones. The magnitude of shear-wave generation is a function of the angle of incidence, reaching its maximum between 45° and 60° (52,53). Also, it has been shown that once a shear wave has been generated in a bone, it can propagate through it and convert back to a longitudinal wave at the second bone–soft tissue interface. This may be useful, for example, in trans-skull treatments (54). The shear wave speed in the skull is close to the longitudinal wave speed in soft tissues and thus the wave distortions induced by the skull are minimized (53,55). The attenuation of shear waves in a skull is frequency-dependent and is several times that of the longitudinal wave in bone being between 94 and 213 Np/m at frequencies between 0.2 and 0.9 MHz (55). It is not known if shear wave generation is an important factor in the wave attenuation at other tissue interfaces.

Nonlinear Propagation

Since sound speed is dependent on the density of the medium, the compression part of the wave travels faster than the rarefaction, resulting in wave distortion (=nonsinusoidal wave). The distorted wave contains higher harmonics, which are attenuated more rapidly than the fundamental frequency (56–58). The wave distortion increases with ultrasound wave pressure amplitude, propagation distance, and frequency. It has been shown that in a sharply focused field, the distortion is minimal in front of the focus where the pressure amplitude of the wave is small. At the focal region, the intensity increases and wave distortion occurs. This distortion results in increased energy absorption and enhanced temperature elevation (59–62). Since the impact of wave distortion increases with frequency and distance traveled, its impact on the temperature elevation, focal-spot location, or its shape is small for most focused ultrasound surgery applications (62,63). However, it has been proposed that pulsed sonications could be used to enhance the focal energy delivery (59,60,64). This may also reduce the amount of energy propagating beyond the focal and target volume, thus decreasing the possibility of undesired hot spots at a bone surface behind the target. The cavitation threshold, however, limits the pressure amplitude and sets the upper boundary for the gains achieved by utilizing nonlinear propagation.

BIOLOGICAL EFFECTS OF ULTRASOUND

Ultrasound interacts with tissue through the particle motion and pressure variation associated with wave propagation. First, all ultrasound waves are continuously losing energy through absorption resulting in an increase in temperature within the tissue. If the temperature elevation is large enough and is maintained for an adequate period, the exposure causes tissue damage. This thermal effect that can be used for tissue coagulation or ablation is similar to that obtained using other heating methods with equal thermal exposure. Second, at high-pressure amplitudes, the pressure wave can cause formation of small gas bubbles that concentrate acoustic energy. Similar focusing of energy can be induced by the oscillation of small bubbles already present. This type of interaction between a sound wave and a gas body is called cavitation and it can cause a multitude of bioeffects from cell membrane permeability changes to complete destruction of tissue. Finally, the mechanical stress and strain associated with wave propagation may sometimes cause direct changes in a biological system. The mechanical interactions between ultrasound and tissue include radiation force and pressure, radiation torque, and streaming (shearing stress). The bioeffects of ultrasound are extensively reviewed (65,66).

Thermal Effects

The thermal effects produced by ultrasound have been utilized in hyperthermia as a cancer therapy as well as in many ultrasound surgery applications. In order to induce thermal tissue damage, the exposure at a given temperature has to exceed a threshold time below which the tissue recovers. The thermal damage threshold depends among other things on tissue type and physiological factors (pH and O_2). A given intensity or power of the ultrasonic field does not necessarily induce a known temperature elevation. The temperature elevation in a tissue depends on the absorption and attenuation coefficients of the tissue, the size and shape of the ultrasound field (thermal conduction effects), and also strongly on the local blood perfusion rate (Fig. 9).

At short exposures in the order of seconds, the blood perfusion effects are small and the heat transference is dominated by thermal conduction (67–69). At longer exposures, the perfusion dominates the heat transfer and thus has a major impact on the actual temperature elevation achieved. All of these tissue parameters (except thermal conduction) vary from tissue to tissue and location to location. Therefore the temperature elevation during an ultrasound exposure has to be measured to ensure that adequate thermal exposure has been achieved.

In order to briefly illustrate the temperature-time relationship, the threshold for tissue necrosis induced by temperature elevations in different studies has been plotted in Figure 10.

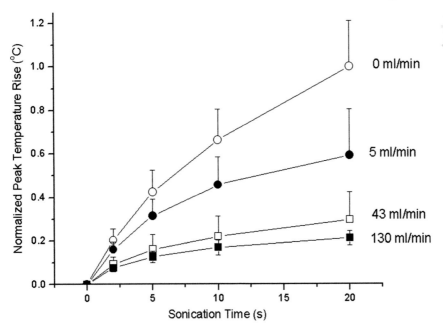

Figure 9 The normalized peak temperature measured in vitro perfused dog kidneys as a function of time for different flow rates into the kidney. *Source*: Adapted from Ref. 67.

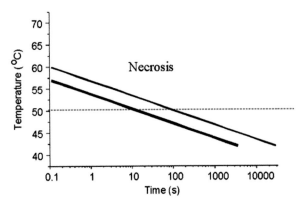

Figure 10 The temperature-time relationship of thermally induced tissue necrosis. *Source*: The two lines bracket the experimental data summarized in Refs. 70,71.

Although the actual temperature threshold varies from tissue to tissue, the threshold is linearly proportional to the log of exposure duration such that a 1°C temperature increase reduces the required exposure duration to half. This relationship is characterized by a thermal dose equation that describes the thermal exposure as the time in minutes at 43°C that achieves an equivalent bioeffect (70,71). To summarize from thermal exposure literature, a thermal dose of 240 minutes at 43°C is sufficient to cause necrosis in all tissues (66,70,71). Similarly, all tissues can survive an exposure of a few minutes at 43°C. There are however many potentially useful thermal effects at exposures that do not cause tissue necrosis, for example, sensitization of tumors to radiation or chemotherapy (71) and the increase of tissue perfusion such that higher quantity of drugs could be delivered in the tissue. Thermal exposures can enhance the blood vessel permeability, release therapeutic agents from liposomal carriers (72,73), and activate drugs or gene therapy (74–76). MRI-guided focused ultrasound can offer highly controllable thermal exposures and thus may provide a method to explore the clinical use of these nonlethal thermal exposures.

Mechanical Effects

To illustrate the effects of direct mechanical forces acting on particles in a biological medium, let us consider the impact of a 1 MHz beam, with an intensity of 100 W/cm^2. Now, the particle displacement, maximum velocity, and acceleration are 0.18 μm, 1.15 m/sec, and 7.4×10^5 gravity, respectively. The maximum displacement occurs over half of the wavelength, which is about 0.75 mm at this frequency (1). Thus, the stress caused by particle displacement is not large, and the direct rupture of cell membranes is unlikely. However, the stimulation of mechanical cell membrane receptors is quite possible. The situation is different if the wave is strongly distorted by nonlinear propagation and a shock wave has been formed. In this case, the particles are under much larger mechanical forces. The beam is also inducing a steady force, the radiation force, on the tissue in the ultrasonic fields. The radiation force in a standing wave field has been found to cause red blood cells, in a vessel of a chick embryo, to align in bands with a spacing of one half of the sonic wavelength (77). In a traveling wave, the radiation force can induce detectable tissue motion. This tissue motion may result in bioeffects. Radiation torque, which tends to produce rotary motion, is closely related to radiation force. Spinning of intracellular organs in ultrasonic fields has been reported (78). Radiation torque causes motion on a cellular level when cell walls, intracellular structures, or gas-filled spaces cause inhomogeneities in the sound field resulting in an imbalance of the macroscopic forces. Acoustic torque can lead to a steady circular flow called acoustic streaming that can induce bioeffects via strong shear forces.

Cavitation

Acoustic cavitation can be defined as the interaction of a sound field with microscopic gas bodies. In order for cavitation to occur in tissue, the presence of small gaseous nuclei, which probably exist in mammalian tissues, is required (79–85). When a medium that can host such cavitation centers is sonicated, the bubbles start to expand and contract in a fashion that is inversely proportional to the acoustical pressure. The pulsation amplitude reaches its maximum value at a frequency near the characteristic frequency corresponding to the volume resonance of the bubbles. The resonance size of the bubbles, in free fluid in a 1 MHz frequency ultrasound field, is only 3.5 µm and decreases with increasing frequency. Smaller bubbles tend to grow toward the resonance size by rectified diffusion, a process in which, during the expansion state, more gas is diffused into the bubble from the surrounding medium than is returned during the compression phase. Most of the current understanding of bubble behavior has been derived from theoretical models of bubbles or experiments in free fluid (80,83,86,87). It is not yet clear how bubbles are influenced by surrounding tissues or blood vessel walls in the body (88–90).

When a bubble oscillates in an ultrasound field, it may intercept and reradiate energy thereby absorbing much more acoustic power than that which would pass through the geometrical cross section of the bubble. This type of bubble oscillation is called stable cavitation and it causes microstreaming of the fluids around a bubble. The highly localized shear stresses may lead to severe cell damage and may be responsible for the increase of cell wall and blood vessel permeability. There is experimental evidence of the generation of these microbubbles in a 0.75 MHz ultrasonic field at intensities as low as $0.68 \, W/cm^2$, with the number of bubbles increasing at higher intensities (91). However, these results have not yet been independently verified. Lele (92) reported stable cavitation with diagnostic intensities at 2.7 MHz, but could not observe any tissue damage due to stable cavitation when the tissue samples were histologically examined. Stable cavitation may be responsible for many of the bioeffects reported when ultrasound contrast agents with preformed gas bubbles are used (93).

At high enough acoustical pressures, the bubble oscillations become highly nonlinear and the bubbles may expand and collapse violently. The transition from stable cavitation to this inertial cavitation occurs with a small increase in pressure amplitude when the threshold has been reached. Again, based on simulation and experimental studies of bubbles in a free fluid, the acoustical pressure of a collapsing bubble can be as high as several thousand atmospheres resulting in a shock wave and temperatures of several thousand degrees of Kelvin. The high temperatures may cause formation of free radicals (–H and –OH), which are chemically active, resulting in a bioeffect. The bubble collapse can completely disintegrate the exposed tissue (92,94), resulting in a homogenized mixture or a fluid-filled cavity. Although mechanical tissue destruction has been known for a long time, it is only recently that it has been investigated as an alternative for thermal tissue coagulation (95–97). The latest results indicate that the method holds significant promise (98).

The threshold pressure for inertial cavitation in free fluids increases as a function of frequency and decreases as the duty cycle and pulse length (99) increase (Fig. 11).

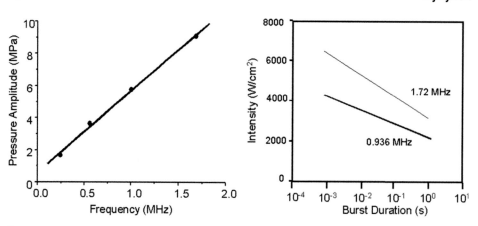

Figure 11 (*Left*) The pressure amplitude threshold for inertial cavitation in in vivo dog thigh muscle as a function of frequency (100). (*Right*) The inertial cavitation intensity threshold as a function of the burst length in in vivo rabbit brain for two different frequencies (101).

In dog muscle tissue, with continuous wave sonication, the threshold pressure amplitude has been found to be approximately 5 to 6 MPa/MHz. This cavitation was associated with a sudden increase in the tissue attenuation that translated to high temperatures at the focus (100). There are large variations in the inertial cavitation thresholds between different tissues and even between locations in the same tissue.

According to animal studies (92,94), the inertial cavitation was associated with hemorrhage and tissue disintegration and the damage was distinguishable from thermal lesions. The location of the tissue damage did not always occur at the site of the maximum intensity but, for example, tissue interfaces in front of the focus could be the initial site of cavitation (100).

Both inertial and stable cavitations cause a significant increase in the absorption of ultrasound in tissue. This results in increased temperature elevation that could potentially be useful in reducing energy transmission beyond the focus (100,102,103) and increasing the volume of focal coagulation (approximately by a factor of 4) (104). This may make treatment times significantly shorter, thus providing a major benefit for the treatment.

The inertial cavitation threshold is significantly reduced in vivo (the threshold can be in the order of 0.5 MPa) when an ultrasound contrast agent bolus containing microbubbles is injected into the blood stream. The bubbles have been shown to increase the energy absorption and the temperature elevation when compared to tissue without the bubbles (105). In addition, it has been shown that the thermal tissue damage temperature threshold during the ultrasound exposure is reduced to approximately half that which was required without the contrast agent. In addition the required time average power was reduced by approximately 90%!

REFERENCES

1. Wells PNT. Biomedical ultrasound. Boston: Academic Press, 1977.
2. Hunt JW. Principles of ultrasound used for generating localized hyperthermia. In: Field SB, Franconi C, eds. Physics and Technology of Hyperthermia. Boston, MA: Martinus Nijhoff Publishers, 1987:354–389.

3. Hynynen K. Biophysics and technology of ultrasound hyperthermia. In: Gautherie M, ed. Methods of External Hyperthermic Heating. New York: Springer-Verlag, 1990:61–115.
4. Nyborg WL. Heat generation by ultrasound in a relaxing medium. J Acoust Soc Am 1981; 70:310–312.
5. Ebbini ES, Cain CA. A spherical-section ultrasound phased array applicator for deep localized hyperthermia. IEEE Trans Biomed Eng 1991; 38:634–643.
6. Clement GT, Sun J, Giesecke T, Hynynen K. A hemisphere array for non-invasive ultrasound brain therapy and surgery. Phys Med Biol 2000; 45(12):3707–3719.
7. Hynynen K, Clement GT, McDannold N, et al. 500-element ultrasound phased array system for noninvasive focal surgery of the brain: a preliminary rabbit study with ex vivo human skulls. Magn Reson Med 2004; 52(1):100–107.
8. Diederich C, Hynynen K. Induction of hyperthermia using an intracavitary multielement ultrasonic applicator. IEEE Trans Biomed Eng 1989; 36:432–438.
9. Hutchinson EB, Buchanan MT, Hynynen K. Design and optimization of an aperiodic ultrasound phased array for intracavitary prostate thermal therapies. Med Phys 1996; 23(5): 767–776.
10. Saleh KY, Smith NB. A 63 element 1.75 dimensional ultrasound phased array for the treatment of benign prostatic hyperplasia. Biomed Eng Online 2005; 4(1):39.
11. Gavrilov LR, Hand JW. Development and investigation of ultrasound linear phased arrays for transrectal treatment of prostate. Ultrason Sonochem 1997; 4(2):173–174.
12. Melodelima D, Salomir R, Chapelon JY, Theillere Y, Moonen C, Cathignol D. Intraluminal high intensity ultrasound treatment in the esophagus under fast MR temperature mapping: in vivo studies. Magn Reson Med 2005; 54(4):975–982.
13. Chopra R, Burtnyk M, Haider MA, Bronskill MJ. Method for MRI-guided conformal thermal therapy of prostate with planar transurethral ultrasound heating applicators. Phys Med Biol 2005; 50(21):4957–4975.
14. Ross AB, Diederich CJ, Nau WH, et al. Curvilinear transurethral ultrasound applicator for selective prostate thermal therapy. Med Phys 2005; 32(6):1555–1565.
15. Hynynen K. The feasibility of interstitial ultrasound hyperthermia. Med Phys 1992; 19: 979–987.
16. Diederich CJ, Khalil IS, Stauffer PR, Sneed PK, Phillips TL. Direct-coupled interstitial ultrasound applicators for simultaneous thermobrachytherapy: a feasibility study. Int J Hyperthermia 1996; 12(3):401–419.
17. He DS, Zimmer JE, Hynynen K, et al. Preliminary results using ultrasound energy for ablation of the ventricular myocardium in dogs. Am J Cardiol 1994; 73:1029–1031.
18. Hynynen K, Dennie J, Zimmer JE, et al. Cylindrical ultrasound transducers for cardiac catheter ablation. IEEE Trans Biomed Eng 1997; 44(2):144–151.
19. Hynynen K, Darkazanli A, Unger E, Schenck JF. MRI-guided noninvasive ultrasound surgery. Med Phys 1993; 20:107–115.
20. O'Neil HT. Theory of focusing radiators. J Acoust Soc Am 1949; 21(3):516–526.
21. Hynynen K, Watmough DJ, Mallard JR. Design of ultrasonic transducers for local hyperthermia. Ultrasound Med Biol 1981; 7(4):397–402.
22. Foster FS, Hunt JW. The focussing of ultrasound beams through human tissue. Acoust Imag 1980; 8:709–718.
23. Beard RE, Magin RL, Frizzell LA, Cain CA. An annular focus ultrasonic lens for local hyperthermia treatment of small tumors. Ultrasound Med Biol 1982; 8(2):177–184.
24. Lalonde RJ, Hunt JW. Optimizing ultrasound focus distributions for hyperthermia. IEEE Trans Biomed Eng 1995; 42(10):981–990.
25. Fjield T, Silcox CE, Hynynen K. Low Profile Lenses for Ultrasound Surgery. Phys Med Biol 1999; 44:1803–1813.
26. Meininger GR, Calkins H, Lickfett L, et al. Initial experience with a novel focused ultrasound ablation system for ring ablation outside the pulmonary vein. J Interv Card Electrophysiol 2003; 8(2):141–148.

27. Khatri D, Hynynen K. Design and evaluation of a 2-D planar therapeutic ultrasound phased array. In: Clement GT, McDannold NJ, Hynynen K, eds. Therapeutic Ultrasound/5th International Symposium on Therapeutic Ultrasound, Boston, Massachusetts, 27–29 October 2005. Melville, NY: American Institute of Physics, 2006.

28. Thurstone FL, von Ramm OT. Electronic beam steering for ultrasonic imaging. In: deVlieger M, ed. Ultrasound in Medicine. NY: American Elsevier Publishing, 1974:43–48.

29. Do-Huu JP, Hartemann P. Annular array transducer for deep acoustic hyperthermia. IEEE Ultrasonics Symp 1981; (81CH1689–9):705–710.

30. Cain CA, Umemura SA. Concentric-ring and sector vortex phased array applicators for ultrasound hyperthermia therapy. IEEE Trans Microwave Theory Tech 1986; (MTT-34): 542–551.

31. Chapelon JY, Faure P, Plantier M, et al. The feasibility of tissue ablation using high intensity electronically focused ultrasound. IEEE Ultrasonics Symp 1993; (93CH3301–9): 1211–1214.

32. Hynynen K, Chung A, Fjield T, et al. Feasibility of using ultrasound phased arrays for MRI monitored noninvasive surgery. IEEE Trans Ultrason Ferroelectr Freq Contr 1996; 43(6): 1043–1053.

33. Daum DR, Hynynen K. A 256 element ultrasonic phased array system for treatment of large volumes of deep seated tissue. IEEE Trans Ultrason Ferroelect Freq Contr 1999; 46(5): 1254–1268.

34. Daum DR, Smith NB, King R, Hynynen K. In vivo demonstration of noninvasive, thermal surgery of the liver and kidney using an ultrasonic phased array. Ultrasound Med Biol 1999; 25(7):1087–1098.

35. Fjield T, Hynynen K. The combined concentric-ring and sector-vortex phased array for MRI guided ultrasound surgery. IEEE Trans Ultrason Ferroelectr Freq Contr 1997; 44(5): 1157–1167.

36. Hutchinson EB, Dahleh MA, Hynynen K. The feasibility of MRI feedback control for phased array hyperthermia treatments. Int J Hyperthermia 1998; 14(1):39–56.

37. Sokka SD, Hynynen KH. The feasibility of MRI-guided whole prostate ablation with a linear aperiodic intracavitary ultrasound phased array [in process citation]. Phys Med Biol 2000; 45(11):3373–3383.

38. Goss SA, Johnson RL, Dunn F. Comprehensive compilation of empirical ultrasonic properties of mammalian tissues. J Acoust Soc Am 1978; 64:423–457.

39. Goss SA, Johnson RL, Dunn F. Compilation of empirical ultrasonic properties of mammalian tissues. II. J Acoust Soc Am 1980; 68:93–108.

40. Duck FA. In: Duck F, ed. Physical Properties of Tissue. London: Academic Press, 1990.

41. Bamber JC, Hill CR. Ultrasonic attenuation and propagation speed in mammalian tissues as a function of temperature. Ultrasound Med Biol 1979; 5:149–157.

42. LeFloch C, Fink MA. Ultrasonic mapping of temperature in hyperthermia: the thermal lens effect. IEEE Ultrasonics Symp 1997; 2:1301–1304.

43. Simon C, VanBaren P, Ebbini ES. Quantitative analysis and applications of noninvasive temperature estimation using diagnostic ultrasound. IEEE Ultrasonics Symp 1997; 2: 1319–1322.

44. Hallaj IM, Cleveland RO, Hynynen K. Simulations of the thermo-acoustic lens effect during focused ultrasound surgery. J Acoust Soc Am 2001; 109(5 Pt 1):2245–2253.

45. Goss SA, Frizzell LA, Dunn F. Ultrasonic absorption and attenuation in mammalian tissues. Ultrasound Med Biol 1979; 5:181–186.

46. Mahoney K, Fjield T, McDannold N, Clement G, Hynynen K. Comparison of modelled and observed in vivo temperature elevations induced by focused ultrasound: implications for treatment planning. Phys Med Biol 2001; 46(7):1785–1798.

47. Mortimer AJ. Physical characteristics of ultrasound. In: Repacholi MH, Benwell DA, eds. Essentials of Medical Ultrasound. Clifton: Humana, 1982.

48. Connor CW, Hynynen K. Patterns of thermal deposition in the skull during transcranial focused ultrasound surgery. IEEE Trans Biomed Eng 2004; 51(10):1693–1706.

49. Fan X, Hynynen K. A theoretical study of the effects of curved tissue layers on the power deposition patterns of therapeutic ultrasound beams. Med Phys 1994; 21:25–34.

50. Frizzell LA, Carstensen E. Shear properties of mammalian tissues at low megahertz frequencies. J Acoust Soc Am 1976; 60:1409–1411.

51. Madsen EL, Sathoff HJ, Zagzebski JA. Ultrasonic shear wave properties of soft tissues and tissue-like materials. J Acoust Soc Am 1983; 74:1346–1355.

52. Chan AK, Sigelmann RA, Guy AW, Lehmann JF. Calculation by the method of finite differences of the temperature distribution in layered tissues. IEEE Trans Biomed Eng 1973; 20(2):86–90.

53. Clement GT, White PJ, Hynynen K. Enhanced ultrasound transmission through the human skull using shear mode conversion. J Acoust Soc Am 2004; 115(3):1356–1364.

54. Clement GT, Hynynen K. Forward planar projection through layered media. IEEE Trans Ultrason Ferroelectr Freq Contr 2003; 50(12):1689–1698.

55. White PJ, Clement GT, Hynynen K. Longitudinal and shear mode ultrasound propagation in human skull bone. Ultrasound Med Biol 2006; 32(7):1085–1096.

56. Carstensen EL, Becroft SA, Law WK, Barber DB. Finite amplitude effects on thresholds for lesion production in tissues by unfocussed ultrasound. J Acoust Soc Am 1981; 70:302–309.

57. Carstensen EL, McKay ND, Dalecki D, Muir TG. Absorption of finite amplitude ultrasound in tissues. Acoustica 1982; 51(2):116–123.

58. Duck FA. Nonlinear acoustics in diagnostic ultrasound. Ultrasound Med Biol 2002; 28(1):1–18.

59. Swindell W. A theoretical study of nonlinear effects with focused ultrasound in tissues: an acoustic Bragg peak. Ultrasound Med Biol 1985; 11:121–130.

60. Hynynen K. Demonstration of enhanced temperature elevation due to nonlinear propagation of focused ultrasound in dog's thigh in vivo. Ultrasound Med Biol 1987; 13:85–91.

61. Hynynen K. The role of nonlinear ultrasound propagation during hyperthermia treatments. Med Phys 1991; 18:1156–1163.

62. Connor CW, Hynynen K. Bio-acoustic thermal lensing and nonlinear propagation in focused ultrasound surgery using large focal spots: a parametric study. Phys Med Biol 2002; 47(11):1911–1928.

63. Watkin NA, ter Haar GR, Rivens I. The intensity dependence of the site of maximal energy deposition in focused ultrasound surgery. Ultrasound Med Biol 1996; 22(4):483–491.

64. Khokhlova VA, Bailey MR, Reed J, Canney MS, Kaczkowski P, Crum LA. Nonlinear mechanisms of lesion formation by high intensity focused ultrasound. In: Clement GT, McDannold NJ, Hynynen K, eds. Therapeutic Ultrasound/5th International Symposium on Therapeutic Ultrasound, Boston, Massachusetts, 27–29 October 2005. Melville, NY: American Institute of Physics, 2006.

65. NCRP Report No. 113. Exposure Criteria for Medical Diagnostic Ultrasound: I. Criteria Based on Thermal Mechanisms. Bethesda, MD: NCRP, 1992.

66. National Council on Radiation Protection and Measurements. Scientific Committee 66 on Biological Effects of Ultrasound. Beou. Exposure Criteria for Medical Diagnostic Ultrasound II—Criteria Based on All Known Mechanisms/Recommendations of the National Council on Radiation Protection and Measurements. Bethesda, MD: National Council on Radiation Protection and Measurements, 2002.

67. Billard BE, Hynynen K, Roemer RB. Effects of physical parameters on high temperature ultrasound hyperthermia. Ultrasound Med Biol 1990; 16:409–420.

68. Kolios MC, Sherar MD, Hunt JW. Blood flow cooling and ultrasonic lesion formation. Med Phys 1996; 23(7):1287–1298.

69. Dorr LN, Hynynen K. The effect of tissue heterogeneities and large blood vessels on the thermal exposure induced by short high power ultrasound pulses. Int J Hyperthermia 1992; 8:45–59.

70. Sapareto SA, Dewey WC. Thermal dose determination in cancer therapy. Int J Radiation Oncology Biol Phys 1984; 10:787–800.

71. Dewhirst MW, Viglianti BL, Lora-Michiels M, Hanson M, Hoopes PJ. Basic principles of thermal dosimetry and thermal thresholds for tissue damage from hyperthermia. Int J Hyperthermia 2003; 19(3):267–294.

72. Magin RL, Niesman MR. Temperature-dependent drug release from large unilamellar liposomes. Cancer Drug Deliv 1984; 1(2):109–117.

73. Needham D, Dewhirst MW. The development and testing of a new temperature-sensitive drug delivery system for the treatment of solid tumors. Adv Drug Deliv Rev 2001; 53(3): 285–305.

74. Moonen C, Madio D, de Zwart J, et al. MRI-guided focused ultrasound as a potential tool for control of gene therapy. Eur Radiol 1997; 7:1165.

75. Bednarski MD, Lee JW, Yuh EL, Li KCP. In vivo target-specific delivery of genetic materials with MR-guided focused ultrasound. Ultrasonics 1998; 30(5):325–330.

76. Silcox CE, Smith RC, King R, et al. MRI-guided ultrasonic heating allows spatial control of exogenous luciferase in canine prostate. Ultrasound Med Biol 2005; 31(7):965–970.

77. Dyson M, Pond JB, Woodward B, Broadbent J. The production of blood cell stasis and endothelial damage in the blood vessels of chick embryos treated with ultrasound in a stationary wave field. Ultrasound Med Biol 1974; 1(2):133–148.

78. Martin CJ, Pratt BM, Watmough DJ. Observations of ultrasound-induced effects in the fish Xiphophorous maculatus. Ultrasound Med Biol 1983; 9(2):177–183.

79. Crum LA, Fowlkes JB. Acoustic cavitation generated by microsecond pulses of ultrasound. Nature 1986; 319:52–54.

80. Apfel RE. Acoustic cavitation: a possible consequence of biomedical use of ultrasound. Br J Cancer 1995; (suppl V):140–146.

81. Carstensen EL, Flynn HG. The potential for transient cavitation with microsecond pulses of ultrasound. Ultrasound Med Biol 1982; 8(6):L720–L724.

82. Fry FJ, Sanghvi NT, Foster RS, Bihrle R, Hennige C. Ultrasound and microbubbles: their generation, detection and potential utilization in tissue and organ therapy—experimental. Ultrasound Med Biol 1995; 21(9):1227–1237.

83. Holland CK, Apfel RE. An improved theory for the prediction of microcavitation threshold. IEEE Trans Ultrason Ferroelectr Freq Contr 1989; 36:204–208.

84. Margulis MA. Sonochemistry of Cavitation. Luxembourg: Gordon and Breach Publishers, 1995.

85. Leighton TG. The Acoustic Bubble. London: Academic Press, 1994.

86. Young IR. Cavitation. New York: McGraw-Hill Book Company, 1989.

87. Kimmel E. Cavitation bioeffects. Crit Rev Biomed Eng 2006; 34(2):105–161.

88. Sassaroli E, Hynynen K. Forced linear oscillations of microbubbles in blood capillaries. J Acoust Soc Am 2004; 115(6):3235–3243.

89. Lindner JR, Kaul S. Delivery of drugs with ultrasound. Echocardiography 2001; 18(4): 329–337.

90. Qin S, Ferrara KW. Acoustic response of compliable microvessels containing ultrasound contrast agents. Phys Med Biol 2006; 51(20):5065–5088.

91. ter Haar GR, Daniels S, Eastaugh KC, Hill CR. Ultrasonically induced cavitation in vivo. Br J Cancer 1982; 45:151–155.

92. Lele PP. Threshold and mechanisms of ultrasonic damage to organized animal tissues. Proceedings of a Symposium on Biological Effects and Characterization of Ultrasound Sources 1977; Rockville, MD, June 1–3, 224–239.

93. McDannold N, Vykhodtseva N, Hynynen K. Targeted disruption of the blood-brain barrier with focused ultrasound: association with cavitation activity. Phys Med Biol 2006; 51(4): 793–807.

94. Vykhodtseva NI, Hynynen K, Damianou C. The effect of pulse duration and peak intensity during focused ultrasound surgery: a theoretical and experimental study in rabbit brain in vivo. Ultrasound Med Biol 1994; 20:987–1000.

95. Smith NB, Hynynen K. The feasibility of using focused ultrasound for transmyocardial revascularization. Ultrasound Med Biol 1998; 24(7):1045–1054.

96. Xu Z, Ludomirsky A, Eun LY, et al. Controlled ultrasound tissue erosion. IEEE Trans Ultrason Ferroelectr Freq Contr 2004; 51(6):726–736.

97. Xu Z, Fowlkes JB, Rothman ED, Levin AM, Cain CA. Controlled ultrasound tissue erosion: the role of dynamic interaction between insonation and microbubble activity. J Acoust Soc Am 2005; 117(1):424–435.

98. Xu Z, Fowlkes JB, Cain CA. A new strategy to enhance cavitational tissue erosion using a high-intensity, initiating sequence. IEEE Trans Ultrason Ferroelectr Freq Contr 2006; 53(8): 1412–1424.

99. Hill CR. Ultrasonic exposure thresholds for changes in cells and tissues. J Acoust Soc Am 1972; 52:667–672.

100. Hynynen K. The threshold for thermally significant cavitation in dog's thigh muscle in vivo. Ultrasound Med Biol 1991; 17:157–169.

101. Vykhodtseva NI, Hynynen K, Damianou C. Histologic effects of high intensity pulsed ultrasound exposure with subharmonic emission in rabbit brain in vivo. Ultrasound Med Biol 1995; 21(7):969–979.

102. Lele PP. Cavitation and its effects on organized mammalian tissues. In: Fry FJ, ed. Ultrasound: Its Applications in Medicine and Biology. Part II. Amsterdam: Elsevier, 1978: 737–741.

103. Holt RG, Roy RA. Measurements of bubble-enhanced heating from focused, MHz-frequency ultrasound in a tissue-mimicking material. Ultrasound Med Biol 2001; 27(10):1399–1412.

104. Sokka SD, King R, Hynynen K. MRI-guided gas bubble enhanced ultrasound heating in in vivo rabbit thigh. Phys Med Biol 2003; 48(2):223–241.

105. McDannold NJ, Vykhodtseva NI, Hynynen K. Microbubble contrast agent with focused ultrasound to create brain lesions at low power levels: MR imaging and histologic study in rabbits. Radiology 2006; 241(1):95–106.

3
Fundamental Principles of Magnetic Resonance Temperature Imaging

R. Jason Stafford and John D. Hazle
Department of Imaging Physics, The University of Texas M. D. Anderson Cancer Center, Houston, Texas, U.S.A.

TEMPERATURE SENSITIVITY OF MAGNETIC RESONANCE IMAGING

Since both the chemical environment and relaxation properties of the nuclei that are the source of the signal in magnetic resonance (MR) are sensitive to Brownian motion and the associated molecular tumbling rates, MR imaging (MRI) techniques are intrinsically sensitive to temperature. Of the many MR parameters that can provide temperature-sensitive contrast, the temperature dependence and sensitivity of several parameters in particular, have proven useful for monitoring temperature changes in soft tissue during delivery of hyperthermia or thermal therapies: the apparent diffusion constant of water (D), the spin-lattice relaxation time (T_1), and the water proton resonance frequency (PRF). The temperature sensitivities associated with each of these parameters are large enough to allow temperature-dependent changes to be observed quantitatively using either direct or indirect measurements using standard MRI devices over a range of temperatures relevant for thermal therapy. The development of these techniques to noninvasively measure temperature changes in tissue has brought renewed interest in using these techniques to enhance the guidance of thermal therapy treatments.

Of the available radiological imaging modalities capable of providing real-time temperature feedback, MRI has the desirable properties of excellent soft-tissue contrast and the ability to provide fast, quantitative temperature imaging in a variety of tissue (1,2). This technology, in concert with the other benefits of MRI for guidance of therapy, led to the investment of significant time and resources to develop specially designed MR suites adapted to the intraoperative and interventional environments (Fig. 1).

Temperature Sensitivity of the Molecular Diffusion Coefficient of Water

Molecular water mobility due to thermal Brownian motion is quantified by the molecular diffusion coefficient of water, which is, by definition, a temperature-dependent process and can be quantified using MRI via the apparent diffusion coefficient (3). A direct relationship exists between temperature and the diffusion coefficient (D) via the Stokes-Einstein relationship:

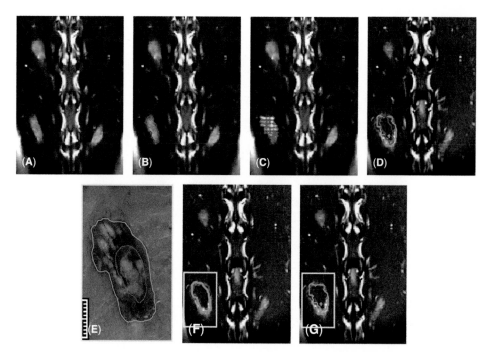

Figure 1 (*See color insert.*) Demonstration of MR guidance for treatment planning, monitoring, and verification of focused ultrasound treatment delivery from a prototype system used to ablate a canine transmissible venereal tumor inoculated in the paraspinal muscle. Subject is imaged and the target region identified using T_2-weighted imaging (**A**). Target (*red*) is then delineated on the treatment planning image (**B**). Complex phase-difference MR temperature imaging using the temperature sensitivity of the proton resonance frequency to visualize a series of 10-second pulsed focused ultrasound treatments, which are applied in raster form across the target to cover the prescribed area (approximately 45 seconds of wait time between consecutive pulses to minimize heating in the near field) (**C**). Contrast-enhanced T_1-weighted imaging results, registered to the treatment plan and MRTI results, verify the treatment delivery by demonstrating hypointense regions where tissue perfusion has shut down (**D**). A pathology photograph of the excised tissue in nearly the same slice shows the estimated region of ablation (*green*) and the tumor (*red*) in (**E**). This tissue section (*yellow*) and the associated estimated damage are overlaid on the contrast-enhanced T_1-weighted image (*green*) to visualize the high degree of correlation between the T_1-weighted verification image, pathology (**F**), and MRTI damage estimates based on a threshold of 57°C (**G**). *Abbreviations*: MR, magnetic resonance; MRTI, magnetic resonance temperature imaging.

$$D \approx D_0 e^{\frac{E_a}{kT}} \tag{1}$$

where E_a is the activation energy of the material (approximately 0.2 eV at 20°C for water), k is Boltzmann's constant (8.617e_5 eV/K), and T is the absolute temperature in Kelvin. From this expression, it can be shown that for a temperature change (ΔT) that is small with respect to the initial temperature (T_0), a corresponding shift in diffusion (ΔD) with respect to the initial diffusion value (D_0) is seen.

$$\Delta T = \frac{kT_0^2}{E_a} \frac{\Delta D}{D_0} \tag{2}$$

Theoretically, this yields a temperature sensitivity of approximately 2.4% for pure water, making it one of the most sensitive MR temperature imaging (MRTI) techniques (4,5). Water mobility is strongly correlated with the degree of hydrogen bonding and the relative ion content of the water (such as sodium, calcium, and potassium). In tissue, mobility of the fast diffusing component is impacted by the tortuosity of the environment from cellular level structures (6), which is significant given the low b-values used for MRTI in order to maintain signal-to-noise ratio (SNR) (generally $\leq 500 \sec/mm^2$) (7). With common diffusion times of 50 msec, root mean square displacement is on the order of 8 vm, which is on the order of the size of the cell, leading to a high probability of intracellular or extracellular water having interaction with some semipermeable structure such as a cell membrane.

In light of this, water mobility in tissue tends to be more complex, resulting in activation energy that is both tissue-dependent and can display some level of anisotropy. Additionally, over time, physiological responses, such as edema, ischemia, cellular swelling, and protein coagulation, can result in local diffusion changes that cannot be separated from the temperature-dependent changes being measured.

Diffusion weighting can be added to virtually any MR pulse sequence by adding a pair of balanced gradients, which lead to a net dephasing of moving spins while stationary spins are refocused. The signal as a function of the diffusion constant is related to the gradient pulse amplitude and timing as

$$S = S_0 e^{-bD}$$

with

$$b = \gamma^2 G^2 \delta^2 \left(\Delta - \frac{\delta}{3} \right) \tag{3}$$

where the b-value is calculated from the known quantities of the gyromagnetic ratio (γ), peak gradient amplitude (G), time between gradient lobes (Δ), and the duration of the diffusion sensitizing gradients (δ) (8). Since acquisition of multiple b-values for extrapolating the diffusion constant (or tensor) takes time, usually only two b-values are used. To help minimize effects of anisotropy, three orthogonal directions can be used, at the cost of imaging time and increased potential motion contamination, to calculate the trace of the diffusion tensor.

Echo-planar imaging (EPI) is widely held to be the current gold standard for rapid diffusion imaging (9,10). However, a wide variety of alternate methods of acquiring diffusion-weighted images using fast spin-echo (FSE), PROPELLER, line scans, and spiral acquisitions are also becoming available. When using sequences that are not fat suppressed, it is important to note that the temperature sensitivity of the diffusion coefficient of fat is different from that of water and will cause measurement errors. For the rates of heating and spatial resolutions associated with temperature monitoring of focused ultrasound ablation, single shot acquisitions are preferred in that they enhance the acquisition speed and minimize the effects of motion, but with compromises in the spatial resolution, SNR, and proclivity to artifacts (4,11). Unfortunately, diffusion methods are extremely sensitive to low SNR, and so techniques that trade off SNR for spatiotemporal resolution, are not feasible for temperature monitoring applications.

It should be noted that new hardware available on most high-field (≥ 1.5 Tesla) scanners, such as high performance gradients with better eddy current compensation, fast phased-array receivers compatible with EPI techniques and parallel imaging techniques, facilitate better resolution, SNR and artifact control for EPI-based diffusion techniques, necessitating a possible re-evaluation of this technique for temperature monitoring of rapid ablations in vivo. That being said, critical in vivo evaluation and validation studies in different tissues are still needed and will be valuable in assessing the appropriateness of the diffusion technique for thermal ablation, particularly at higher field strengths where separation between the fast and slow components of water diffusion may be investigated during application of therapy.

Temperature Sensitivity of the Spin-Lattice Relaxation Time

The first parameter to be used for temperature imaging for therapeutic monitoring was the spin-lattice relaxation time (T_1) (12,13). T_1 is an indicator of how long it takes the nuclear spins to relax back into a state of thermal equilibrium, where the original net magnetization along the longitudinal axis of the static field is regained, after being rotated off the axis. For water protons, the primary mechanism for T_1 relaxation is dipole-dipole interaction. To first order, the T_1 relaxation time is inversely proportional to the correlation time (τc), which can be related to molecular diffusion. The temperature dependence of T_1, like the diffusion coefficient, is extremely sensitive to temperature-dependent Brownian motion (14) and, when the ensemble of correlation times in a voxel are assumed to be similar, is approximately dependent on the temperature according to

$$T_1 \propto T_1(0)e^{\frac{E_a}{kT}} \tag{4}$$

where, in this case, the activation energy is for the T_1 process and, because of this, the T_1 temperature dependence relies critically on the tissue type. An unfortunate limitation of the technique, however, is that T_1 relaxation and its temperature sensitivity are additionally linked to the exchange processes between water in different bound states, making the technique extremely dependent on the tissue environment. As higher temperatures are reached, thermal protein denaturation can cause irreversible T_1 parameter changes due to structural changes in the surrounding proteins. Such changes cannot be separated in any easy fashion from the temperature-dependent changes that are happening concurrently, the result being a loss in the ability to quantitatively track the temperature as thermal coagulation occurs in the region of treatment.

The spin-lattice relaxation time, T_1, increases with increasing temperature. The response to temperature changes is approximately linear for temperatures that do not cause irreversible damage in tissue ($T < 55°C$) (15). As stated, the temperature sensitivity of the technique is highly tissue-dependent, ranging from about $0.8\%°C^{-1}$ to $2.0\%°C^{-1}$ (13,16). The accuracy of the method is heavily dependent on the accuracy of the T_1 measurement, making it the most difficult of the three methods mentioned here to perform accurately with fast imaging techniques.

Tissue T_1 values can be calculated by fitting a multipoint recovery curve to a series of measurement experiments, as is done with inversion recovery and repeated saturation recovery experiments (17). While these techniques do provide the most accurate estimate of T_1, they are also time-consuming, making them poor candidates for thermal ablation MRTI applications. Techniques such as a multiflip angle fast gradient-recalled echo imaging are faster, but yield larger inaccuracies (18). Modern implementations for thermal ablation procedures rely on a long repetition time (TR) baseline image ($TR_0 = \infty$) or a series of magnetization prep pulses followed by a fast, short TR acquisition, such as FSE or fast gradient-recalled echo (2,19,20).

Using an FSE acquisition strategy, a two-point calculation of T_1 can be made from the ratio of the baseline image (S_0) taken at temperature T_0 to the subsequent nth image (S_n) taken at temperature $T_0 + \Delta T$ according to the relation,

$$\frac{S_n}{S_0} = \frac{M_n\left(1 - e^{-\mathrm{TR}/T_1(n)}\right)}{M_0\left(1 - e^{-\mathrm{TR}/T_1(0)}\right)} = \frac{1}{1 + \frac{\Delta T}{T_0}} \cdot \frac{1 - e^{\frac{\mathrm{TR}}{T_1(n) + \alpha \cdot \Delta T}}}{1 - e^{\frac{\mathrm{TR}}{T_1(0)}}} \tag{5}$$

where it is assumed a linear relationship of $T_1(\Delta T) = T_1(0) + \alpha \cdot \Delta T$ exists and the net magnetization available, M, follows a Curie Law for temperature (21). Changes in signal due to temperature-dependent changes in T_2 have also been ignored, which is realistic with choice of a suitably short time to echo (TE). If we restrict $\Delta T < 20°C$ and assume TR $\gg T_1(0)$, the resulting ratio is approximately linear and is given by,

$$\frac{S_n}{S_0} = \frac{\mathrm{TR}_n}{T_1(0) + \alpha \cdot \Delta T} + \frac{1}{2}[0]+ \tag{6}$$

from which the temperature change can be solved for and is given by,

$$\Delta T = \frac{1}{\alpha}\left(\frac{S_n \cdot \mathrm{TR}_n}{S_0} - T_1(0)\right). \tag{7}$$

This is one of the simpler quantitative methods of extracting temperature changes from T_1-weighted MR sequences, although the approximation can be poor for large temperature changes. Implementation can be difficult because both α and $T_1(0)$ are required for quantitative measurement and both are dependent on tissue type ($\alpha\bullet$, which can be positive or negative) (15).

Even when used in conjunction with fast imaging acquisitions, T_1 method is a poor choice for quantitative MRTI monitoring of rapid heat deposition ablation processes because the temperature response quickly becomes nonlinear at higher temperatures, exhibiting hysteresis when irreversible damage has been reached (22). Despite this, T_1-based MRTI is useful for nonquantitative monitoring of tissue temperature changes, particularly when motion causes problems with other techniques. Further, despite limitations, T_1-based MRTI may prove to be the most useful MRTI technique for quantitative measurement of temperature changes in adipose tissue because of the limitations of other methods when it comes to temperature sensitivity and measurement in lipid tissues (23,24). However, because of the difference in temperature sensitivity of lipid and soft-tissue, techniques for separating fat and water, such as Dixon techniques, will be required to avoid inaccurate temperature estimates from partial volume effects.

TEMPERATURE SENSITIVITY OF THE WATER PRF

By far, the most exploited and widely validated quantitative MRTI techniques are based on the temperature sensitivity of the water proton chemical shift (25,26). The shift of the PRF is proportional to temperature over a large range of temperatures (0–100°C), with a sensitivity of -0.01 ppm/°C for bulk water. The effect is relatively insensitive to tissue type with a range of approximately -0.0096 to -0.0113 ppm/°C in tissue (27).

Similar to the previous two methods, the physical basis for the temperature-dependent PRF phenomenon is that a rise in temperature leads to a corresponding increase in molecular Brownian motion. The result of this is that, as temperature rises, hydrogen bonds between local water molecules bend, stretch, and break. However, instead of arising from the increased molecular mobility, like diffusion, the PRF arises from a shift in the molecular shielding of the proton. Decreased net hydrogen bond strength results in an increase in the strength of the covalent bond between the water proton and its oxygen, which better shields the proton from the external magnetic field changing the proton shielding constant ($\Delta\sigma$) and resulting in a resonance frequency shift of the proton (25,28). The degree of hydrogen bonding in water and the measured chemical shift is an approximately linear (29) relationship resulting in a linear shift in the water PRF (Δf) with a change in temperature (ΔT).

$$\Delta f = \gamma \Delta B \cong -\gamma B_0 \left(\Delta\sigma + \frac{2}{3}\Delta\chi \right) \cong \gamma B_0 \alpha \Delta T \tag{8}$$

Where α is referred to as the temperature sensitivity coefficient and is primarily representative of the changes in the shielding constant ($\Delta\sigma$) with some contribution from changes in bulk susceptibility due to temperature ($\Delta\chi$). When carefully measured in biological tissue (4,30,31,32) and agar phantom (32), the magnitude of the temperature sensitivity coefficient of the PRF shift is slightly less than that measured in bulk water, which may be due to effects of hydration layers in the tissue (33), the electrical properties of tissue (34), and non-negligible susceptibility effects (32,35,36).

Using MRI, this temperature-dependent PRF shift can be measured using chemical shift imaging (CSI) techniques to directly measure the frequency shift (37). However, the easiest method for fast, high-resolution estimation of temperature changes due to the PRF shift is based on indirect measurements via relating the difference in phase between subsequent images (37,38) to the frequency shift. Using fast gradient-echo–based techniques (Fig. 2), the accumulated phase difference ($\Delta\phi$) between voxels acquired in two different images due to a temperature-based shift in the resonance frequency (Δf) is given by the expression:

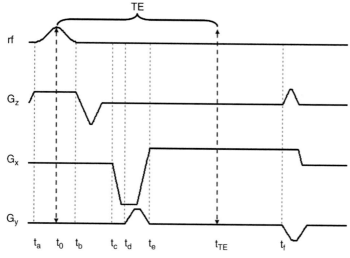

Figure 2 Typical pulse sequence diagram for a RF-spoiled, two-dimensional, fast, gradient-echo sequence used for phase-difference MRTI. A small flip angle (usually ≤30°) excitation pulse is applied under a slice selection gradient (G_z) from $t_a \rightarrow t_b$. Spoiling of the steady state is achieved by cycling the RF phase each TR period. At t_b, G_z polarity is reversed to account for dephasing of the transverse magnetization from $t_0 \rightarrow t_b$ due to G_z. From $t_c \rightarrow t_e$, G_x is turned on to prephase (move to $^-k_{x,max}$ in k-space). The area under G_x over $t_c \rightarrow t_e$ is the same magnitude, and opposite polarity, of the area over $t_e \rightarrow t_{TE}$ to refocus the phase and form the gradient-echo at the echo-time t_{TE} ($k_x = 0$). G_y is applied over $t_d \rightarrow t_e$ and can occur during the period following the G_x prephasing if necessary. End of the readout occurs at t_f. G_z gradient is then applied to dephase residual transverse relaxation. G_x and G_y gradients are applied to rephase spins for the next excitation (return to $k_x = k_y = 0$). By applying G_x for a slightly larger prephasing area, time is saved by no longer needing to ramp G_x for the rephasing period. *Abbreviations*: MRTI, magnetic resonance temperature imaging; RF, radio-frequency; TE, time to echo; TR; repetition time.

$$\Delta = 2\phi \cdot \Delta f \cdot \text{TE} \cong 2\pi \cdot \gamma B_0 \cdot \alpha \Delta T \cdot \text{TE} \tag{9}$$

where γ is the gyromagnetic ratio for the water proton (42.7 MHz/Tesla), B_0 is the magnetic induction of the static field, TE is the echo time of the sequence, and α is the temperature sensitivity coefficient in ppm/°C. The temperature sensitivity is found empirically by plotting the phase difference versus measured temperature (Fig. 3), but tends to be tissue independent.

To extract the temperature change between two images, one only needs the complex phase difference of a reference (S_0) and subsequent MR image (S_1) at a different temperature (Fig. 4):

$$\Delta T = \frac{\Delta \phi}{2\pi \cdot \gamma B_0 \cdot \alpha} \cong \frac{\arg\left(S_0^* S_1\right)}{2\pi \cdot \gamma B_0 \cdot \alpha} \tag{10}$$

Artifacts and inaccuracies in the complex phase-difference PRF technique come from several sources. One limitation is the insensitivity of the lipid chemical shift to temperature. Lipids do not have the strong hydrogen bonding network that gives rise to the temperature-dependent PRF shift seen in water. Therefore, voxels containing both lipid and water exhibit varying temperature sensitivity when complex phase-difference imaging is used. Furthermore, the response will vary as a function of TE. This can produce substantial errors (>10%) in MR thermometry estimates (36,38,39). Therefore, as with the T_1 and diffusion techniques, lipid suppression is critical for accurate MRTI using the temperature-dependent PRF shift.

However, lipids do exhibit a temperature-dependent bulk susceptibility that influences the PRF shift even in the absence of lipid signal (32). Other tissue properties, such as iron content, can also affect the susceptibility. Induced susceptibility effects will then have a tendency to be a function of tissue type as well as orientation of the heating pattern in the field. As previously mentioned, temperature-dependent susceptibilities lead

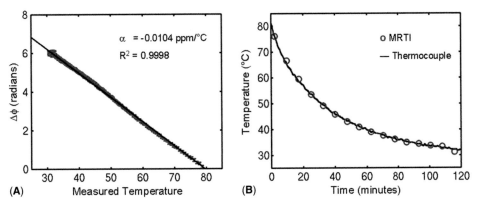

Figure 3 The temperature sensitivity coefficient is empirically determined or verified by plotting the measured phase difference ($\Delta \phi$) from an MRI sequence versus the measured temperature. Case shown is for a deionized water sample imaged during cooling over the range of 30°C to 80°C. A least-squares fit yields a slope of $\alpha = -0.0104 \pm 7.9 \times 10 \times^{-6}$ ppm/°C with a Pearson's $R^2 = 0.9998$ ($n = 300$) (**A**). Once the temperature sensitivity of a material is known, a plot of temperature versus time can be made from the phase-difference data using equation 13 (**B**). *Abbreviations*: MRI, magnetic resonance imaging; MRTI, magnetic resonance temperature imaging.

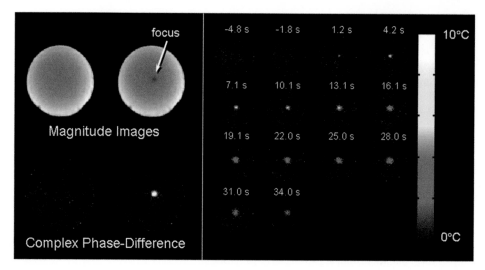

Figure 4 (*See color insert.*) Example output of typical fast gradient-echo MRTI images during focused ultrasound heating of an agar phantom (3 secs per image, 0.7 × 0.7 × 3 mm resolution). A transverse cut of the focus is shown with the reference images (prior to heating) on the left and the postheating images on the right. On magnitude images, the focus becomes dark with increasing temperature, indicative of increasing T_1. The complex phase-difference images demonstrate excellent contrast against the background, with no mean-phase changes measured inside the phantom outside the focal region. The noise in the complex phase-difference images outside the phantom has been masked out based on the SNR of the magnitude image in order to enhance presentation (the phase difference is uniformly distributed between $-\pi$ and π in regions of no signal). *Abbreviations*: MRTI, magnetic resonance temperature imaging; SNR, signal-to-noise ratio.

to phase changes. Using simple phase-difference techniques, these susceptibility-induced phase changes cannot be separated from the PRF generated phase shifts and can result in non-negligible errors (32,35,36), especially in temperature distributions with sharp spatial gradients (27,40). To minimize errors, use of a spherical heating pattern, alignment of cylindrical heating patterns with the main field axis, or generating smaller spatial temperature gradients is helpful. In the case of high lipid content tissue, techniques can be used which attempt to use the lipids for internal reference to minimize error, which is fortunate because fatty tissue can induce its own temperature-dependent susceptibility changes.

Tissue motion is another problem for the complex phase-difference PRF technique, which can limit the usefulness of this technique in some areas of the body. Many approaches have been investigated to limit the errors due to motion, each with their own advantages and limitations. A brief, but excellent, review of motion correction for MRTI can be found in Ref. (41). Respiratory triggering of fast sequences can be used with some sequences at the cost of temporal resolution, but even with novel processing techniques, tend to fail for irregular or deep breathing (42–44). Navigator echoes can also be incorporated into sequences to compensate for translational motion (45). More recently, a brute force postprocessing technique for handling motion-induced changes in the background phase capitalizes upon the fact that the background phase in MR images is spatially slowly varying and so the background phase in the treatment area can be extrapolated using the background phase accurately from the surrounding tissue, resulting in a "referenceless" PRF technique (46). While promising for many regions, this technique is limited by the need to have enough surrounding tissue with which to calculate the phase for extrapolation, problems with rapidly varying phase near boundaries, and the need to modify the acquisition to account for lipid phase. With recent increases in gradient performance and the incorporation of parallel imaging techniques to limit increased acquisition times (47), fast multiecho (48–53) studies may ultimately be necessary for a less motion sensitive estimate of the frequency shift without compromising spatiotemporal resolution.

The PRF shift can be measured directly using MR CSI. CSI offers the benefit of high temperature resolution and the ability to use an internal reference peak, such as lipids, to provide absolute temperature measurements, limit sensitivity to motion artifacts, and correct for susceptibility or inhomogeneity effects (37). The primary disadvantage of using standard CSI techniques is poor spatiotemporal resolution, limiting the ability to directly apply this technique for monitoring rapid heat delivery in a volume.

OTHER TEMPERATURE-SENSITIVE MR TECHNIQUES

The temperature dependence of the spin-spin relaxation time is relatively small compared to the previously mentioned techniques and suffers from long acquisition times and low SNR (54). Temperature sensitivity of other MR parameters, such as magnetization transfer, spin density, and perfusion, have also been investigated, but similarly suffer from acquisition difficulties and low temperature sensitivity, limiting their widespread use (15,55).

However, the introduction of exogenous agents, such as heat-activated liposome-based contrast agents (56–58) or paramagnetic lanthanides (20,59–63), have the advantage of increased sensitivity, the ability to eliminate certain aspects of motion errors during therapy, and the potential for absolute temperature estimation. Unfortunately, in addition to the large doses needed to implement these techniques given current technology, the largest limitation of exogenous agent techniques is the inhomogeneous distribution of material into the target region, rendering them of limited usefulness for quantitative or even qualitative use in therapies where the agent cannot be delivered uniformly throughout the tissue of interest. Despite this limitation, such agents, particularly when targeted or delivered to the specific tissue or site of interest, will likely be of key importance in molecularly targeted thermal therapy techniques in the future where precise, but relatively localized, temperature control will be needed in order to effect a particular response such as increased vascular permeability, gene therapy activation, or drug delivery.

MRTI ACQUISITION STRATEGIES FOR ULTRASOUND ABLATION

The size of volume to be monitored, the size of the heating source, and the rate of heating are all important factors in determining the necessary spatio-temporal resolution and volume coverage needed to monitor a technique (64,65). The needs of technique irradiating a volume over one to several minutes using phased-array or multielement ultrasound heating techniques (Fig. 5) have different sequence requirements than a tightly focused, rapid heating ultrasound technique (Fig. 6).

For tightly focused ultrasound beams, such as those used in extracorporeal focused ultrasound, averaging across the focus can lead to underestimation of the maximum temperature and it is important to adjust your imaging parameters appropriately.

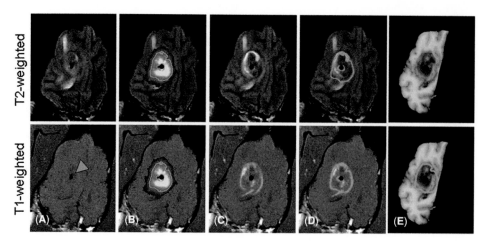

Figure 5 (*See color insert.*) Demonstration of MR-guided ablation of canine transmissible venereal tumors in the brain using a multi-element ultrasound applicator. Phased-array and multielement ultrasound treatments cover larger volumes, usually over longer periods of time. T_1 and T_2-weighted images were acquired for planning and localization of the ultrasound applicator (*arrow*) in the tumor (*Column A*). During therapy, seven planes of MR temperature images were acquired using a multishot echoplanar imaging sequence processed using the complex phase-difference technique described in the text. The central slice of treatment with temperature overlay and estimated region of damage [cumulative equivalent minutes at 43 degrees (CEM 43) $\geq$ 50 minute isodose line in green] are shown on the pretreatment images (*Column B*). T_2-weighted and contrast-enhanced T_1-weighted images acquired after therapy demonstrate the region of damage as assessed by MRI (*Column C*), which correlates strongly with the estimated damage as demonstrated by the overlays in Column D and the gross pathology photographs in Column E. *Abbreviations*: MR, magnetic resonance; MRI, magnetic resonance imaging.

For optimum accuracy, the slice thickness should be oriented along the axial direction of the beam. For instance, assuming an approximately Gaussian distributions of temperature along the longitudinal and transverse axes (a good approximation of the temperature distribution near the focus), for a beam with transverse full-width half maximum (FWHM) = 4 mm and an axial FWHM = 8 mm, transverse plane resolution better than 1.3 mm and a slice thickness •3 mm will keep spatial averaging error of the maximum temperature less than 10%. Switching the slice orientation to obtain a longitudinal view of the beam requires the slice thickness •2 mm to obtain similar accuracy. In addition, very small errors in placement of the imaging slice would have a dramatic effect on the accuracy and sensitivity of your temperature imaging.

Obviously, slice thickness is a very important spatial resolution parameter as it can result in the most detriment to the temperature estimation. When optimizing a protocol, the in-plane resolution should be sacrificed for SNR purposes before the slice thickness. While spatial averaging of in-plane temperature can bias the measurement of the maximum temperature at the focus by several degrees, for reasonably sized lesions, this averaging effect is not nearly as detrimental at the lesion borders as long as the temperature gradient in the region is linear and monotonic within the averaging window. Under these circumstances, the average tends to converge to the actual temperature in the center of the window.

Similar to in-plane resolution, temporal resolution has an averaging affect on the maximum measured temperature at the focus. For rapid heating applications, temporal sampling on the order of three to five seconds is appropriate for maximal $\Delta T/dt \leq 4°C/sec$

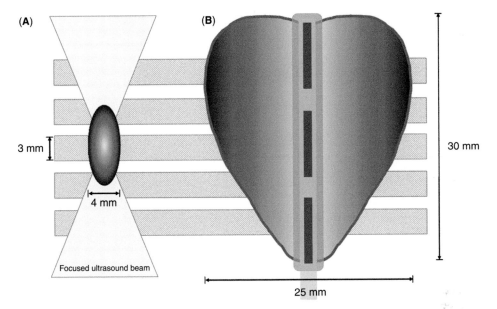

Figure 6 (*See color insert.*) A challenge in temperature-monitoring thermal therapies utilizing ultrasound is conforming the MRTI technique to the geometry and timing. An externally focused high-intensity ultrasound kernel ($\Delta t \sim 10$–20 seconds), such as that shown in (**A**), requires much higher spatiotemporal resolution, while a large, water-cooled, multielement interstitial or transurethral ultrasound applicator such as that shown in (**B**) ($\Delta t \sim 5$–10 minutes) may use relaxed spatiotemporal resolution without penalty but requires more volume coverage to accurately characterize the thermal dose delivered over the region, and may be more likely to incur artifacts from motion or temperature-dependent volume susceptibility. *Abbreviation*: MRTI, magnetic resonance temperature imaging.

(approximately) considering the rate of heating slows as time progresses and is lower at the lesion borders. Aside from averaging, your temporal resolution should reflect the rate of feedback you need to safely monitor your application of energy.

With respect to averaging, the most important factor in minimizing temporal sampling averaging is appropriate trigger timing with respect to the beginning and ending of heating. As long as the heating curve is approximately piecewise linear and monotonic within each averaging window, the average value will tend to better represent the true value of the temperature in the center of the window. The best method for minimizing temporal sampling errors that can seriously degrade damage estimates is to make certain the temporal window for imaging is not centered on a discontinuous heating profile (i.e., whenever possible, do not image during the ramping on or off of the heat source).

For PRF-based techniques, in regions of sufficiently large SNRs, Gaussian distributions of the real and imaginary can be assumed. In this case, the noise in the phase-difference image ($\sigma_{\Delta\phi}$), and hence in the temperature image, can be expressed as (66):

$$\sigma_{\Delta\phi} \cong \frac{\sigma}{A}\sqrt{2} = \frac{\sqrt{2}}{\mathrm{SNR}_A} \tag{11}$$

where A is the magnitude signal, σ is the noise in the magnitude signal, and SNR_A is the SNR of the magnitude image (Fig. 7).

Many find it useful to define a metric as the "phase-difference contrast to phase-difference noise ratio" ($\mathrm{CNR}_{\Delta\phi} = \Delta\phi/\sigma_{\Delta\phi}$) to describe the sensitivity of the technique.

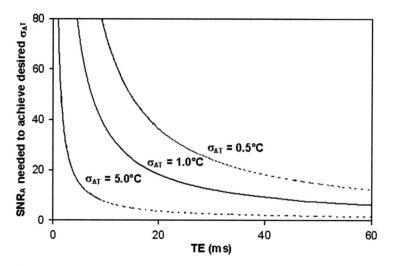

Figure 7 Propagation of error in complex phase-difference MRTI using the PRF shift. The magnitude image SNR necessary to achieve a particular temperature uncertainty ($\sigma_{\Delta T}$) is plotted versus the echo time of the sequence. Note that significantly higher SNR is needed at shorter echo times to keep the uncertainty in the temperature measurement small. *Abbreviations*: MRTI, magnetic resonance temperature imaging; PRF, proton resonance frequency; SNR, signal-to-noise ratio; TE, time to echo.

It can be shown that for a simple gradient-echo type sequence, the optimal choice for TE to balance sensitivity versus noise is the T_2^* of the tissue whereas all other imaging parameters should be chosen to maximize image SNR for the required spatiotemporal resolution (Fig. 8) (49,67).

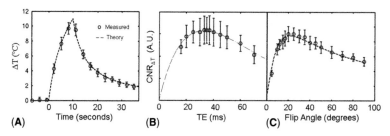

Figure 8 A typical presentation of the temperature change at the focus, ΔT, versus time for focused ultrasound heating in an agar phantom (**A**). Error bars show the uncertainty in the mean ($n = 15$). The measured and theoretical $CNR_{\Delta T}$ curves for a fast gradient-echo-type sequence versus echo time (**B**) and flip angle (**C**) demonstrate the close relationship between theoretical optimization parameters and empirical measurements. The optimal TE in this case is determined to be 32.33 ± 0.85 msec while the measured T_2^* in the phantom over an 80 period was 32.11 ± 1.36 msec. In the case of the flip angle optimization, the effects of slice thickness must be accounted for to properly optimize the SNR. The Ernst angle prediction of the optimal flip angle from the measured T_1 (1087.8 ± 11.2 ms) is $13.24° \pm 0.0012°$ while the optimal flip angle from the measured data is $22.25°$. If the effects of a Gaussian slice profile are accounted for in the fast gradient-echo sequence, the theory produces an optimal flip angle of $20.0° \pm 0.026°$, which is in much better agreement with the measurements. *Abbreviations*: CNR, contrast-to-noise ratio; SNR, signal-to-noise ratio; TE, time to echo.

ADVANCED MR TEMPERATURE IMAGING AND FUTURE DIRECTIONS

As previously mentioned, MRTI techniques should be tailored for the application. Temperature feedback during therapy is a critical component in treatments seeking rapid verification or control of therapy (2,45,68–76).

For PRF-based MRTI using complex phase difference, TE < TR, limiting the ability to obtain an optimal TE for some tissues without sacrificing temporal resolution. Echo-shifted sequences, which allow TE > TR have been employed in the past to facilitate optimal TE $= T_2^*$, but are limited by increased motion sensitivity and the inefficiency of the short TR (even when segmented methods are used) (39,67,77). To address the challenges of obtaining a near-optimal TE, lipid suppression and multiple planes while maintaining the spatiotemporal resolution and SNR of gradient-echo methods, a multishot EPI (78–81) or spiral (82) sequence may be used (Fig. 9).

These segmented acquisition approaches, combined with parallel imaging techniques (47) and respiratory gating, have been used with some success for MRTI in the challenging area of the liver (42,43).

The slice efficiency of the segmented echo-planar sequences can be somewhat reduced by removing the phase encodes in order to generate multiple gradient-echoes, which can be used to map the frequency (83) or generate a spectrum (fast CSI) (37,48, 50). These fast chemical shift acquisitions, in conjunction with appropriate processing, may address many of the limitations associated with the complex phase-difference PRF-based technique by limiting errors due to motion and susceptibility and possibly providing an internal reference for absolute temperature measurement. These techniques, while promising, have thus far been plagued by limitations in spatiotemporal resolution and tremendous process constraints. However, by incorporating modern hardware advancements, such as parallel imaging, and relaxing sampling requirements (i.e., allowing larger echo spacing and reduced total number of echoes), multiplanar techniques

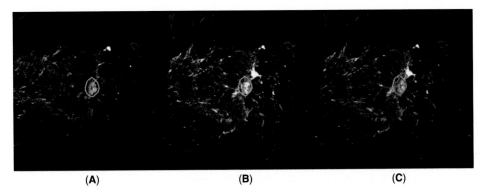

(A)   **(B)**   **(C)**

Figure 9 (*See color insert.*) MR-guided focused ultrasound ablation of breast cancer at The University of Texas M. D. Anderson Cancer Center (unpublished results from 2001). A T_2-weighted image is acquired prior to treatment and used to plan the delivery of therapy (**A**) by outlining the target (*green*). A fat suppressed, multishot EPI sequence (as described in Ref. 80) was used to monitor temperature changes in real time during multiple focused ultrasound pulses. The maximum temperature achieved over the duration of the treatment is plotted cumulatively on top of a T_2-weighted image acquired after the therapy (**B**). Unfortunately, temperature cannot be accurately measured in the fat outside of the glandular tissue, resulting in gaps in the temperature map. The estimated cumulative damage is overlaied on the post-therapy T_2-weighted image (**C**). Note the accumulation of swelling in the region from the procedure. *Abbreviation*: MR, magnetic resonance.

with similar spatiotemporal performance to current single plane gradient-echo techniques can be realized.

CONCLUDING REMARKS

Several investigators have investigated the sensitivity, benefits, and trade-offs of different MRTI techniques (20,84–86). For most applications that require quantitative temperature monitoring with high spatiotemporal resolution, the PRF technique is the most appropriate technique since, with the exception of lipids, it is less sensitive to differences in tissue composition. The primary advantage of the PRF over the other two methods is the high spatiotemporal resolution and accuracy with which measurements can be taken over a variety of system configurations. As MR-guided ultrasound thermal therapy procedures move into the clinical setting, MRTI technology is being adapted to address the specialized needs of each application. Currently, regions of motion and susceptibility as well as extended treatment times are challenges to quantitative MRTIs that do not have robust solutions.

Lastly, it should be noted that now, as precisely controlled and localized delivery of heat into the human body is now slowly becoming a reality, using heat as an energy source capable of inducing localized tissue ablation or for hyperthermia applications is just the beginning of the myriad of potential applications for image-guided thermal therapy. In the future, precise heat delivery can be used as the catalyst or driving energy source for a variety of local chemical reactions, such as drug activation or induction/inhibition of heat shock protein or enzyme activity. Precision heat delivery in vivo, particularly in the tumor microenvironment, will facilitate the advancement of novel molecularly targeted therapies. In order to fully realize the potential for such therapies, a robust suite of complimentary molecular imaging techniques to monitor such therapies in vivo will need to be developed and explored.

REFERENCES

1. Hynynen K, Darkazanli A, Unger E, Schenck JF. MRI-guided noninvasive ultrasound surgery. Med Phys 1993; 20(1):107–115.
2. Cline HE, Schenck JF, Hynynen K, Watkins RD, Souza SP, Jolesz FA. MR-guided focused ultrasound surgery. J Comput Assist Tomogr 1992; 16(6):956–965.
3. Simpson JH, Carr HY. Diffusion and nuclear spin relaxation in water. Phys Rev 1958; 111: 1201–1202.
4. MacFall J, Prescott DM, Fullar E, Samulski TV. Temperature dependence of canine brain tissue diffusion coefficient measured in vivo with magnetic resonance echo-planar imaging. Intern J Hyperther 1995; 11(1):73–86.
5. Le Bihan D, Delannoy J, Levin RL. Temperature mapping with MR imaging of molecular diffusion: application to hyperthermia. Radiology 1989; 171:853–857.
6. Nicholson C, Sykova E. Extracellular space structure revealed by diffusion analysis. Trends Neurosci 1998; 21(5):207–215.
7. Pfeuffer J, Flogel U, Dreher W, Leibfritz D. Restricted diffusion and exchange of intracellular water: theoretical modelling and diffusion time dependence of 1H NMR measurements on perfused glial cells. NMR Biomed 1998; 11(1):19–31.
8. Stejskal EO, Tanner JE. Spin diffusion measurements: spin echoes in the presence of a time-dependent field gradient. J Chem Phys 1965; 48:288–292.
9. Turner R, Le Bihan D, Chesnick AS. Echo-planar imaging of diffusion and perfusion. Magn Reson Med 1991; 19(2):247–253.

10. Turner R, Le Bihan D, Maier J, Vavrek R, Hedges LK, Pekar J. Echo-planar imaging of intravoxel incoherent motion. Radiology 1990; 177(2):407–414.
11. Il'yasov KA, Hennig J. Single-shot diffusion-weighted RARE sequence: application for temperature monitoring during hyperthermia session. J Magn Reson Imag 1998; 8(6): 1296–1305.
12. Parker DL. Applications of NMR imaging in hyperthermia: an evaluation of the potential for localized tissue heating and noninvasive temperature monitoring. IEEE Trans Biomed Eng 1984; 31(1):161–167.
13. Parker DL, Smith V, Sheldon P, Crooks LE, Fussell L. Temperature distribution measurements in two-dimensional NMR imaging. Med Phys 1983; 10(3):321–325.
14. Abragam A. Principles of nuclear magnetism. In: Birman J, ed. The International Series of Monographs on Physics. New York: Oxford University Press, Inc., 1961:324.
15. Young IR, Hand JW, Oatridge A, Prior MV. Modeling and observation of temperature changes in vivo using MRI. Magn Reson Med 1994; 32:358–369.
16. Dikinson RJ, Hall AS, Hind AJ, Young IR. Measurement of changes in tissue temperature using magnetic resonance imaging. J Comput Assist Tomogr 1986; 10(3):468–472.
17. Haacke EM, Brown RW, Thompson MR, Venkatesan R. Magnetic Resonance Imaging: Physical Principles and Sequence Design. New York: John Wiley & Sons, Inc., 1999.
18. Prato FS, Drost DJ, Keys T, Laxon P, Comissiong B, Sestini E. Optimization of signal-to-noise ratio in calculated T1 images derived from two spin-echo images. Magn Reson Med 1986; 3(1):63–75.
19. Matsumoto R, Mulkern RV, Hushek SG, Jolesz FA. Tissue temperature monitoring for thermal interventional therapy: comparison of T1-weighted MR sequences. J Magn Reson Imag 1994; 4(1):65–70.
20. Wlodarczyk W, Hentschel M, Wust P, et al. Comparison of four magnetic resonance methods for mapping small temperature changes. Phys Med Biol 1999; 44(2):607–624.
21. Abragam A. Principles of nuclear magnetism. In: Birman J, ed. The International Series of Monographs on Physics. New York: Oxford University Press, Inc., 1961.
22. Jolesz FA, Bleier AR, Jakab P, Ruenzel PW, Huttl K, Jako GJ. MR imaging of laser-tissue interactions. Radiology 1988; 168(1):249–253.
23. Hynynen K, McDannold N, Mulkern RV, Jolesz FA. Temperature monitoring in fat with MRI. Magn Reson Med 2000; 43(6):901–904.
24. Bohris C, Schreiber WG, Jenne J, et al. Quantitative MR temperature monitoring of high-intensity focused ultrasound therapy. Magn Reson Imag 1999; 17(4):603–610.
25. Hindman JC. Proton resonance shift of water in the gas and liquid states. J Chem Phys 1966; 44(12):4582–4592.
26. McDannold N. Quantitative MRI-based temperature mapping based on the proton resonant frequency shift: review of validation studies. Int J Hyperther 2005; 21(6):533–546.
27. Graham SJ, Chen L, Leitch M, et al. Quantifying tissue damage due to focused ultrasound heating observed by MRI. Magn Reson Med 1999; 41:321–328.
28. Chen L, Bouley DM, Harris BT, Butts K. MRI study of immediate cell viability in focused ultrasound lesions in the rabbit brain. J Magn Reson Imag 2001; 13(1):23–30.
29. Hoffman MM, Conradi MS. Are there hydrogen bonds in supercritical water? J Am Chem Soc 1997; 119:3811–3817.
30. Kuroda K, Chung AH, Hynynen K, Jolesz FA. Calibration of water proton chemical shift with temperature for noninvasive temperature imaging during focused ultrasound surgery. J Magn Reson Imag 1998; 8(1):175–181.
31. Wu T, Kendell KR, Felmlee JP, Lewis BD, Ehman RL. Reliability of water proton chemical shift temperature calibration for focused ultrasound ablation therapy. Med Phys 2000; 27(1): 221–224.
32. De Poorter J. Noninvasive MRI thermometry with the proton resonance frequency method: study of susceptibility effects. Magn Reson Med 1995; 34(3):359–367.
33. Svergun DL, Richard S, Kock MHJ, Sayers Z, Kuprin S, Zaccai G. Protein hydration in solution: experimental observation by x-ray and neutron scattering. Proc Natl Acad Sci 1998; 95:2267–2272.

34. Peters RD, Henkelman RM. Proton-resonance frequency shift MR thermometry is affected by changes in the electrical conductivity of tissue. Magn Reson Med 2000; 43(1): 62–71.

35. Young IR, Bell JD, Hajnal JV, Jenkinson G, Ling J. Evaluation of the stability of the proton chemical shifts of some metabolites other than water during thermal cycling of normal human muscle tissue. J Magn Reson Imag 1998; 8(5):1114–1118.

36. Young IR, Hajnal JV, Roberts IG, et al. An evaluation of the effects of susceptibility changes on the water chemical shift method of temperature measurement in human peripheral muscle. Magn Reson Med 1996; 36:366–374.

37. Kuroda K, Suzuki Y, Ishihara Y, Okamoto K, Suzuki Y. Temperature mapping using water proton chemical shift obtained with 3D-MRSI: feasibility in vitro. Magn Reson Med 1996; 35: 20–29.

38. Kuroda K, Oshio K, Chung AH, Hynynen K, Jolesz FA. Temperature mapping using the water proton chemical shift: a chemical shift selective phase mapping method. Magn Reson Med 1997; 38(5):845–851.

39. de Zwart JA, Vimeux FC, Delalande C, Canioni P, Moonen CT. Fast lipid-suppressed MR temperature mapping with echo-shifted gradient-echo imaging and spectral-spatial excitation. Magn Reson Med 1999; 42(1):53–59.

40. Griffiths DJ. Introduction to Electrodynamics. Upper Saddle River, New Jersey: Simon & Schuster Company, 1989.

41. de Senneville BD, Quesson B, Moonen CT. Magnetic resonance temperature imaging. Int J Hyperther 2005; 21(6):515–531.

42. Weidensteiner C, Quesson B, Caire-Gana B, et al. Real-time MR temperature mapping of rabbit liver in vivo during thermal ablation. Magn Reson Med 2003; 50(2):322–330.

43. Weidensteiner C, Kerioui N, Quesson B, de Senneville BD, Trillaud H, Moonen CT. Stability of real-time MR temperature mapping in healthy and diseased human liver. J Magn Reson Imag 2004; 19(4):438–446.

44. Vigen KK, Daniel BL, Pauly JM, Butts K, Triggered, navigated, multi-baseline method for proton resonance frequency temperature mapping with respiratory motion. Magn Reson Med 2003; 50(5):1003–1010.

45. de Zwart JA, Vimeux FC, Palussiere J, et al. On-line correction and visualization of motion during MRI-controlled hyperthermia. Magn Reson Med 2001; 45(1):128–137.

46. Rieke V, Vigen KK, Sommer G, Daniel BL, Pauly JM, Butts K. Referenceless PRF shift thermometry. Magn Reson Med 2004; 51(6):1223–1231.

47. Bankson JA, Stafford RJ, Hazle JD. Partially parallel imaging with phase-sensitive data: increased temporal resolution for magnetic resonance temperature imaging. Magn Reson Med 2005; 53(3):658–665.

48. Kuroda K, Mulkern RV, Oshio K, et al. Temperature mapping using the water proton chemical shift: self-referenced method with echo-planar spectroscopic imaging. Magn Reson Med 2000; 44(1):167.

49. Chung AH, Hynynen K, Colucci V, Oshio K, Cline HE, Jolesz FA. Optimization of spoiled gradient-echo phase imaging for in vivo localization of a focused ultrasound beam. Magn Reson Med 1996; 36(5):745–752.

50. McDannold N, Hynynen K, Oshio K, Mulkern RV. Temperature monitoring with line scan echo planar spectroscopic imaging. Med Phys 2001; 28(3):346–355.

51. Paliwal V, El-Sharkawy AM, Du X, Yang X, Atalar E. SSFP-based MR thermometry. Magn Reson Med 2004; 52(4):704–708.

52. Scheffler K. Fast frequency mapping with balanced SSFP: theory and application to proton-resonance frequency shift thermometry. Magn Reson Med 2004; 51(6):1205–1211.

53. Ong JT, d'Arcy JA, Collins DJ, Rivens IH, ter Haar GR, Leach MO. Sliding window dual gradient echo (SW-dGRE): T1 and proton resonance frequency (PRF) calibration for temperature imaging in polyacrylamide gel. Phys Med Biol 2003; 48(13):1917–1931.

54. Nelson TR, Tung SM. Temperature dependence of proton relaxation times in vitro. Magn Reson Imag 1987; 5(3):189–199.

55. Hall-Craggs MA. Interventional MRI of the breast: minimally invasive therapy. Eur Radiol 2000; 10(1):59–62.

56. McDannold N, Fossheim SL, Rasmussen H, Martin H, Vykhodtseva N, Hynynen K. Heat-activated liposomal MR contrast agent: initial in vivo results in rabbit liver and kidney. Radiology 2004; 230(3):743–752.

57. Frich L, Bjornerud A, Fossheim S, Tillung T, Gladhaug I. Experimental application of thermosensitive paramagnetic liposomes for monitoring magnetic resonance imaging guided thermal ablation. Magn Reson Med 2004; 52(6):1302–1309.

58. Viglianti BL, Abraham SA, Michelich CR, et al. In vivo monitoring of tissue pharmacokinetics of liposome/drug using MRI: illustration of targeted delivery. Magn Reson Med 2004; 51(6):1153–1162.

59. Hekmatyar SK, Hopewell P, Pakin SK, Babsky A, Bansal N. Noninvasive MR thermometry using paramagnetic lanthanide complexes of 1,4,7,10-tetraazacyclodoecane-alpha,alpha' alpha'',alpha'''-tetramethyl-1,4,7,10-tetraacetic acid (DOTMA4-). Magn Reson Med 2005; 53(2):294–303.

60. Hekmatyar SK, Poptani H, Babsky A, Leeper DB, Bansal N. Non-invasive magnetic resonance thermometry using thulium-1,4,7,10-tetraazacyclododecane-1,4,7,10-tetraacetate [TmDOTA(-)]. Int J Hyperther 2002; 18(3):165–179.

61. Zuo CS, Bowers JL, Metz KR, Nosaka T, Sherry AD, Clouse ME. Tmdotp5-, a substance for NMR temperature measurements in vivo. Magn Reson Med 1996; 36(6):955–959.

62. Aime S, Botta M, Fasano M, et al. A new ytterbium chelate as contrast agent in chemical shift imaging and temperature sensitive probe for MR spectroscopy. Magn Reson Med 1996; 35(5): 648–651.

63. Frenzel T, Roth K, Kossler S, et al. Noninvasive temperature measurement in vivo using a temperature-sensitive lanthanide complex and 1H magnetic resonance spectroscopy. Magn Reson Med 1996; 35(3):364–369.

64. Chung AH, Jolesz FA, Hynynen K. Thermal dosimetry of a focused ultrasound beam in vivo by magnetic resonance imaging. Med Phys 1999; 26(9):2017–2026.

65. Pisani LJ, Ross AB, Diederich CJ, et al. Effects of spatial and temporal resolution for MR image-guided thermal ablation of prostate with transurethral ultrasound. J Magn Reson Imag 2005; 22(1):109–118.

66. Conturo TE, Smith GD. Signal-to-noise in phase angle reconstruction: dynamic range extension using phase reference offsets. Magn Reson Med 1990; 15(3):420–437.

67. de Zwart JA, van Gelderen P, Kelly DJ, Moonen CT. Fast magnetic-resonance temperature imaging. J Magn Reson B 1996; 112(1):86–90.

68. Arora D, Cooley D, Perry T, et al. MR thermometry-based feedback control of efficacy and safety in minimum-time thermal therapies: phantom and in-vivo evaluations. Int J Hyperther 2006; 22(1):29–42.

69. Cline HE, Hynynen K, Hardy CJ, Watkins RD, Schenck JF, Jolesz FA. MR temperature mapping of focused ultrasound surgery. Magn Reson Med 1994; 31(6):628–636.

70. Cline HE, Schenck JF, Watkins RD, Hynynen K, Jolesz FA. Magnetic resonance-guided thermal surgery. Magn Reson Med 1993; 30(1):98–106.

71. Guilhon E, Voisin P, de Zwart JA, et al. Spatial and temporal control of transgene expression in vivo using a heat-sensitive promoter and MRI-guided focused ultrasound. J Gene Med 2003; 5(4):333–342.

72. Hokland SL, Pedersen M, Salomir R, Quesson B, Stodkilde-Jorgensen H, Moonen CT. MRI-guided focused ultrasound: methodology and applications. IEEE Trans Med Imag 2006; 25(6):723–731.

73. Hynynen K, Freund WR, Cline HE, et al. A clinical, noninvasive, MR imaging monitored ultrasound surgery method. Radiographics 1996; 16(1):185–195.

74. Jolesz FA, Hynynen K. Magnetic resonance image-guided focused ultrasound surgery. Cancer J 2002; 8(suppl 1):S100–S112.
75. Quesson B, Vimeux F, Salomir R, de Zwart JA, Moonen CT. Automatic control of hyperthermic therapy based on real-time Fourier analysis of MR temperature maps. Magn Reson Med 2002; 47(6):1065–1072.
76. Salomir R, Palussiere J, Vimeux FC, et al. Local hyperthermia with MR-guided focused ultrasound: spiral trajectory of the focal point optimized for temperature uniformity in the target region [in process citation]. J Magn Reson Imag 2000; 12(4):571–583.
77. Chung YC, Duerk JL, Shankaranarayanan A, Hampke M, Merkle EM, Lewin JS. Temperature measurement using echo-shifted FLASH at low field for interventional MRI. J Magn Reson Imag 1999; 9(1):138–145.
78. Stafford RJ, Price RE, Diederich CJ, Kangasniemi M, Olsson LE, Hazle JD. Interleaved echo-planar imaging for fast multiplanar magnetic resonance temperature imaging of ultrasound thermal ablation therapy. J Magn Reson Imag 2004; 20(4):706–714.
79. Diederich CJ, Stafford RJ, Nau WH, Burdette EC, Price RE, Hazle JD. Transurethral ultrasound applicators with directional heating patterns for prostate thermal therapy: in vivo evaluation using magnetic resonance thermometry. Med Phys 2004; 31(2):405–413.
80. Kangasniemi M, Diederich CJ, Price RE, et al. Multiplanar MR temperature-sensitive imaging of cerebral thermal treatment using interstitial ultrasound applicators in a canine model. J Magn Reson Imag 2002; 16(5):522–531.
81. Hazle JD, Diederich CJ, Kangasniemi M, Price RE, Olsson LE, Stafford RJ. MRI-guided thermal therapy of transplanted tumors in the canine prostate using a directional transurethral ultrasound applicator. J Magn Reson Imag 2002; 15(4):409–417.
82. Stafford RJ, Hazle JD, Glover GH. Monitoring of high-intensity focused ultrasound-induced temperature changes in vitro using an interleaved spiral acquisition. Magn Reson Med 2000; 43(6):909–912.
83. Mulkern RV, Panych LP, McDannold NJ, Jolesz FA, Hynynen K. Tissue temperature monitoring with multiple gradient-echo imaging sequences. J Magn Reson Imag 1998; 8(2):493–502.
84. Quesson B, de Zwart JA, Moonen CT. Magnetic resonance temperature imaging for guidance of thermotherapy. J Magn Reson Imag 2000; 12(4):525–533.
85. Bertsch F, Loffler R, Issels R, Reiser M. A Phantom to Simulate Perfusion Effects in MR Thermometry. Sydney, Australia: International Society for Magnetic Resonance in Medicine, 1998.
86. Depoorter J, Dewagter C, Dedeene Y, Thomsen C, Stahlberg F, Achten E. The proton-resonance-frequency-shift method compared with molecular-diffusion for quantitative measurement of 2-dimensional time-dependent temperature distribution in a phantom. J Magn Reson Series B 1994; 103(3):234–241.

4

Experimental Uses of Magnetic Resonance Imaging–Guided Focused Ultrasound Surgery

Nathan McDannold

Department of Radiology, Brigham and Women's Hospital and Harvard Medical School, Boston, Massachusetts, U.S.A.

INTRODUCTION

The initial experiments involving magnetic resonance imaging (MRI)-guided focused ultrasound surgery (MRIgFUS) were performed in the early 1990s by a collaboration of investigators at the University of Arizona with investigators at Brigham and Women's Hospital and General Electric (1–4). These experiments demonstrated the feasibility of using a focused ultrasound device within an MRI scanner, visualizing the focal heating and detecting the resulting tissue damage. Based on these studies, a prototype computer-controlled MRIgFUS system was developed (5), which was used shortly afterwards in a clinical study to ablate breast fibroadenomas (6). A similar system was developed independently in Germany (7).

Following these initial studies, substantial work involving methods to improve the MRIgFUS device and the treatment monitoring was performed. Key work in this area involved developing MRI-compatible phased arrays (8–13) and driving systems (14) that can be used to increase the focal heating volume and steer the ultrasound beam, and testing and validating MRI-based temperature imaging (15–17) to localize the focal spot (18) and to predict online the ablated zone (19–22). These concepts were integrated into a second-generation MRIgFUS device, the Exablate 2000™, which was produced by InSightec (Haifa, Israel) and was granted Food and Drug Administration approval in the United States in 2004 for the treatment of uterine fibroids (23–25).

The reader is directed to the other chapters in this book for more detailed descriptions of these key concepts involved in MRIgFUS systems. In this chapter, other experimental work with MRIgFUS is reviewed. Different MRI-compatible ultrasound applicators and uses of focused ultrasound within the MRI environment have been developed, and they could have a major impact in the future.

EXPERIMENTAL MRIgFUS DEVICES

In addition to MRIgFUS systems that employ extracorporeal transducers, there has been substantial work developing interstitial, intraluminal, and intracavitary MRIgFUS devices. While these applicators are more invasive, they offer the ability of targeting tissue that is difficult to access with an externally focused beam due to lack of an acoustic window or organ motion. Thermal ablation using other interstitial probes (radiofrequency, microwave, laser, or cryotherapy) has also been an extremely active subject of research in recent years as a less invasive alternative to surgical resection for tumor treatments, and it is poised for widespread use in the clinic (26). Interstitial ultrasound probes may offer significant advantages over these other energy sources, and when coupled to an MRI, they could substantially improve such ablation treatments.

A major advantage of ultrasound is the ability to direct the energy deposition in a particular direction using sectored, multichannel cylindrical applicators (27) or with planar applicators that can be rotated to deliver the acoustic energy in the desired direction (28). Control in the depth direction has been shown possible by using different ultrasound frequencies (29), and applicators can be made at different lengths to heat different sized targets.

MRI-compatible interstitial ultrasound probes have been constructed and tested successfully with online feedback from MRI-based thermometry (30–33). For example, Nau et al. recently reported on experiments that evaluated such probes during thermal ablation of prostate in a dog model (33). The cylindrical transducer was sectored to give a 180° active region. They showed that by implanting multiple probes and by rotating the transducer during sonication, large ablated regions can be produced. They also were able to map the temperature rise online with MRI-based thermometry to predict the extent of the thermal damage. MRI-compatible transurethral applicators with similar designs have also been tested for prostate ablation (34–37). An example of the heating produced by such a device is shown in Figure 1.

MRI-compatible transrectal probes designed for thermal ablation of prostate have also been developed and tested in animals. The ability of these arrays to steer the beam using a phased array and the use of MRI-based treatment planning and thermal feedback could offer a significant improvement over transrectal focused ultrasound devices that have been tested clinically under ultrasound imaging guidance (38,39). Hutchinson et al. designed a linear phased array probe with 57 elements that can steer the focal region along the axis of the probe and in the depth direction. The probe was designed with aperiodic elements to increase element size without increasing grating lobes (40) and can scan the beam during sonication to increase the focal volume (41). Tests of the probe in vivo in rabbit thigh muscle were demonstrated under MRI control (10). Sokka and Hynynen expanded on this design, adding motorized control of the probe to steer the beam laterally (12). Based on in vivo experiments performed in rabbit thigh (Fig. 2), they estimated that they could ablate the entire prostate in about 40 minutes.

MRI-compatible transesophageal probes designed for the treatment of esophageal cancer (42) and transurethral probes designed for the treatment of prostate cancer (34,35,37,43) have also been tested in animals. MRI-compatible transrectal ultrasound applicators designed for hyperthermia treatments have also been investigated (44).

CLOSED-LOOP FEEDBACK CONTROL

As currently implemented clinically, volumes are thermally ablated with an externally located focused ultrasound transducer using relatively short (approximately 10–20 seconds) sonications delivered to multiple overlapping locations while the temperature rise and accumulated thermal dose (45,46) are monitored with MRI. Using short exposures reduces the effects of the tissue perfusion and blood flow (47), which are

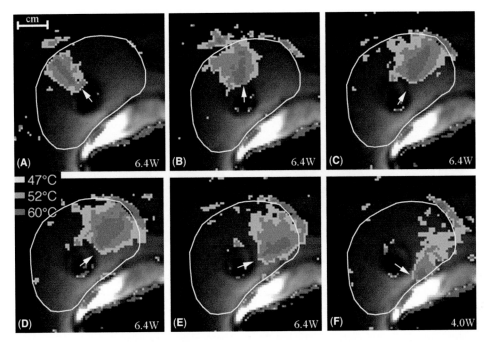

Figure 1 (*See color insert.*) Three transverse MRI-based temperature images showing sonications in canine prostate using an interstitial ultrasound probe. This tubular applicator transmits over a 90° sector. The slices are separated by 6 mm each and are centered at the middle of the heating zone. The red and orange overlays display temperatures greater than 52°C and 47°C, respectively, and the prostate periphery is outlined in white. (**A–C**) Treatment of the left ventral region (6–12 W for 12 minutes). (**D–F**) Treatment of the right ventral region (10–15 W for 12 minutes). *Abbreviation*: MRI, magnetic resonance imaging. *Source*: From Ref. 36. Courtesy of the Institute of Physics Publishing, Bristol, U.K.

unknown for a given target tissue volume and can change in response to heat (48), on the resulting temperature distribution. A delay between sonications is employed to avoid accumulated heating along the ultrasound beam path that occurs when sonications are delivered to neighboring locations (49,50). During these waiting periods, the MRI-derived temperature and thermal dose distribution from the previous sonication are inspected, allowing for adjustment of the sonication parameters and the target locations for the subsequent sonications, ensuring that the entire target volume receives a lethal thermal exposure while surrounding tissues are protected.

This treatment/feedback strategy is fairly conservative in that it does not demand continuous temperature monitoring for extended periods of time and it keeps the thermal deposition well controlled. However, the energy deposition during such sonications may not be ideal, and due to the delay needed between sonications, the treatments can be long for large tumor volumes. In addition, any erroneous heating that may occur during sonication, such as heating above 100°C, mistargeted heating, or heating of surrounding tissue structures, might be missed.

Several automated closed-loop strategies based on MRI-based control have been suggested and implemented successfully in animal experiments. Such techniques can potentially improve upon the human-based control described above that is currently used. The first demonstration of automated feedback was shown using relatively simple methods, such as proportional integral and derivative controllers, that force the

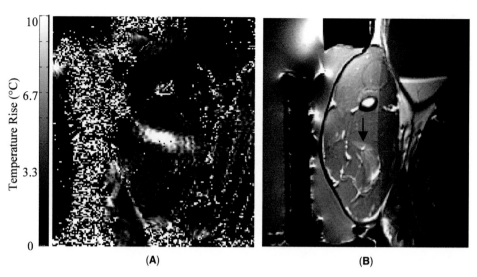

Figure 2 (A) MRI-based temperature image during a high-power sonication (130 W for 30 seconds) into rabbit thigh muscle with an MRI-compatible phased array transrectal applicator. (B) The resulting lesion (indicated by the *arrow*) is seen in T_2-weighted imaging. The bright region to the right of the lesion is a tissue fascia layer. *Abbreviation*: MRI, magnetic resonance imaging. *Source*: From Ref. 12. Courtesy of the Institute of Physics Publishing, Bristol, U.K.

temperature at a single point to follow a predetermined trajectory during long-duration heating with ultrasound (51,52), similar to what was done earlier with invasive temperature measurements (53). Advances to this method, where a physical model of the energy deposition and thermal conduction were taken into account, were reported next (54). Others have suggested methods for automatic control of temperature during short-duration focused ultrasound exposures (55). In addition, control over the thermal dose, instead of the temperature rise, has been proposed (56,57). Automatic feedback based on MRI-based temperature measurements has also been shown for controlling interstitial laser ablation (58) and hyperthermia with a microwave phased array (59,60).

Two-dimensional magnetic resonance (MR) thermometry-based control of ultrasound hyperthermia using phased arrays has also been proposed (61). The most advanced employment of automatic two-dimensional control to date has been shown in papers by Salomir et al., Palussiere et al., and Mougenot et al., who demonstrated in animal experiments real-time, MRI-based temperature feedback control of both the temperature trajectory and the spatial thermal distribution during long-duration focused ultrasound heating (62–64). With this method, the ultrasound transducer is moved so the focal coordinate travels in a double spiral trajectory (Fig. 3). Temperature measurements acquired during the first spiral are used to modify the velocity of the transducer during the second spiral to achieve uniform heating over the target volume. This feasibility of this technique has been shown in vivo animal experiments and with experiments using animals with innoculated tumors (63–64). Alternative sonication trajectories for use in automated MRI-based temperature feedback control have been proposed by Malinen et al. for treatment of breast tumors with a phased array transducer (65).

Another feedback approach has been described by Chopra et al., who have been designing MRI-compatible planar transurethral ultrasound probes for the treatment of prostate cancer (37,43). With these probes, the ultrasound beam propagates radially from a probe inserted in the urethra. This probe is rotated to ablate the entire gland based on

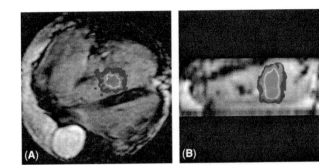
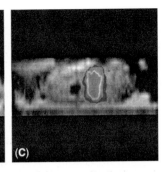

Figure 3 (*See color insert.*) Temperature maps in rabbit thigh muscle in vivo obtained at the end of a spiral trajectory with closed-loop MR thermometry-based control. (**A**) Coronal plane (containing the focal point trajectory); (**B**) sagittal plane; and (**C**) transverse plane. Color levels: blue, 42°C to 45°C; green, 45°C to 48°C; and red, above 48°C. Experimental data were obtained with a $1 \times 1 \times 5$ mm voxel size and were further interpolated to a isotropic matrix (1 mm on each direction). Temperature maps were spatially smoothed by convolution with a Gaussian kernel (2 mm FWHM). *Abbreviations*: FWHM, full-width half maximum; MRI, magnetic resonance. *Source*: From Ref. 64. Courtesy of Wiley-Liss, Inc., Hoboken, NJ.

treatment planning images of the prostate gland. During the treatment, the system chooses the acoustic parameters and rotation rate to conform the ablated zone using control points at the edge of the gland. While this system uses a one-dimensional algorithm to control the temperature at each point, these control points are updated as the probe is rotated, resulting in control of a two-dimensional treatment.

Many of these feedback methods use relatively long, continuous heating produced by a scanned ultrasound beam. While these approaches may be able to decrease the treatment time of MRIgFUS procedures in some cases, such scanning approaches may be limited due to the effects of perfusion and blood flow, which are not known for a given tissue target and can change in response to heat (48). Clinical implantation of these strategies may also be challenging due to issues related to the MRI-based thermometry. Continuous temperature monitoring with MRI-based thermometry can be difficult since it is susceptible to errors due to small patient motion, magnetic field drift (66), and tissue swelling (67,68). Further, care will need to be taken with long sonication durations to avoid pain and thermal damage to bony structures that may lie behind the focal plane. While the ultrasound intensity will be relatively mild in this region, the temperature rise may be significant due to bone's high absorption of ultrasound and the long time required for the bone to cool back to baseline.

NOVEL MRI METHODS TO DETECT TISSUE DAMAGE INDUCED BY MRIgFUS

While standard MRI sequences and imaging with MRI contrast agents have been shown to be sensitive to thermal tissue damage in normal tissue (4,20,69–71), in certain situations alternative methods to detect such damage may be desirable. For example, it may be difficult to distinguish thermal tissue damage from diseased tissues, such as tumors. It may also be desirable to use thermally induced tissue damage as a method to guide and control the procedure as an alternative to MRI-based temperature monitoring. One may also want to detect tissue damage without an MRI contrast agent. Several novel strategies to address these issues have been tested.

MR elastography (MRE) methods such as ultrasound-based methods (72) allow for imaging of mechanical properties of tissues. In this method, the tissue is deformed, typically by either a low-frequency shear wave (73) or a quasistatic compression (74), and the resulting tissue displacement is mapped using motion-sensitive MRI sequences. The resulting images are sensitive to tissue stiffness, since stiffer tissues will be displaced less by the deformation. Since tissue is known to become stiffer after thermal coagulation (75), elastography should be able to detect thermal ablation produced by methods such as focused ultrasound. Using MRE, Wu et al. demonstrated this ability in tissue samples ablated with focused ultrasound (76). The ability to map tissue damage with MRE could allow for treatment evaluation, as the MRIgFUS procedure is ongoing. This group has also demonstrated that the images used to generate the MRE can be used to generate temperature maps, allowing for complementary measures of the treatment progress (77). MRE may be useful if one desires to evaluate the treatment progress before an MRI contrast is administered or to monitor the procedure itself for tissues where MRI-based thermometry is difficult, such as the breast due to its lipid content (66).

Diffusion MRI has also been investigated for detecting MRIgFUS-induced tissue damage in clinical treatments of uterine fibroids (78). Jacobs et al. showed that diffusion-weighted images and the apparent diffusion coefficient were different in ablated regions in the fibroids, suggesting that they could be useful in evaluating the treatments before contrast is used. This information may be useful, since the thermal damage in the fibroids is not always evident in noncontrast T_2-weighted imaging, and if more treatment is necessary, one might not want to administer multiple doses of MRI contrast agent.

Others have investigated contrast kinetics to evaluate thermal tissue damage induced by focused ultrasound. Cheng et al. demonstrated that subtle tissue damage can be investigated by looking at the enhancement kinetics of an MRI contrast agent (79). In that work, the time course of the contrast enhancement was used to estimate two physiological parameters, the vessel permeability (K^{trans}) and leakage space (v_e) (80), which were then compared with standard MR images and histopathology. They found that these estimated parameters showed the extent of subtle tissue damage that surrounds the coagulation necrosis that was not seen in conventional MRI (Fig. 4).

Their data also indicate that these subtle changes when detected immediately after the ablation correlated with the necrosis one week after the treatments. Such measurements may be useful in postablation imaging to evaluate whether further treatment is needed.

Contrast enhancement has also been investigated to determine whether residual tumor exists after MRIgFUS of breast cancer. Gianfelice et al. looked at semiquantitative metrics (increase in signal intensity, maximum difference function, and positive enhancement integral) of the signal intensity profiles of dynamic contrast-enhanced imaging (81). They found a strong correlation in particular between the amount of residual tumor and the maximal increase in signal intensity with the percentage of residual tumor detected in histology performed after post-treatment surgical resection.

MRIgFUS FOR TISSUE AND ACOUSTIC CHARACTERIZATION

The ability of MRIgFUS to heat tissue and monitor the resulting temperature rise under controlled conditions allows for estimation of tissue characteristics. Since these characteristics are not known, such estimates can be then used for treatment planning purposes. For example, Wang et al. suggested a method to measure ultrasound absorption using MRI-based calorimetry (82,83). In this technique, the temperature rise induced by a

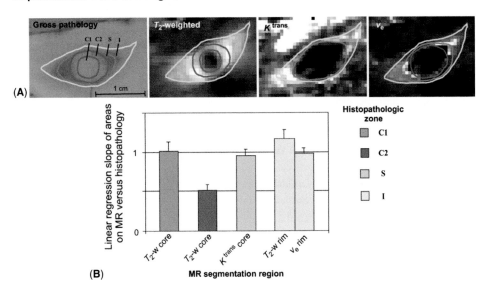

Figure 4 (*See color insert.*) Comparison of histopathologic regions and segmentation areas on MR 40 hours after focused ultrasound heating in rabbit thigh muscle. The MRI information agreed well with the histological findings. (**A**) Contours determined with histopathology overlaid on T_2-weighted MR and maps of estimated contrast kinetics parameters (K^{trans} and v_e) for a sample lesion. Four zones of damage are identified: a core of low signal in T_2-weighted imaging (C1), a center of low K^{trans} (C2), a ring of highest K^{trans} (S), and a region corresponding to the extent of high v_e (I). (**B**) Slope of the regression line fitted to MR versus histology measurements of area for all eight lesions. Error bars represent the 95% confidence interval for the slope (*t*-test). *Abbreviations*: MR, magnetic resonance; MRI, magnetic resonance imaging. *Source*: From Ref. 79. Courtesy of Wiley-Liss, Inc., Hoboken, NJ.

focused ultrasound exposure is mapped with MRI-based thermometry. With knowledge of the ultrasound intensity distribution—which is measured beforehand with hydrophone measurements—one can solve for the ultrasound absorption in the tissue or the phantom. The method was demonstrated in tissue-mimicking phantoms and ex vivo tissue samples embedded in a nonabsorbing agarose phantom (82,83). Measuring thermal conductivity using MRI-based temperature mapping and a heat source produced by focused ultrasound has also been suggested. Cheng et al. demonstrated that if one can assume that the spatial heating distribution is Gaussian, one can use dynamic measurements of the Gaussian radius during short sonications to estimate thermal conductivity of tissue (84). By assuming impulse heating by a short sonication, they show that a plot of the square of the Gaussian radius versus time is linear with a slope proportional to the tissue conductivity. They also suggest a method to use this data along with the temperature decay to estimate tissue perfusion.

The use of MR-based thermometry has also been tested to determine treatment parameters for focused ultrasound surgery. One example of this use is the determination of the cooling time needed between multiple overlapping sonications. This cooling time is needed if one wants to avoid thermal build up that occurs along the ultrasound beam path (49), which can make the treatment difficult to control. In experiments in rabbit thigh muscle, it was shown that this thermal buildup can be quantified using MRI-based thermometry (85). One may also be able to use temperature mapping to determine the correct power level to use during the treatment. The temperature rise is linear with applied acoustic power for the sharply focused transducers used for thermal ablation

(86). By measuring the temperature distribution during a low-power (sublethal) sonication, one can thus estimate the power needed to reach a desired temperature rise or lesion area by simply scaling the power. This ability was demonstrated in experiments in rabbit thigh muscle (87). Such a method could substantially simplify treatment planning, since no knowledge of the tissue parameters is needed to estimate the correct acoustic power level to use.

OTHER EXPERIMENTAL USES OF MRIgFUS

Several other experimental uses of MRIgFUS have been investigated, including drug delivery and gene therapy applications, cavitation-enhanced therapies, and novel clinical applications. The reader is directed to the other chapters of this book for elaboration on these developments.

REFERENCES

1. Cline HE, Schenck JF, Hynynen K, Watkins RD, Souza SP, Jolesz FA. MR-guided focused ultrasound surgery. J Comput Assist Tomogr 1992; 16:956–965.
2. Cline HE, Schenck JF, Watkins RD, Hynynen K, Jolesz FA. Magnetic resonance-guided thermal surgery. Magn Reson Med 1993; 30:98–106.
3. Hynynen K, Damianou C, Darkazanli A, Unger E, Levy M, Schenck JF. On-line MRI monitored noninvasive ultrasound surgery. In: Engineering in Medicine and Biology Society, 1992. Vol. 14. Proceedings of the Annual International Conference of the IEEE. Oct 29–Nov 1, 1992. Vol. 1. 350–351.
4. Hynynen K, Darkazanli A, Unger E, Schenck JF. MRI-guided noninvasive ultrasound surgery. Med Phys 1993; 20:107–115.
5. Cline HE, Hynynen K, Watkins RD, et al. Focused US system for MR imaging-guided tumor ablation. Radiology 1995; 194:731–737.
6. Hynynen K, Pomeroy O, Smith DN, et al. MR imaging-guided focused ultrasound surgery of fibroadenomas in the breast: a feasibility study. Radiology 2001; 219:176–185.
7. Huber PE, Jenne JW, Rastert R, et al. A new noninvasive approach in breast cancer therapy using magnetic resonance imaging-guided focused ultrasound surgery. Cancer Res 2001; 61: 8441–8447.
8. Hynynen K, Chung A, Fjield T, et al. Feasibility of using ultrasound phased arrays for MRI monitored noninvasive surgery. IEEE Trans Ultrason Ferroelectr Freq Contr 1996; 43: 1043.
9. Fjield T, Hynynen K. The combined concentric-ring and sector-vortex phased array for MRI guided ultrasound surgery. IEEE Trans Ultrason Ferroelectr Freq Contr 1997; 44: 1157–1167.
10. Hutchinson EB, Hynynen K. Intracavitary ultrasound phased arrays for prostate thermal therapies: MRI compatibility and in vivo testing. Med Phys 1998; 25:2392–2399.
11. Daum DR, Smith NB, King R, Hynynen K. In vivo demonstration of noninvasive thermal surgery of the liver and kidney using an ultrasonic phased array. Ultrasound Med Biol 1999; 25:1087–1098.
12. Sokka SD, Hynynen K. The feasibility of MRI-guided whole prostate ablation with a linear aperiodic intracavitary ultrasound phased array. Phys Med Biol 2000; 45:3373–3383.
13. Hynynen K, Clement GT, McDannold N, et al. 500-element ultrasound phased array system for noninvasive focal surgery of the brain: a preliminary rabbit study with ex vivo human skulls. Magn Reson Med 2004; 52:100–107.

14. Daum DR, Buchanan MT, Fjield T, Hynynen K. Design and evaluation of a feedback based phased array system for ultrasound surgery. IEEE Trans Ultrason Ferroelectr Freq Contr 1998; 45:431–438.

15. Smith NB, Webb AG, Ellis DS, Wilmes LJ, O'Brien WD. Non-invasive in vivo temperature mapping of ultrasound heating using magnetic resonance techniques. In: Proceedings of the Ultrasonics Symposium. IEEE 1994; (3):1829–1832.

16. Chung AH, Hynynen K, Colucci V, Oshio K, Cline HE, Jolesz FA. Optimization of spoiled gradient-echo phase imaging for in vivo localization of a focused ultrasound beam. Magn Reson Med 1996; 36:745–752.

17. Kuroda K, Chung AH, Hynynen K, Jolesz FA. Calibration of water proton chemical shift with temperature for noninvasive temperature imaging during focused ultrasound surgery. J Magn Reson Imag 1998; 8:175–181.

18. Hynynen K, Vykhodtseva NI, Chung AH, Sorrentino V, Colucci V, Jolesz FA. Thermal effects of focused ultrasound on the brain: determination with MR imaging. Radiology 1997; 204:247–253.

19. McDannold NJ, Hynynen K, Wolf D, Wolf G, Jolesz FA. MRI evaluation of thermal ablation of tumors with focused ultrasound. J Magn Reson Imag 1998; 8:91–100.

20. Vykhodtseva NI, Sorrentino V, Jolesz FA, Bronson RT, Hynynen K. MRI detection of the thermal effects of focused ultrasound on the brain. Ultrasound Med Biol 2000; 26:871–880.

21. McDannold NJ, King RL, Jolesz FA, Hynynen K. Usefulness of MR imaging-derived thermometry and dosimetry in determining the threshold for tissue damage induced by thermal surgery in rabbits. Radiology 2000; 216:517–523.

22. Hazle JD, Stafford RJ, Price RE. Magnetic resonance imaging-guided focused ultrasound thermal therapy in experimental animal models: correlation of ablation volumes with pathology in rabbit muscle and VX2 tumors. J Magn Reson Imag 2002; 15:185–194.

23. Tempany CM, Stewart EA, McDannold N, Quade BJ, Jolesz FA, Hynynen K. MR imaging-guided focused ultrasound surgery of uterine leiomyomas: a feasibility study. Radiology 2003; 226(3):897–905.

24. Hindley J, Gedroyc WM, Regan L, et al. MRI guidance of focused ultrasound therapy of uterine fibroids: early results. AJR Am J Roentgenol 2004; 183:1713–1719.

25. Stewart EA, Rabinovici J, Tempany CM, et al. Clinical outcomes of focused ultrasound surgery for the treatment of uterine fibroids. Fertil Steril 2006; 85:22–29.

26. Dodd GD, Soulen MC, Kane RA, et al. Minimally invasive treatment of malignant hepatic tumors: at the threshold of a major breakthrough. Radiographics 2000; 20:9–27.

27. Nau WH, Diederich CJ, Stauffer PR. Directional power deposition from direct-coupled and catheter-cooled interstitial ultrasound applicators. Int J Hyperther 2000; 16:129–144.

28. Lafon C, Chapelon JY, Prat F, Gorry F, Theillere Y, Cathignol D. Design and in vitro results of a high intensity ultrasound interstitial applicator. Ultrasonics 1998; 36:683–687.

29. Chopra R, Luginbuhl C, Foster FS, Bronskill MJ. Multifrequency ultrasound transducers for conformal interstitial thermal therapy. IEEE Trans Ultrason Ferroelectr Freq Control 2003; 50:881–889.

30. Chopra R, Luginbuhl C, Weymouth AJ, Foster FS, Bronskill MJ. Interstitial ultrasound heating applicator for MR-guided thermal therapy. Phys Med Biol 2001; 46:3133–3145.

31. Kangasniemi M, Diederich CJ, Price RE, et al. Multiplanar MR temperature-sensitive imaging of cerebral thermal treatment using interstitial ultrasound applicators in a canine model. J Magn Reson Imag 2002; 16:522–531.

32. Diederich CJ, Nau WH, Ross AB, et al. Catheter-based ultrasound applicators for selective thermal ablation: progress towards MRI-guided applications in prostate. Int J Hyperther 2004; 20:739–756.

33. Nau WH, Diederich CJ, Ross AB, et al. MRI-guided interstitial ultrasound thermal therapy of the prostate: a feasibility study in the canine model. Med Phys 2005; 32:733–743.

34. Hazle JD, Diederich CJ, Kangasniemi M, Price RE, Olsson LE, Stafford RJ. MRI-guided thermal therapy of transplanted tumors in the canine prostate using a directional transurethral ultrasound applicator. J Magn Reson Imag 2002; 15:409–417.

35. Diederich CJ, Stafford RJ, Nau WH, Burdette EC, Price RE, Hazle JD. Transurethral ultrasound applicators with directional heating patterns for prostate thermal therapy: in vivo evaluation using magnetic resonance thermometry. Med Phys 2004; 31:405–413.

36. Ross AB, Diederich CJ, Nau WH, et al. Highly directional transurethral ultrasound applicators with rotational control for MRI-guided prostatic thermal therapy. Phys Med Biol 2004; 49: 189–204.

37. Chopra R, Burtnyk M, Haider MA, Bronskill MJ. Method for MRI-guided conformal thermal therapy of prostate with planar transurethral ultrasound heating applicators. Phys Med Biol 2005; 50:4957–4975.

38. Bihrle R, Foster RS, Sanghvi NT, Fry FJ, Donohue JP. High-intensity focused ultrasound in the treatment of prostatic tissue. Urology 1994; 43:21–26.

39. Gelet A, Chapelon JY, Bouvier R, et al. Treatment of prostate cancer with transrectal focused ultrasound: early clinical experience. Eur Urol 1996; 29:174–183.

40. Hutchinson EB, Buchanan MT, Hynynen K. Design and optimization of an aperiodic ultrasound phased array for intracavitary prostate thermal therapies. Med Phys 1996; 23: 767–776.

41. Hutchinson EB, Hynynen K. Intracavitary ultrasound phased arrays for noninvasive prostate surgery. IEEE Trans Ultrason Ferroelectr Freq Contr 1996; 43:1032.

42. Melodelima D, Salomir R, Mougenot C, et al. Intraluminal ultrasound applicator compatible with magnetic resonance imaging "real-time" temperature mapping for the treatment of oesophageal tumours: an ex vivo study. Med Phys 2004; 31:236–244.

43. Chopra R, Wachsmuth J, Burtnyk M, Haider MA, Bronskill MJ. Analysis of factors important for transurethral ultrasound prostate heating using MR temperature feedback. Phys Med Biol 2006; 51:827–844.

44. Smith NB, Buchanan MT, Hynynen K. Transrectal ultrasound applicator for prostate heating monitored using MRI thermometry. Int J Radiat Oncol Biol Phys 1999; 43:217–225.

45. Sapareto SA, Dewey WC. Thermal dose determination in cancer therapy. Int J Radiat Oncol Biol Phys 1984; 10:787–800.

46. Chung AH, Jolesz FA, Hynynen K. Thermal dosimetry of a focused ultrasound beam in vivo by magnetic resonance imaging. Med Phys 1999; 26:2017–2026.

47. Billard BE, Hynynen K, Roemer RB. Effects of physical parameters on high temperature ultrasound hyperthermia. Ultrasound Med Biol 1990; 16:409–420.

48. Song CW. Effect of local hyperthermia on blood flow and microenvironment: a review. Cancer Res 1984; 44:4721s–4730s.

49. Damianou C, Hynynen K. Focal spacing and near-field heating during pulsed high temperature ultrasound therapy. Ultrasound Med Biol 1993; 19:777–787.

50. Fan X, Hynynen K. Ultrasound surgery using multiple sonications—treatment time considerations. Ultrasound Med Biol 1996; 22:471–482.

51. Vimeux FC, de Zwart JA, Palussiere J, et al. Real-time control of focused ultrasound heating based on rapid MR thermometry. Invest Radiol 1999; 34:190–193.

52. Smith NB, Merilees NK, Hynynen K, Dahleh M. Control system for an MRI compatible intracavitary ultrasound array for thermal treatment of prostate disease. Int J Hyperther 2001; 17:271–282.

53. Lin WL, Roemer RB, Hynynen K. Theoretical and experimental evaluation of a temperature controller for scanned focused ultrasound hyperthermia. Med Phys 1990; 17:615–625.

54. Salomir R, Vimeux FC, de Zwart JA, Grenier N, Moonen CT. Hyperthermia by MR-guided focused ultrasound: accurate temperature control based on fast MRI and a physical model of local energy deposition and heat conduction. Magn Reson Med 2000; 43:342–347.

55. Vanne A, Hynynen K. MRI feedback temperature control for focused ultrasound surgery. Phys Med Biol 2003; 48:31–43.

56. Arora D, Cooley D, Perry T, Skliar M, Roemer RB. Direct thermal dose control of constrained focused ultrasound treatments: phantom and in vivo evaluation. Phys Med Biol 2005; 50: 1919–1935.

57. Arora D, Cooley D, Perry T, et al. MR thermometry-based feedback control of efficacy and safety in minimum-time thermal therapies: phantom and in-vivo evaluations. Int J Hyperther 2006; 22:29–42.

58. McNichols RJ, Gowda A, Kangasniemi M, Bankson JA, Price RE, Hazle JD. MR thermometry-based feedback control of laser interstitial thermal therapy at 980 nm. Lasers Surg Med 2004; 34:48–55.

59. Behnia B, Suthar M, Webb AG. Closed-loop feedback control of phased-array microwave heating using thermal measurements from magnetic resonance imaging. Concepts Magn Reson 2002; 15:101–110.

60. Kowalski ME, Behnia B, Webb AG, Jin JM. Optimization of electromagnetic phased-arrays for hyperthermia via magnetic resonance temperature estimation. IEEE Trans Biomed Eng 2002; 49:1229–1241.

61. Hutchinson E, Dahleh M, Hynynen K. The feasibility of MRI feedback control for intracavitary phased array hyperthermia treatments. Int J Hyperthermia 1998; 14:39–56.

62. Salomir R, Palussiere J, Vimeux FC, et al. Local hyperthermia with MR-guided focused ultrasound: spiral trajectory of the focal point optimized for temperature uniformity in the target region. J Magn Reson Imag 2000; 12:571–583.

63. Palussiere J, Salomir R, Le Bail B, et al. Feasibility of MR-guided focused ultrasound with real-time temperature mapping and continuous sonication for ablation of VX2 carcinoma in rabbit thigh. Magn Reson Med 2003; 49:89–98.

64. Mougenot C, Salomir R, Palussiere J, Grenier N, Moonen CT. Automatic spatial and temporal temperature control for MR-guided focused ultrasound using fast 3D MR thermometry and multispiral trajectory of the focal point. Magn Reson Med 2004; 52:1005–1015.

65. Malinen M, Huttunen T, Kaipio JP, Hynynen K. Scanning path optimization for ultrasound surgery. Phys Med Biol 2005; 50:3473–3490.

66. De Poorter J. Noninvasive MRI thermometry with the proton resonance frequency method: study of susceptibility effects. Magn Reson Med 1995; 34:359–367.

67. McDannold NJ, Hynynen K, Jolesz FA. MRI monitoring of the thermal ablation of tissue: effects of long exposure times. J Magn Reson Imag 2001; 13:421–427.

68. Daniel BL, Butts K. Deformation of breast tissue during heating; MRI observations of ex vivo radio frequency ablation. In: Proceedings of the Eighth Meeting of the International Society for Magnetic Resonance in Medicine, Denver, CO 2000:1341.

69. Anzai Y, Lufkin RB, Hirschowitz S, Farahani K, Castro DJ. MR imaging-histopathologic correlation of thermal injuries induced with interstitial Nd:YAG laser irradiation in the chronic model. J Magn Reson Imag 1992; 2:671–678.

70. Tracz RA, Wyman DR, Little PB, et al. Comparison of magnetic resonance images and the histopathological findings of lesions induced by interstitial laser photocoagulation in the brain. Lasers Surg Med 1993; 13:45–54.

71. Chen L, Bouley D, Yuh E, D'Arceuil H, Butts K. Study of focused ultrasound tissue damage using MRI and histology. J Magn Reson Imag 1999; 10:146–153.

72. Ophir J, Alam SK, Garra B, et al. Elastography: ultrasonic estimation and imaging of the elastic properties of tissues. Proc Inst Mech Eng [H] 1999; 213:203–233.

73. Muthupillai R, Lomas DJ, Rossman PJ, Greenleaf JF, Manduca A, Ehman RL. Magnetic resonance elastography by direct visualization of propagating acoustic strain waves. Science 1995; 269:1854–1857.

74. Plewes DB, Betty I, Urchuk SN, Soutar I. Visualizing tissue compliance with MR imaging. J Magn Reson Imag 1995; 5:733–738.

75. Righetti R, Kallel F, Stafford RJ, et al. Elastographic characterization of HIFU-induced lesions in canine livers. Ultrasound Med Biol 1999; 25:1099–1113.

76. Wu T, Felmlee JP, Greenleaf JF, Riederer SJ, Ehman RL. Assessment of thermal tissue ablation with MR elastography. Magn Reson Med 2001; 45:80–87.

77. Le Y, Glaser K, Rouviere O, Ehman R, Felmlee JP. Feasibility of simultaneous temperature and tissue stiffness detection by MRE. Magn Reson Med 2006; 55:700–705.

78. Jacobs MA, Herskovits EH, Kim HS. Uterine fibroids: diffusion-weighted MR imaging for monitoring therapy with focused ultrasound surgery—preliminary study. Radiology 2005; 236:196–203.

79. Cheng HL, Purcell CM, Bilbao JM, Plewes DB. Usefulness of contrast kinetics for predicting and monitoring tissue changes in muscle following thermal therapy in long survival studies. J Magn Reson Imag 2004; 19:329–341.

80. Tofts PS, Kermode AG. Measurement of the blood-brain barrier permeability and leakage space using dynamic MR imaging. 1. Fundamental concepts. Magn Reson Med 1991; 17: 357–367.

81. Gianfelice D, Khiat A, Amara M, Belblidia A, Boulanger Y. MR imaging-guided focused ultrasound surgery of breast cancer: correlation of dynamic contrast-enhanced MRI with histopathologic findings. Breast Cancer Res Treat 2003; 82:93–101.

82. Wang Y, Hunt JW, Foster FS, Plewes DB. Tissue ultrasound absorption measurement with MRI calorimetry. IEEE Trans Ultrason Ferroelectr Freq Contr 1999; 46:1192–1200.

83. Wang Y, Plewes DB. An MRI calorimetry technique to measure tissue ultrasound absorption. Magn Reson Med 1999; 42:158–166.

84. Cheng HL, Plewes DB. Tissue thermal conductivity by magnetic resonance thermometry and focused ultrasound heating. J Magn Reson Imag 2002; 16:598–609.

85. McDannold NJ, Jolesz FA, Hynynen K. Determination of the optimal delay between sonications during focused ultrasound surgery in rabbits by using MR imaging to monitor thermal buildup in vivo. Radiology 1999; 211:419–426.

86. Hynynen K. The role of nonlinear ultrasound propagation during hyperthermia treatments. Med Phys 1991; 18:1156–1163.

87. McDannold N, King RL, Jolesz FA, Hynynen K. The use of quantitative temperature images to predict the optimal power for focused ultrasound surgery: in vivo verification in rabbit muscle and brain. Med Phys 2002; 29:356–365.

5
Integrated Therapy Delivery Systems

Kullervo H. Hynynen
Department of Medical Biophysics, University of Toronto and Department of Imaging Research, Sunnybrook Health Sciences Centre, Toronto, Ontario, Canada

Nathan McDannold
Department of Radiology, Brigham and Women's Hospital and Harvard Medical School, Boston, Massachusetts, U.S.A.

INTRODUCTION

The first clinical report (1) that combined magnetic resonance imaging (MRI) guidance and temperature monitoring with focused ultrasound surgery demonstrated feasibility and showed that high focal temperatures (60–90°C) induced by ultrasound can be monitored by magnetic resonance (MR) thermometry. Although the single focused ultrasound systems used in the first clinical studies (1–4) were integrated with the MRI scanner, they were limited due to the small focal spot volume and the range of the mechanical motion of the transducer in the depth direction. The early clinical systems were also limited in their ability to use the MR thermometry. They could visualize single temperature maps, but they did not track the thermal dose distribution (1).

Parallel with the clinical treatments, simulation and experimental studies demonstrated the feasibility and benefits of MRI-compatible ultrasound phased array technology (5–7) and quantitative MR thermometry for guiding the treatments (8–10). This technology together with more advanced software was adopted to the second-generation clinical phased array system that was designed to eliminate the limitations of single focused ultrasound surgery systems. Since this system is the only commercially available clinical MRI-guided focused ultrasound surgery (FUS) system, only it will be reviewed here.

CLINICAL MRI-GUIDED ULTRASOUND PHASED ARRAY SURGERY SYSTEM DESCRIPTION

The first commercial MRI-guided FUS system (Exablate 2000™) was developed by Insightec, Inc. (Haifa, Israel) in collaboration with the investigators at Brigham and Women's Hospital in Boston. The system is based on the clinical experience with the single transducer devices (1,2), simulation studies, and animal experiments (5,6,10–18).

Transducer Array

A spherically curved ultrasound phased array transducer with 208 elements, a 120 mm diameter, and a 160 mm radius of curvature, generates the ultrasound beam at a frequency that can be chosen by the operator, within a range from approximately 0.9 to 1.3 MHz. Each of the transducer elements is driven with an independent radiofrequency (RF) signal with computer-controlled phase and amplitude. The focus can be moved electronically (by adjusting the phases of the driving RF-signals) along the axial direction between 5 cm (skin depth) and 20 cm without the need of mechanically moving the transducer (Fig. 1).

The RF-drivers are located in the base of the MR-table with the power supply and controlling computer outside of the shielded magnet room.

Treatment Table

The sonication system is built into a standard MRI table that can be quickly docked into a standard 1.5 T magnet. Thus, the same magnet can easily be used for routine clinical imaging and FUS. Currently, this system can only be used with MRI scanners from General Electric. The transducer array is mounted in a mechanical two-dimensional positioning system that can move it in the plane of the MRI table. In addition, the transducer array can be tilted approximately 20° in two directions. Motion in each direction is induced by a computer-controlled piezoelectric motor. Rotary encoders are used to provide position feedback to assure accurate movement. The whole transducer assembly together with the positioning device is sealed in a plastic chamber filled with degassed deionized water (Fig. 2).

The ultrasound beam propagates up out of the table through a thin plastic window that permanently seals the chamber. A gel pad is placed on top of this window and acoustic coupling to the skin ensured with a layer of degassed water or acoustic gel. For breast tumor treatments, a water circulation system is integrated with the unit. This system circulates chilled water through tubing that surrounds the breast and serves to cool the skin to avoid skin burns that have occurred in some trials (19).

Safety Monitoring

The system includes three panic buttons that allow the patient, the operator, or a nurse who is in the MRI room with the patient to stop any sonication due to patient discomfort or other unforeseen event. While the patient is sedated during treatment, she is awake and routinely converses with the treatment team on her comfort level. Her feedback is essential to a safe treatment, as she can let the treatment team know whether there is heating on the skin. For the uterine treatments, she also can convey heating in the pelvis or rectum, or if there is sacral nerve pain. For the breast treatments, it is important to know about pain in the chest wall. By informing the staff of such heating, the treatment parameters can be adjusted. In our experience, one can typically adjust the parameters adequately to relieve the pain without compromising treatment.

Cavitation and Ultrasound Reflection Detection

In addition to the 208 elements, the array has central elements that are used for monitoring of the treatment. One of the center elements of the array is connected to a filtering and amplifier board for the detection of ultrasound emission at frequencies below the fundamental driving frequency. The spectrum of the detected signal is displayed

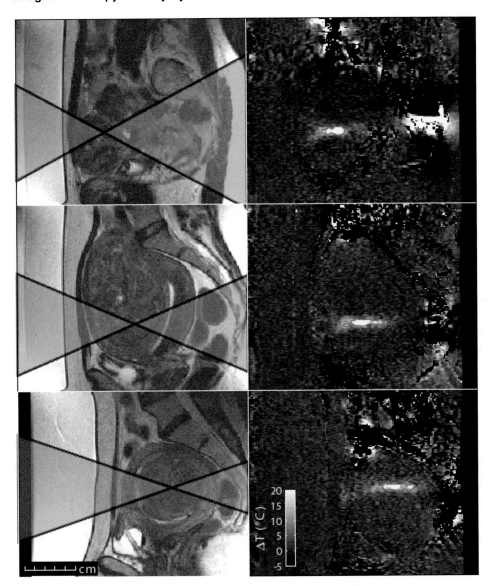

Figure 1 (*See color insert.*) Anatomical T_2-weighted MR images (*left*) and MRI-derived temperature maps of three sonications delivered at different depths into uterine fibroids (*right*). The temperature maps were acquired at peak temperature rise and were oriented through the center of the ultrasound focus parallel to the direction of the ultrasound beam. Temperature changes were estimated from phase-difference FSPGR images. Contours indicate regions that reached a thermal dose of at least 240 equivalent minutes at 43°C. The path of the ultrasound beam path is superimposed on the anatomical images. *Abbreviations*: FSPGR, fast spoiled gradient-echo sequence; MR, magnetic resonance; MRI, magnetic resonance imaging.

online during the ultrasound exposures for monitoring of cavitation (gas bubble formation or activity) or boiling. When these events occur, a broadband ultrasound signal is detected (20). One of these elements is also used to detect reflections in the ultrasound beam path. Before the high-power sonications, a low-level short pulse is delivered, and the A-mode signal detected by the element is displayed for the user. Poor acoustic coupling, for

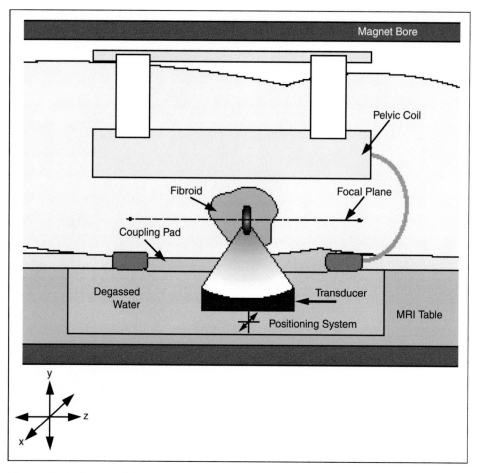

Figure 2   A diagram of the second-generation phased array focused ultrasound system.

example, due to gas in the beam path, is detected as a reflected signal and warns the operator before the start of the sonication, who can then stop sonication using one of the panic buttons.

Treatment Planning

Images in three orthogonal orientations (axial, sagittal, and coronal) are acquired by the MRI scanner and transferred to the treatment computer for treatment planning. These images show the location of the ultrasound array, thus allowing verification and realignment of the coordinate systems (Fig. 3).

Using the system software, the user contours the skin surface on a contiguous set of axial MR images to aid the system to determine the tissue attenuation effects on the focal intensity. Then the treatment depth is selected and the target volume is outlined in the coronal images. The outlined volume is displayed in the axial and sagittal images to aid in the planning. The software fills the outlined target volume with multiple sonication locations. The degree of the overlap of the focal spots can be chosen during treatment planning. Tightly packed targets are chosen to ensure that all tissue in the targeted volume is fully treated. This is used, for example, in cancer treatments. Loosely packed targets,

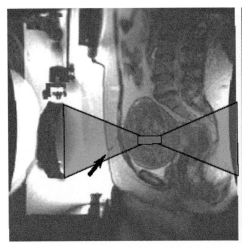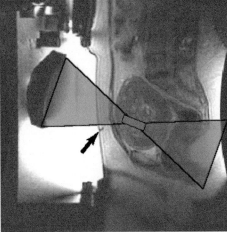

Figure 3   Focused ultrasound beam path superimposed on T_2-weighted images used for treatment planning. (*Left*) Without angling the transducer, the beam path went through a scar (*arrow*). (*Right*) With angling, the scar can be avoided.

where the predetermined coagulated tissue volumes are not overlapping, can also be chosen (typically for debulking large benign tumors, such as uterine fibroids). During the planning, the user interface displays the outline of the beam path for the whole sonicated volume or each spot. These beam outlines are used by the operator to avoid bone or gas that will have undesirable effect on the energy deposition (except, of course, in the treatments of bone tumors) (Fig. 3) (21,22).

   The planning software determines the initial value for the power and the pattern of the sonications (Fig. 4).

   This software uses the ultrasound field distribution at the depth of the focus and then solves for the temperature distribution using the bioheat transfer equation (23). Based on these simulations and earlier animal experiments, look-up tables were developed to provide initial power settings for the sonications. The simulation methods are based on algorithms reported earlier (5,24). The operator can interactively modify this plan by moving the individual focal spot locations and controlling the sonication frequency and power and the focal spot size and location.

Sonications

The sonications are directed to a desired depth by controlling the phase and amplitude of the RF-signal driving each element of the transducer array such that all of the waves are in the same phase at the desired location. This method is described in detail elsewhere (25,26). The system is also designed to allow for control over the focal spot size. In these treatments, the focal volume is increased by scanning the focus electronically during the sonication along a predetermined pattern, as described in Refs. (13,27). Five different scanning patterns can be chosen from to change the size and/or shape of the coagulated tissue volume.

MR Imaging

A custom-made array coil was developed by USA Instruments to improve the signal to noise ratio for the pelvic treatments. This coil has an open loop that is fixed on top of the

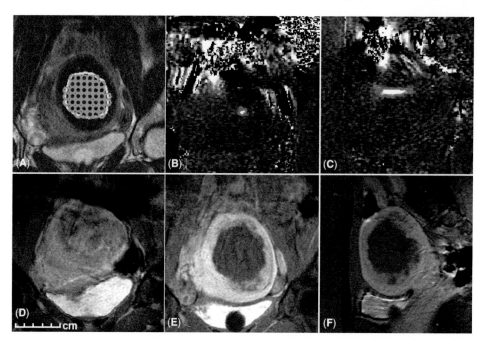

Figure 4 (*See color insert*.) MR images of a uterine fibroid acquired before, during, and after focused ultrasound surgery. (**A**) T_2-weighted images used for treatment planning. The planned sonication locations and outline of the target volume are shown. The targets were chosen so that no area closer than 15 mm from the outer edge of the uterus was ablated. The treatment plan was adjusted during treatment based on thermal dosimetry acquired during each sonication. (**B** and **C**) Temperature maps acquired during two sonications. The contours indicate the regions that achieved a thermal dose of 240 equivalent minutes at 43°C. (**D–F**) Contrast-enhanced T_1-weighted images acquired before (**D**) and after (**E** and **F**) focused ultrasound. The dark areas in **E** and **F** show the area with a coagulated blood supply, indicating a successful treatment. (**A–E**, coronal imaging in the focal plane; **C** and **F**, sagittal imaging along ultrasound beam.)

water bath and a flexible part that wraps around the back of the patient, which contains two additional coils. For more superficial tumors in the breast, a single-loop receiver-only coil is used. The sonications are performed through the coil opening.

MRI examinations are performed on a 1.5 T standard whole body system (Signa, GE Medical System, Milwaukee, Wisconsin, U.S.A.), although it is expected that the system is soon available also for the 3 T magnet. For the localization and targeting, standard T_2-weighted fast spin-echo images are acquired in axial, coronal, and sagittal directions. The ultrasound system is interfaced with the MRI scanner and controls the MRI scanning and accesses the images for treatment planning and monitoring (Fig. 4). Currently, treatment planning with contrast-enhanced images is not approved, as that is an off-label use of the contrast agent. This is a substantial problem for treating breast cancer, which may be hard to delineate with noncontrast MRI. Currently, the use of contrast for treatment planning is undergoing tests for breast cancer (28).

Temperature Monitoring with MRI

The temperature elevations during sonications are monitored by obtaining temperature-sensitive MR images. The ultrasound system software automatically prescribes and executes the temperature imaging. As in the initial clinical study (1), the temperature-dependent proton-resonant frequency shift (29) is calculated using a fast spoiled gradient echo sequence. The first image is triggered prior to the start of the sonication so that the second image acquisition starts when the ultrasound beam is turned on. A series of images are acquired during the sonication and after the power is turned off to map the temperature history of the sonicated tissue volume. The scanner is programmed to reconstruct the magnitude and real and imaginary images for each of these time points. The real and imaginary parts are used to calculate the phase difference between the two time points as described in Refs. (18,30). The proton-resonant frequency change is estimated by dividing the phase change by 2π TE, where TE (the echo time) is the time that the phase in the MR image develops. The magnitude images are used to detect any bulk motion during the sonications. Any motion that destroys image subtraction results in unreliable temperature maps. Such motions may also require repeating the treatment planning. Also, if a large motion is detected in the real-time imaging during sonication, the operator can halt the sonication.

The temperature dependence of the proton-resonant frequency has been shown to be linear above the coagulation threshold (31–33). A problem with the proton-resonant shift thermometry is that it does not detect the temperature elevation in fat (34,35). This also causes uncertainty in the temperature measurement if the voxel contains mixture of fat and other soft tissues. In these cases, special measures such as fat suppression are needed to obtain accurate temperature measurements. Another problem is the gas in the image that distorts the magnetic field and the temperature image. This can happen in the ultrasound field when temperatures in excess of 100°C are induced and cause tissue boiling. This distorts the temperature image at the focus but good estimation of the temperature can be obtained outside of the boiling tissue such that the induced tissue damage can be accurately predicted. Similarly, induction of inertial cavitation bubbles and their use to enhance tissue heating do not prevent accurate lesion size prediction (36).

The ultrasound system workstation automatically prescribes and triggers the temperature-sensitive MRI sequences during the sonications. The imaging plane is determined by the operator either to be across the focus (coronal) or along the beam path (axial or sagittal) by selecting the appropriate option in the user interface display. The imaging plane follows the location of the ultrasound focus automatically from location to location without operator input to the MRI scanner. After the sonication, the images are automatically transferred to the ultrasound system workstation that performs near real-time temperature elevation and thermal dose calculations and display. In the system that is currently Food and Drug Administration (FDA) approved, the temperature and dose distributions are displayed within seconds after the sonication is completed. A more advanced system is currently undergoing FDA review, which displays each temperature map immediately after each image acquisition.

The system uses the time-temperature profile for each MR voxel to calculate a map of the accumulated thermal dose induced by the temperature exposure (10,18). The boundary of an isothermal dose value of 240 minutes at the reference temperature of 43°C is selected to predict the size of the coagulated tissue (12). The voxels that reach this threshold are colored on temperature images. The cumulative thermal dose from all sonications is displayed on top of the treatment plan after each exposure. For sonications monitored along the beam direction, the dose is estimated in the coronal plane by assuming radial symmetry of the beam. This dose contour can be used to determine where additional sonications should be placed to reach complete dose coverage of the target volume. In uterine fibroids, it has been found that the thermal dose underpredicts the resulting nonperfused volume observed in post-treatment contrast-enhanced imaging

(37,38). In some cases, regions that were obviously not heated at all become nonperfused. A likely explanation of this underprediction is that the ablation is occluding blood vessels (39), resulting in secondary tissue damage via ischemia. It should be noted that these nonperfused regions are contained within the fibroid itself, so this phenomena is likely a net benefit, as it increases the ablated volume.

Treatment Execution

After the treatment planning, a low-energy test pulse with the beam aimed in a single location in the target volume is delivered. The temperature rise during such sonications can be detected even for sonications that do not produce damage (40). The temperature imaging is performed across the beam at the focal depth. The power is increased until the temperature elevation at the focus is visible on the temperature sensitive image. The location of the actual temperature elevation is then indicated to the system to precisely align the MRI and ultrasound beam coordinate systems. After this, the same alignment procedure is repeated while performing the temperature imaging along the axis of the beam.

When the test pulse is located in the planned position, the complete target volume is sonicated with a series of high-power bursts, typically 10 to 20 seconds in duration. A new location adjustment can be made after any of the sonications. The initial sonication power, frequency, duration, and focal spot size are predicted by the system software. The operator can adjust these sonication parameters based on the measured temperature and thermal dose values so that predetermined volume of tissue coagulation can be achieved with each sonication. During the volume sonications, the temperature imaging direction is selected either along or across the beam axis (Fig. 4). After the completion of the planned sonications, the system allows the operator to add sonications to any location that did not receive adequate thermal exposure. During each sonication, a series of phased images are obtained together with regular magnitude images. The fast spoiled gradient echo magnitude images provide anatomical information and the patient anatomy can be clearly seen. These images are used to determine if the patient moves during or between sonications and that the temperature elevation is induced in the desired tissue volume. This is critical safety feature during ultrasound surgery when awake patients are treated.

In addition, since the thermal coagulation of the fibroid tissue is not painful, feedback from the patient is used to determine normal tissue heating. For example, if the patient experiences sensations in their back during sonications in the uterine fibroid treatments (due to thermal stimulation of nerves located next to the pelvic bone that is heated by diverging beam beyond the focus), the parameters can be adjusted to reduce the exposure of the nerves. This adjustment can be changing the angle of the ultrasound beam, increasing the ultrasound frequency, or decreasing the focal volume and sonication power. With this patient feedback combined with quantitative temperature mapping, a reliable temperature rise can be achieved that is high enough to produce thermal coagulation, but not high enough to produce boiling or pain (38).

Treatment Effect Verification

To ensure that the target volume was sufficiently treated, contrast-enhanced imaging is performed to show the areas that were coagulated. For contrast-enhanced images, T_1-weighted imaging is started before intravenous injection of the gadolinium-based contrast agent and continued after the injection to demonstrate areas of lack of contrast enhancement, indicating coagulation of the blood supply (Fig. 4) (41).

FUTURE DIRECTIONS

The latest clinical studies evaluated the feasibility of deep tissue surgery using a second-generation MRI-guided focused ultrasound system that utilizes a large-scale ultrasound phased array applicator for electronic focal spot depth and volume control. The research demonstrates that the phased array could significantly increase the focal spot size and allow larger targets to be treated. In the first-generation system with a single element transducer, the targeted volume was approximately $0.1\,cm^3$ per sonication. With the second-generation system, volumes up to approximately $1\,cm^3$ per sonication can be coagulated. The results also show that the focal spot depth could be electronically controlled up to 12 cm deep. In addition, the temperature information derived from the MR thermometry was shown to be a reasonable estimate of the treatment effect in the tissue. Therefore, MRI-guided focused ultrasound offers online control of the thermal exposure in the target and surrounding tissues to assure safe and effective thermal coagulation of tissue in a clinical setting. It is anticipated that the future phased array systems would have a large number of elements thus reducing and eliminating the need for mechanical motion. This will allow fast focal spot positioning needed for optimal and automated treatment delivery (42–47) but will require array and driving hardware development. The optimal utilization of bubble-enhanced heating (36,48–50) will most likely require phased array applicators resulting in an increase in the focal spot size and reduction in the treatment time. The treatment planning software will likely be extended to utilize the MRI information to calculate the wave propagation through the heterogeneous tissues and determine the phase and amplitude corrections needed to provide desired focusing (51).

Several methods that allow for temperature monitoring in moving organs are also being investigated (52–54), which could allow for monitoring of focused ultrasound treatments in organs such as liver and kidney. If this motion-robust imaging is combined with real-time tracking of the organ location and a phased array transducer that can rapidly steer the focal point, one could treat these moving organs while the patient is breathing freely. Previous tests of focused ultrasound ablation of such organs have been performed in patients under general anesthesia (55,56) or during breath-holds (57).

There are experimental devices that integrate the MRI thermometry and ultrasound delivery in a closed-loop feedback system that allows potentially faster energy delivery. For example, spiral scanning to increase the treated tissue has been demonstrated in animals (43,44). Similarly, a transurethral system with rotational element scanning while controlling the temperature automatically had been shown to be effective in treating prostate tissue in animals (58). Both of these systems utilize longer sonications (minutes) while using the MRI thermometry to determine the completeness of the coagulation thus reducing the overall treatment time. According to a simulation study, similar result can be achieved by fast but optimized sonication patters with a multielement phased array (59). All of these studies show that in the future, the MRI-guided focused ultrasound systems will potentially be even more integrated where the online MRI thermometry is used by the software to control and alter the treatment execution such that the target volume is precisely coagulated with the minimal exposure to the surrounding tissues. This will no doubt result in faster and better treatments in the future.

MRI-guided focused ultrasound systems will develop, making it feasible to treat more targets that can be reached by the ultrasound beam without being blocked by bone or gas. In addition, there will be development of site-specific devices to treat targets not reachable via the external route. As an example, intracavitary arrays may be developed for prostate (60), cardiac ablation (61), and esophageal tumor treatments (62). It may also be that interstitial or catheter-based ultrasound sources (58,63–67) will become clinically available and preferred method for some treatments. All of these approaches will have their own registration and control challenges that need to be solved for reliable clinical treatment execution.

REFERENCES

1. Hynynen K, Pomeroy O, Smith DN, et al. MR imaging-guided focused ultrasound surgery of fibroadenomas in the breast: a feasibility study. Radiology 2001; 219(1):176–185.
2. Gianfelice D, Khiat A, Boulanger Y, Amara M, Belblidia A. Feasibility of magnetic resonance imaging-guided focused ultrasound surgery as an adjunct to tamoxifen therapy in high-risk surgical patients with breast carcinoma. J Vasc Interv Radiol 2003; 14(10): 1275–1282.
3. Gianfelice D, Khiat A, Amara M, Belblidia A, Boulanger Y. MR imaging-guided focused US ablation of breast cancer: histopathologic assessment of effectiveness—initial experience. Radiology 2003; 227(3):849–855.
4. Huber PE, Jenne JW, Rastert R, et al. A new noninvasive approach in breast cancer therapy using magnetic resonance imaging-guided focused ultrasound surgery. Cancer Res 2001; 61(23): 8441–8447.
5. Fjield T, Hynynen K. The combined concentric-ring and sector-vortex phased array for MRI guided ultrasound surgery. IEEE Trans Ultrason Ferroelectr Freq Contr 1997; 44(5):1157–1167.
6. Daum DR, Hynynen K. A 256 element ultrasonic phased array system for treatment of large volumes of deep-seated tissue. IEEE Trans Ultrason Ferroelect Freq Contr 1999; 46(5): 1254–1268.
7. Daum DR, Smith NB, King R, Hynynen K. In vivo demonstration of noninvasive, thermal surgery of the liver and kidney using an ultrasonic phased array. Ultrasound Med Biol 1999; 25(7):1087–1098.
8. Kuroda K, Oshio K, Chung A, Hynynen K, Jolesz FA. Temperature mapping using water proton chemical shift: chemical shift selective phase mapping method. Magn Reson Med 1997; 38:845–851.
9. Cline HE, Hynynen K, Hardy CJ, Watkins RD, Schenck JF, Jolesz FA. MR temperature mapping of focused ultrasound surgery. Magn Reson Med 1994; 30:98–106.
10. Chung A, Jolesz FA, Hynynen K. Thermal dosimetry of a focused ultrasound beam in vivo by MRI. Med Phys 1999; 26(9):2017–2026.
11. Damianou C, Hynynen K. Focal spacing and near-field heating during pulsed high temperature ultrasound hyperthermia treatment. Ultrasound Med Biol 1993; 19:777–787.
12. Damianou C, Hynynen K, Fan X. Evaluation of accuracy of a theoretical model for predicting the necrosed tissue volume during focused ultrasound surgery. IEEE Trans Ultrason Ferroelectr Freq Contr 1995; 42:182–187.
13. Daum DR, Hynynen K. Thermal dose optimization via temporal switching in ultrasound surgery. IEEE Trans Ultrason Ferroelectr Freq Contr 1998; 45(1):208–215.
14. Daum DR, Hynynen K. Theoretical design of a spherically sectioned phased array for ultrasound surgery of the liver. Eur J Ultrasound 1999; 9(1):61–69.
15. Fan X, Hynynen K. A study of various parameters of spherically curved phased arrays for noninvasive ultrasound surgery. Phys Med Biol 1996; 41:591–608.
16. Fan X, Hynynen K. Ultrasound surgery using multiple sonications—treatment time considerations. Ultrasound Med Biol 1996; 22(4):471–482.
17. McDannold N, Hynynen K, Wolf D, Wolf G, Jolesz F. MRI evaluation of thermal ablation of tumors with focused ultrasound. J Mag Res Imag 1998; 8(1):91–100.
18. McDannold N, Jolesz FA, Hynynen K. The use of MRI in vivo to monitor thermal build-up during focused ultrasound surgery. Radiology 1999; 211:419–426.

19. Gianfelice D, Khiat A, Amara M, Belblidia A, Boulanger Y. MR imaging-guided focused ultrasound surgery of breast cancer: correlation of dynamic contrast-enhanced MRI with histopathologic findings. Breast Cancer Res Treat 2003; 82(2):93–101.

20. Coakley A. Acoustical detection of single cavitation events in a focussed field in water at 1 MHz. J Acoust Soc Am 1971; 49:792–801.

21. Hynynen K. Hot spots created at skin-air interfaces during ultrasound hyperthermia. Int J Hyperther 1990; 6:1005–1012.

22. Hynynen K, DeYoung D. Temperature elevation at muscle-bone interface during scanned, focused ultrasound hyperthermia. Int J Hyperther 1988; 4:267–279.

23. Pennes HH. Analysis of tissue and arterial blood temperatures in the resting human forearm. J Appl Physiol 1948; 1(2):93–122.

24. Damianou C, Hynynen K. The effect of various physical parameters on the size and shape of necrosed tissue volume during ultrasound surgery. J Acoust Soc Am 1994; 95:1641–1649.

25. Cain CA, Umemura SA. Concentric-ring and sector vortex phased array applicators for ultrasound hyperthermia therapy. IEEE Trans Microwave Theory Tech 1986; MTT-34: 542–551.

26. Fjield T, Fan X, Hynynen K. A parametric study of the concentric-ring transducer design for MRI guided ultrasound surgery. J Acoust Soc Am 1996; 100:1220–1230.

27. Wan H, VanBaren P, Ebbini ES, Cain CA. Ultrasound surgery: comparison of strategies using phased array systems. IEEE Trans Ultrason Ferroelectr Freq Contr 1996; 43(6): 1085–1098.

28. Furusawa H, Namba K, Thomsen S, et al. Magnetic resonance-guided focused ultrasound surgery of breast cancer: reliability and effectiveness. J Am Coll Surg 2006; 203(1):54–63.

29. Ishihara Y, Calderon A, Watanabe H, Okamoto K, Suzuki Y, Kuroda K. A precise and fast temperature mapping using water proton chemical shift. Magn Reson Med 1995; 34: 814–823.

30. Chung A, Hynynen K, Cline HE, Colucci V, Oshio K, Jolesz F. Optimization of spoiled gradient-echo phase imaging for in vivo localization of focused ultrasound beam. Magn Reson Med 1996; 36(5):745–752.

31. Hynynen K, Freund W, Cline HE, et al. A clinical noninvasive MRI monitored ultrasound surgery method. Radiographics 1996; 16(1):185–195.

32. Kuroda K, Chung A, Hynynen K, Jolesz FA. Calibration of water proton chemical shift with temperature for noninvasive temperature imaging during focused ultrasound surgery. J Mag Res Imag 1998; 8:175–181.

33. Peters RD, Hinks RS, Henkelman RM. Ex vivo tissue-type independence in proton-resonance frequency shift MR thermometry. Magn Reson Med 1998; 40:454–459.

34. De Poorter J. Noninvasive MRI thermometry with the proton resonance frequency method: study of susceptibility effects. Magn Reson Med 1995; 34(3):359–367.

35. De Zwart JA, Vimeux FC, Delalande C, Canioni P, Moonen CT. Fast lipid-suppressed MR temperature mapping with echo-shifted gradient-echo imaging and spectral-spatial excitation. Magn Reson Med 1999; 42(1):53–59.

36. Sokka SD, King R, Hynynen K. MRI-guided gas bubble enhanced ultrasound heating in in vivo rabbit thigh. Phys Med Biol 2003; 48(2):223–241.

37. Tempany CM, Stewart EA, McDannold N, Quade BJ, Jolesz FA, Hynynen K. MR imaging-guided focused ultrasound surgery of uterine leiomyomas: a feasibility study. Radiology 2003; 226(3):897–905.

38. McDannold N, Tempany CM, Fennessy FM, et al. Uterine leiomyomas: MR imaging-based thermometry and thermal dosimetry during focused ultrasound thermal ablation. Radiology 2006; 240(1):263–272.

39. Hynynen K, Colucci V, Chung A, Jolesz FA. Noninvasive artery occlusion using MRI guided focused ultrasound. Ultrasound Med Biol 1996; 22(8):1071–1077.

40. Hynynen K, Vykhodtseva NI, Chung A, Sorrentino V, Colucci V, Jolesz FA. Thermal effects of focused ultrasound on the brain: determination with MR Imaging. Radiology 1997; 204: 247–253.

41. Hynynen K, Darkazanli A, Damianou C, Unger E, Schenck JF. The usefulness of contrast agent and GRASS imaging sequence for MRI guided noninvasive ultrasound surgery. Invest Radiol 1994; 29:897–903.

42. Smith NB, Merilees NK, Hynynen K, Dahleh M. Control system for an MRI compatible intracavitary ultrasound array for thermal treatment of prostate disease. Int J Hyperther 2001; 17(3):271–282.

43. Vimeux FC, De Zwart JA, Palussiere J, et al. Real-time control of focused ultrasound heating based on rapid MR thermometry. Invest Radiol 1999; 34(3):190–193.

44. Mougenot C, Salomir R, Palussiere J, Grenier N, Moonen CT. Automatic spatial and temporal temperature control for MR-guided focused ultrasound using fast 3D MR thermometry and multispiral trajectory of the focal point. Magn Reson Med 2004; 52:1005–1015.

45. Malinen M, Huttunen T, Hynynen K, Kaipio JP. Simulation study for thermal dose optimization in ultrasound surgery of the breast. Med Phys 2004; 31(5):1296–1307.

46. Arora D, Minor MA, Skliar M, Roemer RB. Control of thermal therapies with moving power deposition field. Phys Med Biol 2006; 51(5):1201–1219.

47. Arora D, Cooley D, Perry T, et al. MR thermometry-based feedback control of efficacy and safety in minimum-time thermal therapies: phantom and in-vivo evaluations. Int J Hyperther 2006; 22(1):29–42.

48. Hynynen K. The threshold for thermally significant cavitation in dog's thigh muscle in vivo. Ultrasound Med Biol 1991; 17:157–169.

49. Curiel L, Chavrier F, Gignoux B, Pichardo S, Chesnais S, Chapelon JY. Experimental evaluation of lesion prediction modelling in the presence of cavitation bubbles: intended for high-intensity focused ultrasound prostate treatment. Med Biol Eng Comput 2004; 42(1):44–54.

50. McDannold NJ, Vykhodtseva NI, Hynynen K. Microbubble contrast agent with focused ultrasound to create brain lesions at low power levels: MR imaging and histologic study in rabbits. Radiology 2006; 241(1):95–106.

51. Liu H-L, McDannold N, Hynynen K. Focal beam distortion and treatment planning in abdominal focused ultrasound surgery. Med Phys 2005; 32(5):1270–1280.

52. De Zwart JA, Vimeux FC, Palussiere J, et al. On-line correction and visualization of motion during MRI-controlled hyperthermia. Magn Reson Med 2001; 45(1):128–137.

53. Vigen KK, Daniel BL, Pauly JM, Butts K. Triggered, navigated, multi-baseline method for proton resonance frequency temperature mapping with respiratory motion. Magn Reson Med 2003; 50(5):1003–1010.

54. Rieke V, Vigen KK, Sommer G, Daniel BL, Pauly JM, Butts K. Referenceless PRF shift thermometry. Magn Reson Med 2004; 51(6):1223–1231.

55. Wu F, Wang ZB, Zhu H, et al. Extracorporeal high intensity focused ultrasound treatment for patients with breast cancer. Breast Cancer Res Treat 2005; 92(1):51–60.

56. Wu F, Wang ZB, Chen WZ, et al. Advanced hepatocellular carcinoma: treatment with high-intensity focused ultrasound ablation combined with transcatheter arterial embolization. Radiology 2005; 235(2):659–667.

57. Visioli AG, Rivens IH, ter Haar GR, et al. Preliminary results of a phase I dose escalation clinical trial using focused ultrasound in the treatment of localised tumours. Eur J Ultrasound 1999; 9(1):11–18.

58. Chopra R, Burtnyk M, Haider MA, Bronskill MJ. Method for MRI-guided conformal thermal therapy of prostate with planar transurethral ultrasound heating applicators. Phys Med Biol 2005; 50(21):4957–4975.

59. Malinen M, Huttunen T, Kaipio JP, Hynynen K. Scanning path optimization for ultrasound surgery. Phys Med Biol 2005; 50(15):3473–3490.

60. Sokka SD, Hynynen K. The feasibility of MRI-guided whole prostate ablation with a linear aperiodic intracavitary ultrasound phased array [In Process Citation]. Phys Med Biol 2000; 45 (11):3373–3383.

61. Yin X, Epstein LM, Hynynen K. Noninvasive transesophageal cardiac thermal ablation using a 2-D focused, ultrasound phased array: a simulation study. IEEE Trans Ultrason Ferroelectr Freq Control 2006; 53(6):1138–1149.

62. Melodelima D, Salomir R, Mougenot C, et al. Intraluminal ultrasound applicator compatible with magnetic resonance imaging "real-time" temperature mapping for the treatment of oesophageal tumours: an ex vivo study. Med Phys 2004; 31(2):236–244.
63. Hynynen K, Davis KL. Small cylindrical ultrasound sources for induction of hyperthermia via body cavities or interstitial implants. Int J Hyperther 1993; 9:263–274.
64. Nau WH, Diederich CJ, Ross AB, et al. MRI-guided interstitial ultrasound thermal therapy of the prostate: a feasibility study in the canine model. Med Phys 2005; 32(3):733–743.
65. Nau WH, Diederich CJ, Shu R. Feasibility of using interstitial ultrasound for intradiscal thermal therapy: a study in human cadaver lumbar discs. Phys Med Biol 2005; 50(12): 2807–2821.
66. Diederich CJ, Nau WH, Ross AB, et al. Catheter-based ultrasound applicators for selective thermal ablation: progress towards MRI-guided applications in prostate. Int J Hyperther 2004; 20(7):739–756.
67. Pisani LJ, Ross AB, Diederich CJ, et al. Effects of spatial and temporal resolution for MR image-guided thermal ablation of prostate with transurethral ultrasound. J Magn Reson Imag 2005; 22(1):109–118.

6
Treatment Planning

Gregory T. Clement

Department of Radiology, Brigham and Women's Hospital and Harvard Medical School, Boston, Massachusetts, U.S.A.

INTRODUCTION

Treatment planning in radiation therapy refers to the stages before clinical operation in which the beam strength, distribution, target windows, and predicted doses are calculated on a per-patient basis. Such planning has become a standard part of radiation oncology and is the primary role of medical physicists. Although many procedures have resulted in documented treatment strategies (1), standardized treatment guidelines have yet to be established in focused ultrasound therapies.

In principle, the process of focusing ultrasound into deep tissue to induce temperatures high enough to ablate tissue is straightforward. It can be achieved with a single, spherically curved radiator operating at frequencies approximately between 0.5 and 10 MHz, with most procedures performed around 1 MHz. The intensity achieved at the focus varies with the procedure in the range of 103 to 104 W/cm^2, sustained for 1 to 30 seconds. The main requirement is that the frequency be high enough to allow significant energy absorption at the focus, yet not so high as to cause appreciable energy loss in the region between the transducer and the focus. Unfortunately, tissue inhomogeneities can distort the intended focal point and make the temperature rise at the focal point very hard to predict. For this reason, magnetic resonance (MR) targeting and monitoring has been critical to provide insight on the behavior of the therapeutic ultrasound field. The addition of more advanced prediction in the pretreatment stages of therapy offers a way to go beyond simply providing quality assurance and, in fact, may allow treatment within volumes otherwise unreachable.

A number of aspects of traditional radiation planning stages can be expedited in magnetic resonance imaging (MRI)-guided focused ultrasound surgery (MRIgFUS) due to the immediate availability of an imaging modality, allowing relaxed requirements for immobilization and altogether eliminating the need for certain steps such as marking. Presently, integrated MRI is being employed for treatment planning in order to register patient location to the ultrasound transducer and focused beam. In this manner, the operator may visually assess the ultrasound path via a graphic overlay and verify that no critical structures are traversed (Fig. 1).

In this procedure, computer algorithms indicate the volume of tissue that will potentially be exposed to ultrasound radiation during treatment. The actual treatment volume and the size of the ablated area will have dependency on several controlled parameters, including the sonication time, the focal depth, transducer geometry, transducer

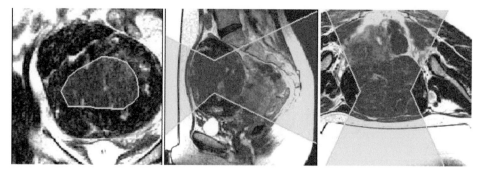

Figure 1 Geometric outline of the intended treatment volume (*left*) and regions potentially traversed by the ultrasound beam (*center* and *right*). The graphic can be used to rapidly check for sensitive areas over the volume as well as aid in the initial positioning of the transducer relative to the target.

efficiency, and element configuration. They also depend on the lesser-known acoustic properties of the tissues within the ultrasound beam.

While the recent clinical results using MRI and MRI-based thermometry to guide focused ultrasound surgery (FUS) have been promising, large variations in focal temperature distribution have been reported (2). These results indicate that the implementation of more advanced treatment planning techniques will be essential if therapeutic ultrasound procedures are to be fully realized. The observed variations are the result of a number of factors including tissue composition and heterogeneity as well as the size and shape of the ultrasound beam. Significant tissue inhomogeneity leads to focal beam distortion, which can restrict the ability to focus energy in deep-seated tissues. It is, however, possible to restore a distorted focus (3,4) by means of planning algorithms specifically tailored to ultrasound propagation.

This chapter covers the necessary steps for comprehensive treatment planning. Unlike its better-established counterpart in radiotherapy, the integration of FUS with MRI offers the ability to perform the planning in a short period, allowing the possibility of combining planning and treatment stages into a single session. Procedures include an imaging and registration stage, followed by tissue identification and segmentation, modeling of the acoustic and thermal fields within the relevant region, identification of sensitive areas, beam modification, and finally, quantitative prediction of the optimized ultrasound beam.

FIELD MODELING

The initial planning step involves predicting the overall ultrasound path as it propagates through the body. Calculating this path requires a priori knowledge of the acoustic properties and orientation of all tissues in front of the transducer as well as accurate registration between the transducer and the body. While all major tissues have been characterized (5), many tissues, and bone in particular (6), can be highly patient-specific. Some tissues, such as the breast, also have a significant degree of heterogeneity with poorly defined boundaries and interleaved regions of fat and other tissues.

Both registration and tissue identification can be performed with information from computed tomography (CT) or MR images. However, CT has the additional ability to offer three-dimensional (3D) density information given the reconstructed X-ray intensity in Hounsfield units. This spatially dependent density, ρ, can be used to calculate the speed of sound, c, and the acoustic impedance ($\sim\rho \cdot c$). Moreover, the 3D maps created from CT do not require further segmentation to distinguish between tissue types. While CT measurement is vital for accurate modeling through highly heterogeneous structures such as bone (3,7), MR may be sufficient for less complex structures. Future MR developments may also allow automated tissue identification that could eliminate the need for CT maps in soft tissues. With MRI, interfaces may be manually selected via an interface or, given sufficient contrast between tissue types, the segmentation process may be automated (4).

The acoustic properties of tissues may be altered by the onset of cavitation (8), as well as self-induced changes in acoustic properties due to a dependence on tissue temperature. The former effect has been broadly studied in vivo and shown to both enhance heating and affect lesion shape and location (9), and a FUS protocol that induces and then uses gas bubbles at the focus to enhance the ultrasound absorption and ultimately create larger lesions in vivo. In the context of field modeling, a cluster of cavitating bubbles has a shielding effect, scattering energy and moving the planned focus forward toward the transducer. Thermal lensing is caused by temperature changes that rise or, in the case of fat, lower the sound speed, causing the area to act as a lens. The effect has been reported to result in a 1 to 2 mm error introduced into the planned focal location (10).

Given knowledge of the medium, accurate modeling of ultrasound must stem from an equation that sufficiently describes the response of the tissue to the impending ultrasound energy. Thermal and viscous losses are not only appreciable but play the central role in thermal ablation. Nonlinear effects indicating that the tissue's displacement can no longer respond linearly with pressure are clearly present in high-intensity therapeutic beams. Yet, in modeling the field propagation, nonlinearities can often be neglected due to the relatively short distances traversed and the high gain of the focused beam. Nonlinear wave propagation can lead to enhanced heating by transfer of energy in to higher harmonic frequencies of the driving frequency (11). These higher frequencies have a higher absorption coefficient and thus are more readily converted into thermal energy.

Equally important to model selection is the application of a valid method for solving the relevant equation. The preferred method is dependent on the complexity of the tissue being modeled, with a general trade-off between accuracy and computation time. The key is to select a method that is sufficiently accurate to within a given tolerance, without becoming computationally exhaustive. Properly selected near-real-time planning is now attainable for many problems in therapeutic ultrasound. Even for relatively coarse but rapid methods, the computation error is generally significantly smaller than the uncertainty of the acoustic properties of the tissues being considered. In this respect, placing exhaustive attention on reducing computational error is analogous to sanding jagged wood with fine sandpaper.

Major methods of modeling propagation include finite element modeling (FEM) (12), finite difference (FD) (13), temporal or spatial planar projection (spectral) (14), full wave vector domain modeling (k-space) (15), and integral solutions. In the FD approach, the values on a given mesh can be used to produce a discrete version of a spatial derivative. These derivatives are obtained in terms of differences at the grid points. For instance, in three dimensions, a discrete version of the wave equation (linear or nonlinear), which can be solved on a cubic grid of size, may be derived directly from the definition of a derivative. In treatment planning, the grid can represent any type of tissue structure within the propagating ultrasound beam. This is in contrast to the finite element approach, where a fitting function such as a polynomial is obtained for the regions between the points, and the coefficients of the fitting function are determined by the values at specified nodes. In each case, the spatial derivative can be used to iterate the solution in time, but in FD, the definition of the time derivative is used to infer the solution at some point in time. The method, properly implemented, will provide a complete solution in space and time for an arbitrary tissue structure. However, this method can be quite computationally intensive and may become numerically unstable for improperly selected time steps.

Particular attention will be paid to the spectral and wave vector methods, based on computational advantages, discussed below, and their ability to easily incorporate real data. That is, simulations generally start with an ideal source distribution of uniformly radiating transducer elements. With spectral and wave vector algorithms, it is straight-forward to start with a source distribution consisting of actual pressure field measurements, which may be projected backward to the transducer surface. In a treatment planning study conducted in vivo, the spectral planar projection method used with a laboratory-measured source distribution was shown to significantly improve the ability to predict temperature rise (16).

Spectral planar projection techniques have strong parallels with Fourier optics (17) and use Fourier integral solutions of the overlying wave equation to reduce the problem to a Helmholtz equation. For homogeneous tissues, the knowledge of the field in a single plane is sufficient to specify the field everywhere in the tissue. A transfer function propagates the field in the spatial frequency domain between a specified plane and a new plane, which does not need to be parallel to the final plane. The transfer function is dependent only upon the frequency of the ultrasound, making it particularly advantageous to most therapeutic techniques, which generally use a continuous wave (CW) or near-CW mode. For example, given an initial plane, a full treatment volume may be described in under than a minute using a presently standard (2 GHz Pentium, 1 MB RAM) desktop computer. A similar result may be acquired using the above-mentioned FEM or FD approaches, but requiring much greater processing time ($>10^2 \times$) due to the fact that a single complex number can represent an entire infinite plane wave in the wave vector-frequency domain, as opposed to a requirement in space time of storing and tracking the instantaneous behavior of a wave over 3D space for each time step.

Specular reflection (14) may readily be added to projection techniques as well as the inclusion of shear modes of vibration (18). At typical therapeutic frequencies between 0.5 and 2 MHz shear wave attenuation is too high to be appreciable in tissue, however such waves can be as large or even larger than standard longitudinal modes in bone. Consideration of shear waves becomes necessary in new procedures, such as transskull treatment, that utilize the bone as a treatment window.

Where applicable, the spectral model has clear advantages and has already been applied to the complex problem of transskull propagation (3). The primary limitations of the spectral model arise from regions of significant heterogeneity or a large degree of curvature between the sections of tissue being considered. The primary assumption is that for a given layer, the local boundary conditions are those for horizontally layered media with no curvature. Similar assumptions have been considered in underwater acoustics, where cylindrical shells have been modeled as flat plates. The solutions are known to be valid when the wavelength of waves is smaller than the radius of curvature. Following this criterion, the layered-projection method is valid for the propagation of a field through a curved surface, provided the surface is sufficiently smooth relative to the highest relevant wave number. In practice, the field will be projected to a plane near the surface and then divided into a series of virtual sources. The spectral method can be used if first the planar approximation agrees to at least within ¼ λ or less depending upon the desired tolerance of the maximum spatial frequency k. That is, a continuous surface must be present whose surface varies by less than ¼ λ over the section of the beam being considered. Second, scattering due to inclusions smaller than the ultrasound wavelength becomes impractical to model. Thus in regions containing objects on the order of or smaller than the imaging wavelength, the planar spectral model is at its limit, and the k-space approach becomes preferable. Alternative methods such as variable grid finite-difference time-domain (FDTD) or FEM can also be applied, but they are slow and require large amounts of physical memory.

The k-space method allows the medium to be expressed in terms of space-varying density and sound speed. Such an approach was followed by Mast et al. (19), who have studied 3D models for wave propagation in fluid-like inhomogeneous tissues. The method operates as a spectral model to the extent that its operations are performed in wave vector space but advances the waveform in small finite time steps, dt. In this manner, the waveform "feels" its way forward in time determining the field with each step and then replacing this newly calculated field as the initial value. Such operations bring the possibility of variable timescale techniques, with larger steps used if the waveform is within a homogeneous region. In the limiting case where the region is completely homogeneous, the method is equivalent to the temporal planar projection method (20).

Although it can be both computationally exhaustive and time-intensive, direct solution of the Rayleigh–Sommerfeld integral is the most straightforward and still most utilized method for calculating fields. The integral is strictly valid for the case of a planar, baffled radiator. However, a number of studies have been performed showing how this approach may be used to perform acoustic field calculations in inhomogeneous media with curved interfaces for high-frequency ultrasound (21). However, under certain conditions, measurable error is present not only near the transducer but also at the ultrasound focus (22). Layered integral approaches have been described for therapy (23,24), but generally break down as the curvature becomes large. Further, to stay computationally feasible, the method generally considers only the forward-propagating wave, potentially neglecting localized regions of high intensity caused by reflected waves.

For the purpose of treatment planning, the ideal method for a particular situation is the one that provides the fastest calculation while staying within an acceptable degree of accuracy. In MRIgFUS, tissue geometry can be acquired from initial MR images in order to outline the tissue boundaries, while literature values of tissue properties (5) can be used as an input for the calculation program. Once the field is calculated over its entire route through the patient, including any appreciable backscattered energy, the resultant field has several direct applications in planning. The most direct application is the identification of potential problematic regions within the focused beam. In addition to avoiding sensitive areas, gas interfaces produce strong reflections and can result in undesired heating at the interface. After identification, compensation for such interfaces is possible by shaping the beam to avoid the interface. A simple version of this method is currently used clinically in uterine fibroid treatments, as illustrated in Figure 1. In this case, the beam is simply assumed to lie within conic volumes extending from the focus toward and away from the transducer. Surgical planning algorithms perform beam steering using standard beam-shading techniques, where a null pressure is planned in the region with air, using information from MRI. If the air lies directly within the beam path, associated array elements are turned off and addition planning is performed without these elements.

A second application is the calculation of the acoustic intensity at and away from the treatment target. Figure 2 shows both an idealized and a distorted focus.

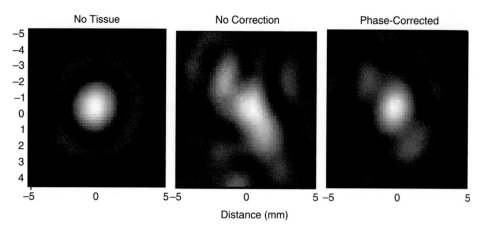

Figure 2 Ultrasound field distribution across the focus in water (*left*) and with a part of abdominal wall in front of the focus (*center*). Phase aberration correction was able to restore the focus and increase the amplitude at the intended target location (*right*).

This measurement gives a quantitative prediction of the treatment location, and how much it deviates from an idealized case. It is stressed, however, that knowledge of intensity alone has been shown to be a poor predictor of damage (2). For this purpose, the intensity is better utilized in the third and most critical application of the field calculation: the prediction of the time-dependent temperature rise and the thermal dose (25), a parameter that describes the overall exposure as a function of time and temperature. Accurate dose prediction is highly dependent upon the ability to accurately predict the heat transfer from acoustic to thermal energy. In this respect, much can be utilized from treatment planning in hyperthermia (26). A full treatment of thermal dose prediction is presented in the next section.

A final application for field modeling involves compensation for wave front distortion. Individual elements of an ultrasound phased array may be propagated forward to the intended focus, providing amplitude and phase information. Alternatively, a theoretical point source may be positioned at the focus and then the wave propagated through the tissue to the transducer array. The phase and amplitude at each phased-array element will be recorded and will be used to drive the phased array to focus to the intended target. For thermal treatment planning, the acoustic pressure amplitude distribution will be calculated throughout the sonicated volume and then used in the thermal simulation program.

THERMAL DOSE

Thermal predictions for focused ultrasound build upon a body of work that has been studied beyond a decade for use in hyperthermia applications (26–29). The traditional starting point for thermal dose calculation is the Pennes bioheat transfer equation (30):

$$\rho C_t \frac{\partial T}{\partial t} = \kappa \nabla^2 T - w C_b (T - T_a) + Q$$

where Q provides the heat introduced by ultrasound. The equation is shown here with spatially dependent density ρ, temperature T, arterial temperature T_a, specific heat C_t, thermal conductivity κ, and perfusion w. The equation is nearly always immediately simplified to neglect perfusion terms. Combined with variation in tissue characteristics, the actual temperature profile has been very difficult to predict in vivo in the planning stage. This inability has necessitated the clinical use of online temperature monitoring such as MRI. Fortunately, recent advances in heat transfer modeling combined with improved perfusion measurement techniques using dynamic contrast-enhanced CT and MRI (31) promise to greatly improve the ability to plan thermal dose. In particular, discrete vasculature thermal modeling technique (32) takes into account the thermal behavior of individual blood vessels. Modeling of the bioheat equation is generally more straightforward and may be reduced to a series of ordinary differential equations and solved via the Runge-Kutta iterative method, FDTD, or spectral methods (Fig. 3). A series of numeric and experimental studies have investigated such modeling for treatment planning (12,16,33,34).

Once temperature is predicted as a function of position and time, the thermal dose may be calculated. The notion of thermal dose was born out of empirical observation showing a basic relationship between toxic effect on cells in vitro and in vivo dependent upon both temperature and time. A convention of using 43°C as a reference temperature has been adopted allowing an "equivalent" time to be calculated for temperatures away from this value:

$$t_{43} = \sum_{t=0}^{t=t_f} R^{43-T} \Delta t$$

where T is the average temperature over the time step Δt and R is 0.5 above 43°C and 0.25 below 42°C. In vivo examination of the thermal dose has shown its ability as a predictor of thermal damage (2).

ABERRATION CORRECTION

The central problem in treatment planning lies in predicting the behavior of the ultrasound field after passing through tissue layers. These layers can cause significant

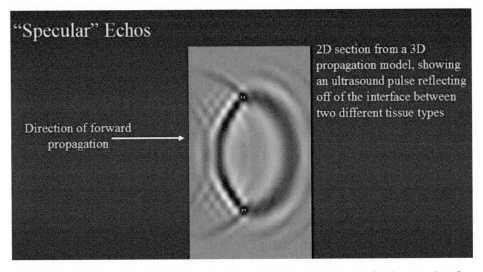

Figure 3 Planar section of a 3D image showing a 0.5 MHz pulsed beam reflecting at an interface with a tissue at higher speed of sound. *Abbreviations*: 2D, two-dimensional; 3D, three-dimensional.

reflection, diffraction, and absorption of the field. In order to correct for these aberrations, an array of ultrasound transducers can be assembled and driven in such a manner that restores a focus. Using a modeling method discussed above, each element in an array is separately simulated using thickness, density, and orientation information obtained from CT or MRI images. These algorithms require precise knowledge of the orientation of the tissue relative to individual array elements using the images. For example, an error of only 0.4 mm represents a ¼-wavelength of a typical 1 MHz signal in tissue. In this application, the primary purpose of the algorithm is to predict the amplitude and phase of the ultrasound radiated by each element at the intended focal point.

To reconstruct a distorted focus, the calculated pressure phase is then compared with the phase expected if the tissues were homogeneous. The phase change caused by the tissues is recorded and used for correcting the driving phase of the transducer array. The driving phase of each element is adjusted by an amount

$$\Delta\phi = \arg\left[P(r)/P_0(r)\right]$$

where P is the acoustic pressure at the intended focal point in the tissue and P_0 is the acoustic pressure expected at the same point in homogeneous tissue. Similarly, a large element could be divided into M sections for propagation, with the driving phase adjusted by

$$\Delta\phi = \arg\left(\sum_{m=1}^{M} P_m(r)/P_0(r)\right).$$

An example of the ability to correct distortion in soft tissue is presented in Figure 2. The field was acquired using a combined 104-element annular-sector phased-array transducer to correct for distortion encountered by a focused ultrasound wave when propagated through tissue layers at 1.5 MHz. Prior to ultrasound measurements, the tissue samples were imaged in a standard 1.5 T MRI system to provide information on the thickness and composition of the tissue interfaces. Tissue samples were excised from pigs, immediately after they were sacrificed. These samples consisted of skin, fat, and tissue layers and with a thickness of approximately 40 mm. Ultrasound measurements were conducted in a tank filled with degassed deionized water. The intensity plots shown were acquired using a 0.075 mm diameter polyvinylidene difluoride hydrophone positioned normal to the axis of symmetry of the transducer array. The hydrophone was scanned over a plane to produce the plots using a stepping motor–controlled 3D positioning system. In the example, significant beam distortion was corrected by phase adjustment and the relative peak amplitude squared was observed to increase by 1.4× the value in the uncorrected case.

This straightforward phase adjustment can be surprisingly powerful and is even used to focus ultrasound through the skull. Clement and Hynynen (3) are using the approach with a layered wave vector-frequency domain model, which propagates ultrasound from a hemisphere-shaped transducer through the skull using input from CT scans of the head. The algorithm calculates the driving phase of each element as described above to maximize the signal at the intended focus. In practice, a stereotaxic reference frame must be affixed to the skulls in order to provide accurate registration between the CT images, MRI, and the transducer. Figure 4 demonstrates the method, which can be utilized in noninvasive ultrasound brain surgery and therapy.

The above method concerns only phase adjustment without concern of the signal amplitude. It is altogether reasonable to assume that beam focusing may be further enhanced through the introduction of amplitude correction in such a way that the acoustic

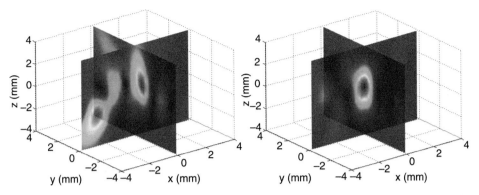

Figure 4 Sections of the three-dimensional ultrasound field about the focus through an ex vivo human skull before (*left*) and after (*right*) a treatment-planning model consisting of planar projection followed by phase correction.

pressures from individual transducer array elements are adjusted to be normalized at the focus. In fact, for the case of transcranial planning, a recent study (35) indicated a small (6%) mean reduction in sidelobe intensity relative to the focal intensity and a reduction (2%) in the full-width-at-half-maximum (FWHM) of the ultrasound beam at the focus. However, these slight improvements came at the expense of large intensity loss at the focus due to the fact that the amplitude correction method necessitates "higher" attenuation in regions that transmit "less" energy. The same study also considered a second correction method that distributed amplitudes such that windows transmitting more energy were exposed with higher ultrasound intensities. In this case, sidelobes also decreased slightly (3%) with no change in the FWHM at the focus. However, the acoustic intensity at the focus also remained the same. Overall, it may be concluded that amplitude correction may offer measurable, but small gains in the focal quality.

SUMMARY

Ultrasound phased arrays and MRI are both already integral parts of FUS treatment. It is seemingly inevitable that treatment devices will be increasingly utilized to their full potential by implementing planning stages for safety assurance, correction of beam aberration, and optimization of thermal dose. Numerous approaches are possible, but successful planning will depend on developing sensible methods and theory. Practical considerations include obtaining accurate knowledge of the thickness and internal structure of tissues and precise registration between all points within the tissue and the ultrasound array. Theoretical considerations involve finding a model as uncomplicated as possible—keeping the problem computationally feasible—without oversimplification of the problem.

The growing number of therapeutic applications and available treatment systems provide clear motivation for the eventual standardization of the planning stages of ultrasound therapy. Such measures would offer consistency and improved quality assurance and the ability to accurately compare treatment data between institutions and systems. Although it is premature to state the optimal modeling methods for a given procedure, a growing body of clinical data will help to center upon ideal planning tools.

Even with improved planning, patient-specific variation in tissue geometry and composition will require monitoring for all stages of treatment. However, implementation of the planning stages will both expand and improve the abilities of MRIgFUS.

REFERENCES

1. Knoos T, Wieslander E. Review of today's treatment planning algorithms. Radiother Oncol 2004; 73:S68.
2. McDannold N, King RL, Jolesz FA, Hynynen K. The use of quantitative temperature images to predict the optimal power for focused ultrasound surgery: in vivo verification in rabbit muscle and brain. Med Phys 2002; 29(3):356–365.
3. Clement GT, Hynynen K. A noninvasive method for focusing ultrasound through the human skull. Phys Med Biol 2002; 47:1219–1236.
4. Liu HL, McDannold N, Hynynen K. Focal beam distortion and treatment planning in abdominal focused ultrasound surgery. Med Phys 2005; 32(5):1270–1280.
5. Duck FA. Physical Properties of Tissue. London: Academic Press, 1990.
6. Clement GT, Hynynen K. Correlation of ultrasound phase with physical skull properties. Ultrasound Med Biol 2002; 28(5):617–624.
7. Aubry JF, Tanter M, Pernot M, Thomas J-L, Fink MA. Experimental demonstration of noninvasive transskull adaptive focusing based on prior computed tomography scans. J Acoust Soc Am 2003; 113(1):84–93.
8. Hynynen K. The threshold for thermally significant cavitation in dog's thigh muscle in vivo. Ultrasound Med Biol 1991; 17:157–169.
9. Sokka SD, King R, Hynynen K. MRI-guided gas bubble enhanced ultrasound heating in in vivo rabbit thigh. Phys Med Biol 2003; 48:223–241.
10. Connor CW, Hynynen K. Bio-acoustic thermal lensing and nonlinear propagation in focused ultrasound surgery using large focal spots: a parametric study. Phys Med Biol 2002; 47(11): 1911–1928.
11. Hynynen K. Demonstration of enhanced temperature elevation due to nonlinear propagation of focussed ultrasound in dog's thigh in vivo. Ultrasound Med Biol 1987; 13(2):85–91.
12. Malinen M, Huttunen T, Kaipio JP. Thermal dose optimization method for ultrasound surgery. Phys Med Biol 2003; 48(6):745–762.
13. Hallaj IM, Cleveland RO. FDTD simulation of finite-amplitude pressure and temperature fields for biomedical ultrasound. J Acoust Soc Am 1999; 105(5):L7–L12.
14. Clement GT, Hynynen K. Forward planar projection through layered media. IEEE Trans Ultrason Ferroelectr Freq Contr 2003; 50:1689–1698.
15. Mast TD, Souriau LP, Liu D-LD, Tabei M, Nachman AI, Waag RC. A k-space method for large-scale models of wave propagation in tissue. IEEE Trans Ultrason Ferroelectr Freq Contr 2001; 48(2):341–354.
16. Mahoney K, Fjield T, McDannold N, Clement GT, Hynynen K. Comparison of modeled and observed in vivo temperature elevations induced by focused ultrasound: implications for treatment planning. Phys Med Biol 2001; 46:1785–1798.
17. Goodman JW. Introduction to Fourier Optics. 1st ed. New York: McGraw-Hill, 1968.
18. Clement GT, White PJ, Hynynen K. Enhanced ultrasound transmission through the human skull using shear mode conversion. J Acoust Soc Am 2004; 115(3):1356–1364.
19. Mast TD, Hinkelman LM, Metlay LA, Orr MJ, Waag RC. Simulation of ultrasonic pulse propagation, distortion, and attenuation in the human chest wall. J Acoust Soc Am 1999; 106 (6):3665–3677.
20. Clement GT, Liu R, Letcher SV, Stepanishen PR. Temporal backward planar projection of acoustic transients. J Acoust Soc Am 1998; 103(4):1723–1726.
21. Fan X, Hynynen K. A study of various parameters of spherically curved phased arrays for noninvasive ultrasound surgery. Phys Med Biol 1996; 41(4):591–608.

22. Sapozhnikov OA, Sinilo TV. Acoustic field produced by a concave radiating surface with allowance for the diffraction. Acoust Phys 2002; 48(6):720–727.

23. Fan X, Hynynen K. The effects of curved tissue layers on the power deposition patterns of therapeutic ultrasound beams. Med Phys 1994; 21:25–34.

24. Sun J, Hynynen K. Focusing of therapeutic ultrasound through a human skull: a numerical study. J Acoust Soc Am 1998; 104:1705–1715.

25. Sapareto SA, Dewey WC. Thermal dose determination in cancer therapy. Int J Radiat Oncol Biol Phys 1984; 10:787–800.

26. Lagendijk JJW. Hyperthermia treatment planning. Phys Trans Med Biol 2000; 45(5): R61–R76.

27. Anhalt DP, Hynynen K, Roemer RB. Patterns of changes of tumour temperatures during clinical hyperthermia: implications for treatment planning, evaluation and control effect of phase errors on field patterns generated by an ultrasound phased-array hyperthermia applicator. Int J Hyperther 1995; 11(3):425–436.

28. McGough RJ, Kessler ML, Ebbini ES, Cain CA. Treatment planning for hyperthermia with ultrasound phased arrays. IEEE Trans Ultrason Ferroelectr Freq Contr 1996; 43(6): 1074–1084.

29. Roemer RB. Engineering aspects of hyperthermia therapy. Annu Rev Biomed Engineer 1999; 1:347–376.

30. Pennes HH. Analysis of tissue and arterial blood temperatures in the resting human forearm. J Appl Physiol 1948; 1(2):93–122.

31. Padhani AR. Dynamic contrast-enhanced MRI in clinical oncology: current status and future directions. J Magnet Reson Imag 2002; 16(4):407–422.

32. Kotte ANTJ, van Leeuwen GMJ, Lagendijk JJW. Modeling the thermal impact of a discrete vessel tree. Phys Med Biol 1999; 44(1):57–74.

33. Lin WL, Liauh CT, Chen YY, Liu HC, Shieh MJ. Theoretical study of temperature elevation at muscle/bone interface during ultrasound hyperthermia. Med Phys 2000; 27(5):1131–1140.

34. Malinen M, Huttunen T, Kaipio JP, Hynynen K. Scanning path optimization for ultrasound surgery. Phys Med Biol 2005; 50(15):3473–3490.

35. White J, Clement GT, Hynynen K. Transcranial ultrasound focus reconstruction with phase and amplitude correction. IEEE Trans Ultrason Ferroelectr Freq Contr 2005; 52(9): 1518–1522.

7

Current and Future Clinical Applications of Magnetic Resonance Imaging–Guided Focused Ultrasound Surgery

Ferenc A. Jolesz
Department of Radiology, Brigham and Women's Hospital and Harvard Medical School, Boston, Massachusetts, U.S.A.

Clare M.C. Tempany
Division of MRI, Department of Radiology, Brigham and Women's Hospital and Harvard Medical School, Boston, Massachusetts, U.S.A.

INTRODUCTION

The application of acoustic energy for tumor treatment is not a new idea. More than a half century ago, focused ultrasound surgery (FUS) was already considered viable as a "surgical" technique for treating deeply embedded soft-tissue tumors noninvasively. Despite this early recognition of its potential, FUS has not been widely accepted as a real alternative to invasive surgery. The reason is not the limitation of FUS technology but the inadequacy of image guidance and the control of energy deposition. We believe strongly that the integration of FUS with magnetic resonance imaging (MRI) represents a major step toward a noninvasive image-guided therapy substitute that can replace most of the existing tumor surgery methods. MRI-guided focused ultrasound (MRIgFUS) surgery that has been developed during the last decade (1,2) provides accurate targeting of focused sound waves that can be directed to destroy tumor tissue within MRI-detected tumor margins. MRI not only provides tumor localization with high sensitivity but also monitors temperature distribution in "real time," effectively generating "temperature maps" of the targeted surgical field during treatment. In turn, this allows the FUS delivery of thermal energy at safe, therapeutically effective doses "without" damaging collateral normal tissue. The integration of MRI and FUS creates an image-guided therapy delivery system with which real-time, image-controlled, noninvasive soft-tissue coagulation is feasible, and from which a wide range of clinical applications may ultimately develop.

THE DEVELOPMENT OF THE TECHNOLOGY

In conventional invasive surgeries, the surgeon is using hands for execution and eyes to remove or repair diseased or damaged tissue. For this hand-eye coordinated surgical procedure, the operator uses the eye for direct visualization of the extent of the disease, which is a rather crude and unsatisfactory method to define tumor margins. To be able to visualize the surgical area of interest, the surgeon must manually dissect or cut through normal tissue. In the process, the nontargeted, intervening tissue may be damaged; this "invasion" of normal-tissue integrity can cause serious complications and impede recovery.

An "ideal surgery," on the other hand, should result in complete treatment (removal or repair) without causing any damage to the collateral tissue, even when the target is deep inside the body. Such an ideal and essentially noninvasive process would eliminate the obvious inadequacy of human visual targeting and control as well as the invasive instrumental access. Conceptually, this requires unobstructed three-dimensional (3D) visualization of the targeted tissue and the surrounding normal anatomy by using an imaging method. Targeted delivery of energy and deposition of the tissue-killing energy dose within the target also requires image-based, real-time monitoring and control of the energy delivery process. This requirement necessitates the image-based detection of either the deposited energy itself or its effect on the tissue or both. If all the requirements of image guidance (localization, targeting, monitoring, and control) can be accomplished, the real-time feedback (closed loop control) can be established. This was first demonstrated for the real-time MRI-based control of FUS (3) and of interstitial laser therapy (4).

Advances in medical imaging such as diagnostic ultrasound (US), X ray–based computed tomography (CT), and MRI have revolutionized our ability to reach accurate and timely diagnoses and provide noninvasive 3D views into the patient's body for safely executing various image-guided interventions. These collective advances in imaging science and image-guided therapy now enable the physician to visualize both normal anatomical structures and diseased tissue before, during, and after treatment for localization, targeting, and follow-up. Various imaging methods are used to complement direct visualization during open surgeries and minimally invasive interventions. In the last decade, interventional and intraoperative MRI emerged as the best choice for image guidance (5–8). This is due to the inherent tissue contrast provided by MRI that allows the accurate localization of the target lesion and its border definition. In addition, temperature-sensitive MRI methods are used to monitor thermal ablations (9). Thermal ablations can be applied using various minimally invasive probes (e.g., optical laser fiber, radiofrequency needle, or microwave antenna) to deposit heat in deep-lying tumors; intraprocedural MRI is also utilized to monitor and control cryoablation (10).

One of the most attractive methods of thermal ablation is, however, the completely noninvasive tissue destruction by acoustic energy that converts to heat during absorption. While other methods are only minimally invasive because of the use of percutaneous needles and needle-like probes, FUS is completely noninvasive with no percutaneous probes required. The US waves penetrate through soft tissue and can be focused to small focal volumes with dimensions of a few millimeters. The acoustic energy absorption at the focal spot leads to tissue temperature elevations with such sharp thermal gradients that the boundaries of the treated volume are sharply demarcated without damage to the overlying or surrounding adjacent tissues. No other probe-delivered heating methods can achieve similar, well-controlled, deep thermal ablation.

Thus, the concept of "ideal surgery" ensures that only the targeted tumor tissue is removed or destroyed and there is no associated injury of the adjacent normal tissue. Although, it has been known for sometime that FUS can in fact be this "ideal surgery," (11) it was not competitive with traditional surgery because of the lack of appropriate image guidance and thermal control. A fully developed image-guided therapy delivery system should correctly localize tumor margins, find acoustic energy trajectories, carefully select acoustic windows, monitor energy deposition in real time, and accurately control the deposited thermal dose within the entire targeted tumor volume. Only this "closed-loop" image-guided FUS system can truly satisfy the requirements for ideal surgery.

The most obvious imaging method for FUS is diagnostic US imaging. Eventually, diagnostic US did indeed become the primary localization and targeting method for FUS, but because temperatures still could not be accurately monitored, this method of noninvasive soft-tissue ablation has not gained true widespread acceptance. US imaging is not yet applicable for the real-time detection of tissue temperature changes and the confirmation of thermally induced tissue changes. It is possible that eventually US will provide some kind of temperature monitoring. However, the current lack of temperature sensitivity is not the only shortcoming of US-based image guidance. The other major shortcoming is the lack of its ability to detect tumor margins for accurate target definition and it is unlikely that diagnostic US will ever be comparable to MRI in this respect.

Because of these shortcomings, the successful implementation of an image-guided FUS has centered on the development of a noninvasive imaging system that can achieve good anatomic resolution, high sensitivity to tumors, and accurate monitoring and control of treatment outcomes in real time.

While the temperature sensitivity of MRI was well known, the original idea to use MRI monitoring and control for thermal therapies came only in the early 1980s, when the concept of MRI-guided hyperthermia (12–14) and interstitial laser therapy (15,16) was described. In a series of publications our team at the Brigham and Women's Hospital described that during both interstitial laser ablation therapy and cryoablation real-time monitoring is necessary for assessment of ongoing thermal effects in tissue (15–18). This preliminary work showed that MRI can display the location and distribution of the temperature elevation and accurately depict the extent of thermal damage, as confirmed at histological examination (19).

There were two critical findings that preceded the development of MRIgFUS. In a series of experiments, the static magnetic field of an MRI system was used as a component of an electromagnetic (EM) transducer for generating acoustic pressure waves. It suggested that the integration of an acoustic pressure wave generator with MRI and magnetic resonance (MR) control can provide a novel combination of technologies for the treatment of solid soft-tissue tumors (20). The other important finding was that MRI temperature monitoring can be used to develop a real-time feedback that can control all types of thermal ablations (16,21)

The Boston team initially described MRI-guided thermal ablations (Jolesz and Bleier, Higuchi, Matsumoto, etc.) (16–19,21), and then, recognizing that the optimal image-guided thermal ablation method is MRIgFUS, began work with General Electric's (GE) corporate research (Cline H) on the development of this new technology. The Brigham research team and GE were looking for a research partner with experience with therapeutic US. In 1990, GE invited the University of Arizona group to the Corporate Research Center where Jolesz presented the original idea of MRIgFUS.

The first description of the temperature monitoring–based MRIgFUS system was published in 1992 (22). This paper described the MRI-compatible US transducer technology developed at the University of Arizona [already tested in vivo (23,24) and was the basis for the development of the first therapy system by GE]. Initially, a prototype experimental system was constructed to assess MRI thermal monitoring ability and the MRI localization of the heat zone in muscle; later, the first clinical system was built (3,22,25). In 1993, Hynynen et al. published a paper describing the feasibility of MRI-compatible US transducers and demonstrated changes in MRI parameters seen in vivo during an FUS treatment (23,24). The results were consistent with those seen after treatment with other thermal ablation methods. The feasibility of using the T_1-weighted images to visualize the locations of the temperature elevation at the focal spots in vivo muscle and tumor tissue was also demonstrated with their experimental hydraulic positioning system (23,24,26).

Accurate targeting and control initially requires the detection of thermal changes below the level of tissue destruction or before the actual ablation begins. Fortunately, with temperature-sensitive MRI, the sonication beam can be localized at power levels that are below the threshold for thermal damage of the tissue (27). Temperature imaging based on the proton resonance frequency shift is the best method to obtain the temperature distribution and change during sonication and to calculate the thermal dose distribution and volume resulting from multiple sonications. MRI thermometry is applicable for monitoring the thermal exposure and allows real-time control of the sonication parameters to optimize clinical treatments (28–31). Since the temperature rise induced by a FUS beam scales linearly with power, the temperature maps acquired during subthreshold sonications can be used to determine the power necessary to produce thermal tissue damage with a desired size.

THE THERAPY DELIVERY SYSTEM FOR MRIgFUS SURGERY

MRIgFUS surgery effectively combines two technologies (MRI and US) into a breakthrough, noninvasive image-guided therapy delivery system that fulfills the requirements of the "ideal surgery." By using a precisely focused, high-power acoustic beam, the tissue destruction is limited to the focus. In fact, before the sound waves are concentrated at the focus point, they propagate through the tissue without damaging it. Further, at the focus, the intensified acoustic energy beam raises the tissue temperature to a range where tissue is coagulated by protein denaturation and capillary bed destruction.

MRI, with its excellent sensitivity for imaging soft-tissue tumors, is preferable over other imaging modalities for localizing 3D tumor margins and targeting tumor volumes. In addition, MRI is also capable of measuring temperature changes inside the body with accuracy in the range of $\pm 3°C$ at 1.5 T field strengths—or with even greater accuracy at higher field strengths. Because of its excellent temperature sensitivity, the focal point can be visualized and localized well before any irreversible tissue damage is induced at about 20°C above normal body temperature. Moreover, MRI's ability to capture the temperature change enables the physician to delineate temperature maps and tumor volume and apply this quantitative information in real time to allow for "closed loop" therapy (1,2).

This noninvasive real-time closed loop ablation methodology is unique to MRIgFUS. The following is a list of the key advantages: (*i*) MRI provides excellent tumor localization, much improved over direct visualization at open surgery. This is because it provides 3D volumetric tumor definition and can see "beyond the surface"; (*ii*) MRI can be used for planning the trajectory of the acoustic beams by finding an optimal acoustic window for safe passage of the US beam; (*iii*) MRI can accurately localize the higher temperature focal spot by temperature-sensitive imaging and verify its position within the target (and thus, damage to normal tissue is averted). If the position is not correct, it can quickly be adjusted before any therapeutic energy is delivered; and (*iv*) MRI can detect tissue coagulation during and at the end of the procedure through the use of MR thermometry, and with intravenous (i.v.) contrast, the occlusion of tumor vascularity.

Successful design, testing, and development of a clinical MRIgFUS system is a significant engineering challenge. The MRI environment is frequently hostile to and sometimes incompatible with electronic and electromechanical systems. For example, the magnetic field inside a 1.5 T MRI is 150,000 times stronger than the earth's magnetic field and twice this number in a 3 T scanner. The challenge in designing an MRIgFUS system is dual: First, MRI uses very low EM signals generated in the body to reconstruct the anatomy, and any external EM interference could easily destroy the MR image. Second, the static and dynamic EM fields of the MRI can influence the FUS component, including beam-forming electronics and high-accuracy robotic systems to such an extent they will fail to function.

Following the early implementation of the technique (3,25,32) and after the development of a prototype workstation at the Brigham and Women's Hospital by McDannold et al., InSightec (Haifa, Israel) developed the first commercial MRIgFUS therapy delivery system known as the ExAblate® 2000. This system is the first of its kind that had real-time closed loop control for MRIgFUS. Currently, both Philips and Siemens Medical Systems are developing MRIgFUS surgery but those systems are not commercially available.

CLINICAL APPLICATIONS OF MRIgFUS

The first 50 years of FUS technology have been very interesting but clinically disappointing (33). Without appropriate image guidance, the method did not live up to the initial high expectations. The technique was first used for destruction of portions of the central nervous system (CNS) (34) and has been extensively tested for so-called "trackless" brain surgery in both animals and humans (35,36). Since its introduction, FUS has been investigated as an alternative method to invasive surgery and radiation therapy and considered for many clinical applications including benign and malignant prostate disease and tumors of the liver, kidney, breast, bone, uterus, and pancreas. These clinical investigations and the related extensive literature have been described in several review papers (37–40).

The introduction of MRIgFUS represents a new and extremely promising chapter in the history of FUS technology. After preliminary feasibility testing of the first integrated MRI-FUS therapy delivery system by a team of Brigham and Women's and GE researchers, the first clinical application, ablation of benign breast fibroadenomas, was selected.

Breast Fibroadenoma

The treatment of benign breast tumors was chosen to test feasibility of MRIgFUS. There were several compelling reasons: firstly, the breast is easily accessible to the US beam, with no bone or gas obstructing the acoustic window to the tumor. Secondly, breast MRI defines focal fibroadenoma well, especially after i.v. Gadolinium. Thirdly, these lesions are benign but can be very symptomatic. In a feasibility study, 11 fibroadenomas in 9 women were treated with MRIgFUS under local anesthesia using MRI-based temperature monitoring. Of the 11 lesions treated, 8 demonstrated complete or partial lack of contrast material uptake after treatment on T_1-weighted images (41).

After the transfer of technology from GE to InSightec (Haifa, Israel), there were significant further improvements made to the technology that resulted in the development of the previously described ExAblate 2000 system and the continuation of clinical trials for benign tumors now in the pelvis, namely uterine leiomyomas or fibroids.

Uterine Fibroid

The clinical trials and clinical practice of MRIgFUS for treatment of symptomatic uterine leiomyomas will be covered in a separate chapter. In this section, the experience will be reviewed briefly. Prior to FUS treatment, the initial proof of concept came from the work in MRI-guided laser ablation of benign uterine fibroids, which demonstrated a 30% to 40% decrease of tumor volume and associated symptomatic relief at three-months to one-year follow-up. (42). Based on these preliminary studies, initial Phase I/II trials of the ExAblate 2000 device for this treatment began. The first paper by Tempany et al. reported the initial results in nine women, with symptomatic leiomyomas, all scheduled for hysterectomy. They all agreed to undergo MRIgFUS prior to surgery. Thermal lesions were created within target fibroids using an MRIgFUS therapy system. The developing lesion was monitored using real-time MR thermometry, which was used to assess treatment outcome in real time to change treatment parameters and achieve the desired outcome. In six cases, the leiomyoma received full therapeutic doses, and 98.5% of the sonications were visualized. Focal necrotic lesions were seen in all cases on MRI, and five were pathologically confirmed after hysterectomy. Thus, it was demonstrated that MRIgFUS can successfully cause thermal coagulation and necrosis in uterine leiomyoma and is feasible and safe, without serious consequences (43). Following this, a Food and Drug Administration (FDA)–approved multicenter trial was initiated by InSightec.

In October 2004, the FDA approved the use of MRIgFUS for the treatment of uterine fibroids treatment (44–47). MRIgFUS offers the patient a noninvasive alternative to hysterectomy or myomectomy—invasive surgical procedures that often result in postoperative complications and lengthy recuperation times. By contrast, MRIgFUS treatment is performed on an outpatient basis and allows the woman to resume her normal daily activities within a couple of days. Although the specific clinical application in this instance treats a benign disease (uterine fibroids), the procedure is quite challenging, involving deep abdominal treatment within a complex pelvic anatomy in which there are several critical organs (bowel, uterus, nerves, and urinary bladder) that must be protected from damage. To date, 2200 patients have been treated with MRIgFUS. The accrued results demonstrate significant improvement in more than 80% of the patients at 12 months, and very good durability at 24 months, with approximately 20% of the patients looking for alternative treatments at 24 months.

MRIgFUS TREATMENT OF CANCER

FUS has been investigated as a tool for the treatment of cancer for many decades but is only now beginning to emerge as a potential alternative to conventional therapies. FUS treatments follow a surgical concept and strategy. In oncologic surgery, the tumor or index lesion should be correctly localized and the target well defined. If the target definition is incorrect, the surgical approach is doomed to fail, as the tumor resection margins will be positive and tumor will be left behind after resection. The applications of FUS for tumor ablation rely of the sensitivity of MRI to define tumor margins. This critical delineation of the tumor's extent may be better than the surgeon's visual and tactile ability during open surgery but is inevitably still not perfect. If MRI does not correctly define the boundary of the tumor, then the FUS will essentially become, as is often the case in many surgeries, a tumor debulking procedure. In such a case of incomplete tumor removal, the treatment has to be combined with radiation or chemotherapy; it is anticipated the MRIgFUS in which image guidance replaces visual assessment will be an improvement over conventional tumor surgery but it is still not a magic solution or cure for cancer.

Breast Cancer

The first Phase I trial for breast cancer treatment first with the GE system and then with the InSightec system was done by Gianfelice et al. (48–50). To test the feasibility of breast cancer treatment by MRIgFUS, two breast cancer cases were performed at the Brigham in Women's Hospital with the original GE prototype system. The treatments were followed by mastectomy. Using a Siemens prototype system in Germany, a single treatment was attempted (51).

In the first study (48–50), before undergoing tumor resection, 12 patients with invasive breast carcinomas were treated with multiple sonications that were monitored with temperature-sensitive MRI. The effectiveness of the treatment was determined by histopathological analysis of the resected mass that was performed to determine the volumes of necrosed and residual tumor. FUS ablation was well tolerated by the patients, and with the exception of minor skin burns in two patients, no complications occurred. More the 90% of the tumor volume was treated and the residual tumor was identified predominantly at the periphery of the tumor mass. This indicated the need to increase the total targeted area (i.e., with an increased number of sonications). In a later more-complete study (and with the use of improved technology), 24 female patients were treated by MRIgFUS. Following MRIgFUS they received adjunct chemotherapeutic (tamoxifen). Percutaneous biopsy was performed after six-month followup, and if residual tumor was present, a second MRIgFUS treatment session was initiated, followed by repeat biopsy one month later. Overall, 19 of 24 patients had negative biopsy results after one or two treatment sessions. In a later study (48–50), gadolinium contrast was used for targeting and there was further improvement of tumor volume coverage by FUS. In breast cancer, the role of MRIgFUS is to replace conventional lumpectomy and the desired outcome is a total coagulation of the tumor. The most current data indicate the rate of recurrence is significantly higher in patients treated by lumpectomy only, as compared to patients treated with lumpectomy and radiation therapy administered as an adjuvant therapy following surgery. "The medical community should therefore view lumpectomy as a debulking tool." A surgery panel convened in the summer of 2003 concluded that total coagulation of breast carcinomas should reach or exceed 95%. To date, the ExAblate 2000 has been used to treat 150 breast cancer patients. In the most recent cohort of 30 patients treated in Japan, the pathology results were 97% ± 3% tumor destruction (52). Based on this data, an extended Phase II Investigational Device Exemptions (IDE) protocol is slated to begin during Q2/2006. This protocol will include treatment by MRIgFUS, follow-up MRI to assess treatment outcome, lumpectomy, and pathological assessment of the excised tissue.

Liver Cancer

Liver metastases and increasingly hepatocellular carcinomas, in conjunction with the worldwide pandemic of hepatitis c, are now important and common causes of death, which otherwise have relatively poor treatments available for them, which vary from quite toxic in terms of chemotherapy to the very invasive with surgery. The potential, therefore, of minimally invasive work in this field is highly desirable and could help a great many patients. Many patients with liver disease have associated coagulation defects that may or may not be easily treatable while minimally invasive or noninvasive procedures are a substantial improvement in terms of morbidity in comparison to surgery. Thermal ablations provide a potential alternative to surgery in the treatment of primary or metastatic liver cancer (53–55).

Percutaneous radiofrequency, microwave, laser ablation, and cryotherapy have all been utilized to treat livers malignancies successfully.

Several investigations used US image guidance for high-intensity focused ultrasound (HIFU) procedures used to treat liver lesions. This essentially noninvasive approach is a very preferable alternative to the more invasive surgeries that are required to achieve similar outcomes.

Most of the work has been done in China and some is from Oxford, U.K. where they evaluated the safety and performance of the device (40,56). All these studies described their results as extremely promising.

There are several technical problems with liver FUS therapy that should be resolved before the advantages of MRI guidance are realized (57). Without motion compensation, the phase subtraction–based temperature measurement does not work; therefore, currently, ExAblate treatments are performed only inpatient with general anesthesia and without respiratory motion during sonications. Also, in the current phased-array arrangement, MRIgFUS cannot reach lesions behind ribs or lung and is confined at the moment to treatment of low liver lesions that peak out from below the rib line or to left lobe lesions that can be accessed with conventional application through the epigastrium. It is anticipated that improvements in the phased-array transducer technology eventually will allow access to lesions between ribs.

Prostate Cancer

There have been multiple efforts to evaluate the feasibility of HIFU for the treatment of localized prostate cancer in a population of potentially curable patients (58,59). Current results with the US-guided EDAP system (EDAP/TMS, Vaulx-en-Velin, France) show that HIFU is a treatment option achieving similar results to those of other nonsurgical treatments for prostate cancer (60).

MRI has a significant advantage in defining the extent and type of local prostate cancer. It is anticipated that the combination of MRI-based diagnosis and MRI-controlled FUS therapy will provide a competitive advantage over radical prostatectomy in the treatment of prostate cancer.

Renal Tumors

Renal-cell carcinomas are relatively slow growing and very frequently asymptomatic for the majority of their time course. They are found increasingly commonly at quite early stages due to the widespread use of cross-sectional imaging, particularly screening CT. This has resulted in more patients seeking minimally invasive treatments such as thermal ablations rather than the more invasive and aggressive surgical procedures that are available. "Nephron-sparing" approaches are very important for patients with either single kidney or chronic renal failure. Multiple papers are now available describing the use of radiofrequency, cryotherapy, or laser approaches for the destruction of renal masses using minimally invasive procedures, which show very good early promise when the whole mass of the tumor can be treated (61). MRI-guided percutaneous cryoablation of renal tumors can be done safely and effectively (62).

HIFU treatment of renal carcinomas was attempted by US image guidance (63).

Many of the same problems that are encountered in MRIgFUS of the liver apply equally to renal procedures. The kidney is an even more mobile organ than the liver and has much greater respiratory excursion than the liver; so control of this motion is absolutely crucial in the undertaking of such a process. We believe that similar procedures to those described in the liver, however, should be able to treat renal masses, particularly the lower pole or exophytically located.

Bone

Metastatic bone tumors develop in 50% to 60% of cancer patients and are often very painful, generating micro- or macrofractures in the bones. Many patients with bony metastatic deposits have continuing disabling pain despite the use of other conventional therapies such as radiotherapy, chemotherapy, hormonal manipulation, and analgesics. Further palliative therapeutic options for this group of patients are, therefore, highly desirable to improve the way we treat these patients. The percutaneous delivery of thermal ablative energy directly into skeletal metastases is evolving as a very effective new modality in the palliation of painful tumors. The majority of the studies in this area have been carried out using radiofrequency electrodes as the source of heat although studies using cryotherapy and laser fibers are also published in the literature with similar promising overall results (64,65).

Callstrom and Charboneaeu (66) have reported on a study of 62 patients who had severe pain secondary to bony metastases. All their patients were treated with percutaneous radiofrequency ablation and 95% of their patients experienced a significant drop in pain scores that continued to improve over 24 weeks of follow-up, and this improvement was associated with a very significant fall in the opiate usage in this group. These studies indicate that there is substantial gain to be achieved in the palliation of painful metastases using MRIgFUS. They also concluded that the tumor interface with normal bone should always be treated for best pain relief. and if the thermal ablation is limited to the center of the tumor, very little gain is achieved in terms of pain improvement. These suggest that pain relief is primarily due to the coagulation of nerve fibers and not the soft-tissue tumor itself.

MRIgFUS can ablate soft-tissue tumors in the bone but also has the potential to provide very effective pain palliation in a single treatment that can be repeated in the case of pain recurrence. Diagnostic US cannot be used for targeting and monitoring in bones since US is absorbed and or reflected by bones, preventing visualization.

Bone absorbs US very avidly, which explains why it disrupts US beams, making treatment of lesions obscured by bones so problematic, as described above. This ability of bone, however, can be utilized to carry out thermal ablation treatments by targeting the abnormal areas with FUS and depositing energy in to these areas to raise the temperatures sufficiently to cause tissue destruction. This process suggests that we may be able to utilize FUS as a modality to treat bone lesions palliatively.

Patients are currently being treated under a Phase I protocol in various sites using the InSightec system. The initial results are promising with relatively quick improvements in pain scores in most patients without the patient having to undergo any form of interventional procedure. MR is simply used to target the FUS deposition so a very effective, easy, and accurate way of depositing the heat is achieved.

This form of therapy has great potential and can be combined with radiation and provide improved pain relief, particularly for very painful metastases, which are refractory to other therapies.

Brain Tumor

Invasive open craniectomies or brain surgery typically entails attempts to resect and remove deep-seated target lesions by cutting or dissecting through normal brain—a surgical course that frequently results in damage to intervening tissues. Given this, a completely noninvasive treatment alternative capable of treating targeted brain tissue without injuring normal brain could prove extremely attractive. Therefore, the use of FUS as an "ideal" brain surgery method has been under investigation for some time (11,34–36).

Considering the preponderance and widespread use of MRI in clinical neuroimaging, which allows the display of the lesion and all surrounding structures in 3D, an MR-based image-guided therapy would be ideal. The combination of high-resolution 3D brain imaging with the ability of MRI for thermal monitoring, resulting in MRIgFUS for treatment of brain tumors has become a primary goal for many investigators in the last decade. Utilization of therapeutic US in the brain has been seriously limited by the commonly accepted view that these exposures would require that a piece of the skull bone be removed to allow the US beam to propagate into the brain. As US beams do not normally pass through bone, rather are deflected by it, the skull posed a considerable barrier to the potential of transcranial FUS treatments.

However, in 1998, after experimental studies, it was demonstrated that transcranial delivery of therapeutic US into the brain is feasible (67). Using phased-array transducers surrounding the skull, the phase shifts caused by the uneven cranial bone thickness can be compensated for by thickness measurements generated from X-ray CT data. These phase corrections allow a sharp focus to be generated at various (relatively lower) frequencies. A prototype MRI-compatible FUS phased-array system for trans-skull brain tissue ablation (Hemispherical 500-element US phased array operating at frequencies of 700–800 kHz) was developed by InSightec and the Brigham and Women's Hospital Focused Ultrasound Laboratory (68). The device was then modified to operate in the orientation that will be used in the clinic and successfully tested in phantom experiments.

ExAblate® 3000

A system for the MRI-guided and monitored FUS thermal surgery of brain through intact skull was developed by InSightec and tested in rhesus monkeys (69) and in three patients at the Brigham and Women's Hospital. The US beam is generated by a 512-channel phased-array system (Exablate 3000, InSightec, Haifa, Israel) that is integrated within a 1.5 T MR scanner. The MRI thermometry was shown to be useful in detecting the tissue temperature distribution next to the bone, and it should be used to monitor the brain surface temperature. The effect of thermal lesions for brain edema was also investigated (70,71).

An FDA IDE-approved Phase I clinical trial centered on brain-tumor treatments through the intact skull. This research is currently being conducted solely at the Brigham and Women's Hospital in Boston but will expand to multiple U.S. sites later. Initial cases involve inoperable malignant brain tumors, but in the future, benign tumors will also be considered. MRIgFUS lesions can also be used for functional neurosurgery for the treatment of epilepsy, movement disorders, and other CNS diseases.

APPLICATION OF MRIgFUS FOR NON-NEOPLASTIC DISEASES
Arthritic Joints

There is also the potential for treatment of these painful joints. As shown in animal experiments, it is possible to perform synovectomy noninvasively using MRIgFUS

(72). This noninvasive FUS method can be used to treat patient with arthritis who do not respond to drug treatment.

Vascular Occlusion

The histological examinations indicate that not only do the treated tumor cells show coagulative necrosis but small tumor vessels are also severely damaged by the HIFU treatment. The damaged tumor vessels might play a critical role in secondary tumor cell death by decreasing tissue perfusion (73). Highly perused nontumorous tissues such as the renal cortex can also be coagulated from outside the body with FUS and MRI can be used to guide and monitor this procedure. Arterial occlusion was achieved by FUS energy deposition in rabbit arteries (74,75). In some cases, hemorrhage or vessel rupture was caused by the sonication. This condition should be avoided during noninvasive FUS surgery (76).

Acoustic hemostasis can be used to prevent diffuse tissue hemorrhage after trauma or surgical incisions. Liver hemorrhage, the major cause of death in hepatic trauma, is especially difficult to control. By using FUS, liver hemorrhage can be reduced to a slow oozing of blood. The mechanism of hemostasis appears to be coagulative necrosis of small blood vessels (77). Hemorrhage of punctured major blood vessels (femoral artery and vein, axillary artery, carotid artery, and jugular vein) was also interrupted by HIFU treatment and the vessels were patent after the procedure (78).

Slow-flow arterial venous malformations (AVMs) are often extremely problematic and long lasting and recurrent problems for patients. Surgery is frequently disfiguring and unsuccessful and embolization procedures are of a variable success. We anticipate that improvements in FUS technology should allow much greater power deposition to be achieved within individual slow-flow AVMs that should be able to overcome some of the problems. Much of the vascular flow of these lesions, which is very slow is responsible for the difficulty with which heat can be deposited within them but if FUS could be utilized successfully to treat such abnormalities, it could be a very successful and useful way of taking the treatment of this type of lesion forward. Cavernous hemangioma of brain and other organs is a disease that can be treated by MRIgFUS in the future.

It is also possible to use FUS to create lesions in cardiac valves. Mitral and aortic valve perforation was achieved in animal experiments and this extracorporeal treatment procedure may prove useful for valvulotomy or valvuloplasty (79).

Cavitation-Based Clinical Applications

The interaction between the acoustic beam and tissue results in several mechanisms such as reflection, refraction, scatter, absorption, propagation, and cavitation. Cavitation aside, the primary tissue heating mechanism is absorption generated by molecular vibrations that are induced, in turn, by the acoustic beam—creating, in essence, a pressure wave and intermolecular friction. The vibration amplitude depends, however, on the pressure amplitude and, hence, is significantly higher at the focus where the pressure is the highest, implying a higher temperature rise at the focus. The difference in temperature rise between the focus volume and the surrounding tissue depends on the specific acoustic design; and generally, this difference is very significant.

By using short bursts at high-pressure amplitudes, thermal effects can be minimized or eliminated, and the nonthermal effects of cavitation can be used. Various mechanical effects have been observed with such exposures. Cavitation can disrupt the blood-brain barrier (BBB) (80–82), cause selective vascular damage, generate tissue necrosis, and produce complete tissue disintegration (76,83). The disruption of atherosclerotic plaques and thrombi are also thought to be cavitation-mediated events (84). Finally, high-amplitude FUS beams can also be distorted to create shock waves at the focus, which might influence cell-membrane permeability that can be used for gene delivery to cells (85–89).

Cavitation effects can be further amplified by injecting preformed microbubbles into the vasculature. While these bubbles have been developed for imaging, they have also been shown to reduce the power required for inducing tissue effects by at least two orders of magnitude. It may also be possible to include therapeutic agents in the shell of the micro bubbles so that they break and release their contents in the target location when exposed to US (90).

Percutaneous catheter-delivered US energy appears promising in peripheral vessels to reduce arterial stenoses and recanalize complete arterial obstructions (91). US and microbubbles are capable of recanalizing acute arteriovenous graft thromboses (84).

If MRIgFUS can recanalize obstructed blood vessels using extracorporeal beams, there is enormous potential for this technique for treating stroke and maybe even coronary occlusion.

Gene Therapy

As a result of the human genome project and continuing advances in molecular biology, many therapeutic genes have been discovered. Gene therapy is a promising approach to the treatment of many forms of disease, including cancer. US-mediated transfection appears to be a promising method for gene transfer into mammalian cells (92,93).

Gene therapy as a form of molecular medicine is expected to have a major impact on medical treatments in the future. However, the clinical use of gene therapy today is hampered by inadequate gene delivering systems to ensure sufficient, accurate, and safe DNA uptake in the target cells in vivo. Of critical concern in its implementation is the ability to control the location, duration, and level of expression of the therapeutic gene. MRIgFUS has a potential to accomplish gene therapy with spatiotemporal control. Because US waves can be focused on different anatomical locations in the human body without significant adverse effects, the control of DNA transfer by FUS is a promising in vivo method for spatial regulation of gene-based medical treatments (94–96).

BBB Opening

The BBB is a persistent obstacle for the local delivery of macromolecular therapeutic agents to the CNS. Many drugs that show potential for treating CNS diseases cannot cross the BBB, and there is a need for a noninvasive targeted drug delivery method that allows local therapy of the CNS using larger molecules. In the presence of intravenously injected microbubbles (routinely used as US imaging contrast agents), low US powers and pressure amplitudes can cause BBB transient disruption. This method may have potential for targeted delivery of macromolecules in the brain (97,98). Local BBB opening is an advantageous approach for targeted drug delivery to the brain. The cellular mechanisms of such transient barrier disruption are largely unknown. Several mechanisms of transcapillary passage are possible after sonications: (*i*) transcytosis; (*ii*) endothelial cell cytoplasmic openings—fenestration and channel formation; (*iii*) opening of a part of tight junctions; and (*iv*) free passage through the injured endothelium (with the higher power sonications). These mechanisms could be considered in further development of the strategy for drug delivery to brain parenchyma (99).

Our ongoing research shows that BBB can be reproducibly opened by localizing the cavitation-generated, mechanical stresses to the blood vessel walls by injecting preformed gas bubbles into the blood stream just prior to the sonications. Since the microbubbles are intravascular, any adverse effects to the adjoining brain tissue should be minimal. The opening is reversible and the power levels used are orders of magnitude lower than that required for generating tissue ablation or the tissue damaging cavitation threshold. Because this technique allows the procedure to be performed in a clinical MRI scanner, the images can be used online to aim and monitor the US exposures. Thus, MRIgFUS can target an image-specified tissue volume anywhere in the brain—a feature very desirable for both molecular targeting and molecular imaging of the brain. This controlled opening of the BBB at a desired location would permit novel, noninvasive methods of treating brain tumors and interrogate brain function by using various chemical probes. Specifically, it would provide targeted access for chemotherapy and gene therapy and allow the use of large, molecular-sized peptides, neuroactive proteins, and various antibodies (93,100,101).

Using animal experiments, we demonstrated that Herceptin®, a humanized anti-HER2 (c-erbB2) monoclonal antibody, can be locally and noninvasively delivered into the CNS through the BBB under image guidance by using an MRIgFUS BBB disruption technique. The amount of Herceptin delivered in the target tissue had a good correlation with the extent of the barrier opening monitored by MRI, making it possible to indirectly estimate the amount of delivered Herceptin by MRI (100,101).

CONCLUSION

Without the ability of MRI to localize the tumor margins and without MRI-based temperature-sensitive imaging, correct targeting and closed-loop control of energy deposition is not possible. These are the reasons that the original US-guided FUS technology is inadequate and has not become widespread for most clinical applications. Given these limitations, FUS initially appeared to have a narrow application area and was not able to compete with other surgical or ablation methods. Today, MRIgFUS has become a safe and effective alternative to probe-delivered thermal ablations and minimally invasive surgery. Moreover, it has the potential to replace treatments that use ionizing radiation such as radiosurgery and brachytherapy. Although the cost of integrating MRI systems with complex and expensive phased arrays is high, this expenditure will largely be offset by eliminating costly hospitalization and anesthesia and by reducing complications. In effect, an investment in this emerging technology will ultimately redound to the benefit of the health care delivery system and, most important, to the patient. The MRIgFUS system provides a safe, repeatable treatment approach for benign tumors (e.g., uterine fibroid and breast fibroadenoma) that do not require an aggressive approach. MRIgFUS can also be used for debulking cancerous tissue. It has already been tested as a breast cancer treatment; its application for other malignancies in the brain, liver, bone, and prostate is under development. MRIgFUS offers an attractive alternative to conventional surgery because it incorporates intraoperative MRI, which provides far more precise target definition than is possible with the surgeon's direct visualization of the lesion. MRIgFUS is undeniably the most promising interventional MRI method in the field of image-guided therapy today. It is applicable not only in the thermal coagulative treatment of tumors but also in several other medical situations for which invasive surgery or radiation may not be an effective treatment option. The future use of FUS for treating vascular malformation or functional disorders of the brain is also exciting. It is uniquely applicable for image-guided therapy using targeted drug delivery methods and gene therapy. Further advances in this technology will no doubt improve energy deposition and reduce treatment times. In the near future, FUS will offer a viable alternative to conventional surgery and radiation therapy; in the longer term, it may also enable a host of targeted treatment methods aimed at eradicating or arresting heretofore-intractable diseases such as certain brain malignancies and forms of epilepsy (2).

Despite this potential, many individual problems in the widespread application of MRIgFUS remain. Motion, predominately due to respiration, is problematic because it is often inconsistent and the movement of the upper abdominal organs in response to respiration for instance is usually not entirely consistent, making exact targeting difficult. Ribs overlying the path of the FUS would disrupt the beam, preventing accurate application of destructive energy and marked vascularity of a target in the tissue may prevent an easy visualized tissue response. MRIgFUS is the ultimate noninvasive tumor treatment method. It requires, however, correct localization and targeting with MRI. Future improvement of MRI technologies will result in better definition of tumor margins and more accurate localization of targeted tissue. With further advances in acoustic technology, especially with phased arrays with greater numbers of elements, treatment sessions will be shorter and the number of anatomic locations that will be amenable to therapy will increase. Ultimately, MRIgFUS will replace a substantial number of invasive and minimally invasive surgical procedures and also radiation therapy applications. The possibility of repeat treatment without tissue toxicity and the ability of real-time control make MRIgFUS a major alternative to ionizing radiation-based methods. MRIgFUS is a disruptive technology that will eliminate the need for many invasive approaches to benign tumors. In combination with new drugs and improvements in MRI, effective, multiple, repeatable treatments of tumors will be enabled, without the current comor-bidities. This may generate a paradigm shift in cancer treatment, effectively transforming cancer into malignant chronic disease.

Although MRIgFUS technology is still in its infancy, this revolutionary imaging technology has already been established as a viable, noninvasive treatment for uterine fibroids, breast carcinomas, certain brain malignancies, and bone tumors. With additional research, we will no doubt develop MRIgFUS applications for CNS and vascular diseases, targeted drug delivery, gene therapy, and more. The integration of MRI and FUS surgery has resulted in real-time, image-controlled, closed loop–feedback based, noninvasive therapy delivery systems. Moreover, MRI has the ability to control tissue heating and the deposition of thermal dose. This feature significantly improves the safety and efficacy of FUS in the treatment of tumors. The major advantage of MRI guidance over other imaging modalities is its ability to achieve accurate targeting while avoiding thermal injury of normal tissues. Over the next decade, MRIgFUS will almost certainly replace several invasive open surgeries and will likely supplant minimally invasive approaches as the preferred treatment approach.

REFERENCES

1. Jolesz FA, Hynynen K. Magnetic resonance image-guided focused ultrasound surgery. Cancer J 2002; 8(suppl 1):S–100.
2. Jolesz FA, Hynynen K, McDannold N, et al. MR imaging-controlled focused ultrasound ablation: a noninvasive image-guided surgery. Magn Reson Imag Clin N Am 2005; 13(3): 545–560.
3. Hynynen K, Freund WR, Cline HE, et al. A clinical, noninvasive, MR imaging-monitored ultrasound surgery method. Radiographics 1996; 16(1):185–195.

4. Zientara GP, Saiviroonporn P, Morrison PR, et al. MRI monitoring of laser ablation using optical flow. J Magn Reson Imag 1998; 8(6):1306–1318.

5. Jolesz FA. Interventional and intraoperative MRI: a general overview of the field. J Magn Reson Imag 1998; 8(1):3–7.

6. Jolesz FA, Nabavi A, Kikinis R. Integration of interventional MRI with computer-assisted surgery. J Magn Reson Imag 2001; 13(1):69–77.

7. Jolesz FA, Talos IF, Schwartz RB, et al. Intraoperative magnetic resonance imaging and magnetic resonance imaging-guided therapy for brain tumors. Neuroimag Clin N Am 2002; 12(4):665–683.

8. Jolesz FA. Future perspectives in intraoperative imaging. Acta Neurochir Suppl 2003; 85: 7–13.

9. McDannold NJ, Jolesz FA. Magnetic resonance image-guided thermal ablations. Top Magn Reson Imag 2000; 11(3):191–202.

10. Silverman SG, Tuncali K, vanSonnenberg E, et al. MR imaging-guided percutaneous cryotherapy of liver tumors: initial experience. Radiology 2000; 217(3):657–664.

11. Lele PP. Production of deep focal lesions by focused ultrasound—current status. Ultrasonics 1967; 5:105–112.

12. Parker DL, Smith V, Sheldon P, Crooks LE, Fussell L. Temperature distribution measurements in two-dimensional NMR imaging. Med Phys 1983; 10(3):321–325.

13. Dickinson RJ, Hall AS, Hind AJ, Young IR. Measurement of changes in tissue temperature using MR imaging. J Comp Ass Tomogr 1986; 10:468–472.

14. Le B, Levin D. Temperature mapping with MR imaging of molecular diffusion: application to hyperthermia. Radiology 1989; 171(3):853–857.

15. Jolesz FA, Bleier AR, Jakab P. MR imaging of laser-tissue interactions. Radiology 1988; 168 (1):249–253.

16. Jolesz FA, Bleier AR, Lauter RS. Laser surgery benefits from guidance by MR. Diagn Imag (San Franc) 1990; 12(9):103–108.

17. Matsumoto R, Selig AM, Colucci VM, et al. Interstitial Nd:YAG laser ablation in normal rabbit liver: trial to maximize the size of laser-induced lesions. Lasers Surg Med 1992; 12(6): 650–658.

18. Higuchi N, Bleier AR, Jolesz FA, et al. Magnetic resonance imaging of the acute effects of interstitial neodymium:YAG laser irradiation on tissues. Invest Radiol 1992; 27(10): 814–821.

19. Matsumoto R, Oshio K, Jolesz FA. Monitoring of laser and freezing-induced ablation in the liver with T1-weighted MR imaging. J Magn Reson Imag 1992; 2(5):555–562.

20. Jolesz FA, Jakab PD. Acoustic pressure wave generation within an MR imaging system: potential medical applications. J Magn Reson Imag 1991; 1(5):609–613.

21. Jolesz FA, Moore GJ, Mulkern RV, et al. Response to and control of destructive energy by magnetic resonance. Invest Radiol 1989; 24(12):1024–1027.

22. Cline HE, Schenck JF, Hynynen K, et al. MR-guided focused ultrasound surgery. J Comput Assist Tomogr 1992; 16(6):956–965.

23. Hynynen K, Darkazanli A, Unger E, et al. MRI-guided noninvasive ultrasound surgery. Med Phys 1993; 20(1):107–115.

24. Hynynen K, Darkazanli A, Damianou C, Unger E, Schenck JF. Tissue thermometry during ultrasound exposure. Eur J Urol 1993; 23(suppl 1):12–16.

25. Cline HE, Schenck JF, Hynynen K, et al. MR temperature mapping of focused ultrasound surgery. Magn Reson Med 1994; 31(6):628–636.

26. Darkazanli A, Hynynen K, Unger EC, Schenck JF. MRI monitoring of ultrasound surgery. J Magn Reson Imag 1993; 3(3):509–514.

27. Chung AH, Hynynen K, Colucci V, et al. Optimization of spoiled gradient-echo phase imaging for in vivo localization of a focused ultrasound beam. Magn Reson Med 1996; 36 (5):745–752.

28. Chung AH, Jolesz FA, Hynynen K, et al. Thermal dosimetry of a focused ultrasound beam in vivo by magnetic resonance imaging. Med Phys 1999; 26(9):2017–2026.

29. McDannold N, Hynynen K, Jolesz F. MRI evaluation of thermal ablation of tumors with focused ultrasound. J Magn Reson Imag 1998; 8(1):91–100.

30. McDannold NJ, Jolesz FA, Hynynen K. Determination of the optimal delay between sonications during focused ultrasound surgery in rabbits by using MR imaging to monitor thermal buildup in vivo. Radiology 1999; 211(2):419–426.

31. McDannold N, King RL, Jolesz FA, Hynynen K. The use of quantitative temperature images to predict the optimal power for focused ultrasound surgery: in vivo verification in rabbit muscle and brain. Med Phys 2002; 29(3):356–365.

32. Cline HE, Schenck JF, Waykins RD, Jolesz FA, Hynynen K. Magnetic resonance-guided thermal surgery. Magn Reson Med 1993; 30(1):98–106.

33. Kremkau FW. Cancer therapy with ultrasound: a historical review. J Clin Ultrasound 1979; 7 (4):287–300.

34. Fry WJ, Barnard JW, Fry RF, Krumins RF, Brennan JF. Ultrasonic lesions in the mammalian central nervous system. Science 1955; 122(3168):517–518.

35. Lele PP. A simple method for production of trackless focal lesions with focused ultrasound: physical factors. J Physiol 1962; 160:494–512.

36. Fry WJ, Fry FJ. Fundamental neurological research and human neurosurgery using intense ultrasound. IRE Trans Med Electron 1960; ME-7:166–181.

37. Madersbacher S, Marberger M. High-energy shockwaves and extracorporeal high-intensity focused ultrasound. J Endourol 2003; 17(8):667–672.

38. Kennedy JE, ter Haar GR, Cranston D. High intensity focused ultrasound: surgery of the future? Br J Radiol 2003; 76(909):590–599.

39. Kennedy JE. High-intensity focused ultrasound in the treatment of solid tumours. Nat Rev Cancer 2005; 5(4):321–327.

40. ter Haar GR. High intensity focused ultrasound for the treatment of tumors. Echocardiography 2001; 18(4):317–322.

41. Hynynen K, Pomeroy O, Jolesz FA, et al. MR imaging-guided focused ultrasound surgery of fibroadenomas in the breast: a feasibility study. Radiology 2001; 219(1):176–185.

42. Law P, Gedroyc WM, Regan L. Magnetic resonance-guided percutaneous laser ablation of uterine fibroids. J Magn Reson Imag 2000; 12(4):565–570.

43. Tempany CM, Stewart EA, McDannold N, Quade BJ, Jolesz FA, Hynynen K. MR imaging-guided focused ultrasound surgery of uterine leiomyomas: a feasibility study. Radiology 2003; 226(3):897–905.

44. McDannold N, Tempany CM, Fennessy FM, et al. Uterine leiomyomas: MR imaging-based thermometry and thermal dosimetry during focused ultrasound thermal ablation. Radiology 2006; 240(1):263–272.

45. So MJ, Fennessy FM, Zou KH, et al. Does the phase of menstrual cycle affect MR-guided focused ultrasound surgery of uterine leiomyomas? Eur J Radiol 2006; 59(2):203–207.

46. Stewart EA, Rabinovici J, Tempany CM, et al. Clinical outcomes of focused ultrasound surgery for the treatment of uterine fibroids. Fertil Steril 2006; 85(1):22–29.

47. Fennessy FM, Tempany CM. MRI-guided focused ultrasound surgery of uterine leiomyomas. Acad Radiol 2005; 12(9):1158–1166.

48. Gianfelice D, Khiat A, Amara M, et al. MR imaging-guided focused ultrasound surgery of breast cancer: correlation of dynamic contrast-enhanced MRI with histopathologic findings. Breast Cancer Res Treat 2003; 82(2):93–101.

49. Gianfelice D, Khiat A, Amara M, Belblidia A, Boulanger Y. MR imaging-guided focused US ablation of breast cancer: histopathologic assessment of effectiveness—initial experience. Radiology 2003; 227(3):849–855.

50. Gianfelice D, Khiat A, Amara M, et al. Feasibility of magnetic resonance imaging-guided focused ultrasound surgery as an adjunct to tamoxifen therapy in high-risk surgical patients with breast carcinoma. J Vasc Interv Radiol 2003; 14(10):1275–1282.

51. Huber PE, Jenne JW, Rastert R, et al. A new noninvasive approach in breast cancer therapy using magnetic resonance imaging-guided focused ultrasound surgery. Cancer Res 2001; 61 (23):8441–8447.

52. Furusawa H, Namba K, Thomasen S, et al. Magnetic resonance-guided focused ultrasound surgery of breast cancer: reliability and effectiveness. J Am Coll Surg 2006; 203(1):54–63.

53. Silverman SG, Tuncali K, vanSonneberg E, et al. MR Imaging-guided percutaneous tumor ablation. Acad Radiol 2005; 12(9):1100–1109.

54. Goldberg SN, Bonn J, Dodd G, et al. Society of Interventional Radiology Interventional Oncology Task Force: interventional oncology research vision statement and critical assessment of the state of research affairs. J Vasc Interv Radiol 2005; 16(10):1287–1294.

55. Goldberg SN. Science to practice: can we differentiate residual untreated tumor from tissue responses to heat following thermal tumor ablation? Radiology 2005; 234:317–318.

56. Kennedy JE, Wu F, ter Haar GR, et al. High-intensity focused ultrasound for the treatment of liver tumours. Ultrasonics 2004; 42(1–9):931–935.

57. Jolesz FA, Hynynen K, McDannold N, Freundlich D, Kopelman D. Noninvasive thermal ablation of hepatocellular carcinoma by using magnetic resonance imaging-guided focused ultrasound. Gastroenterology 2004; 127(5 suppl 1):S242–S247.

58. Poissonnier L, Chapelon JY, Rouviere O, et al. Control of prostate cancer by transrectal HIFU in 227 patients. Eur Urol 2006; 51:381–387.

59. Gianduzzo TR, Eden CG, Moon DA. Treatment of localised prostate cancer using high-intensity focused ultrasound. BJU Int 2006; 97(4):867–868.

60. Poissonnier L, Gelet A, Chapelon JY, et al. Results of transrectal focused ultrasound for the treatment of localized prostate cancer (120 patients with PSA < or + 10ng/ml. Prog Urol 2003; 13(1):60–72.

61. Deane LA, Clayman RV. Review of minimally invasive renal therapies: needle-based and extracorporeal. Urology 2006; 68(1 suppl):26–37.

62. Tuncali K, Morrison PR, Tatli S, Silverman SG. MRI-guided percutaneous cryoablation of renal tumors: use of external manual displacement of adjacent bowel loops. Eur J Radiol 2006; 59(2):198–202.

63. Kohrmann KU, Michel MS, Gaa J, et al. High intensity focused ultrasound as noninvasive therapy for multilocal renal cell carcinoma: case study and review of the literature. J Urol 2002; 167(6):2397–2403.

64. Groenemeyer DH, Schirp S, Gevargez A. Image-guided percutaneous thermal ablation of bone tumors. Acad Radiol 2002; 9(4):467–477.

65. Carrino JA, Blanco R. Magnetic resonance—guided musculoskeletal interventional radiology. Semin Musculoskeletal Radiol 2006; 10:159–174.

66. Callstrom MR, Charboneau JW, Goetz MO, et al. Image-guided ablation of painful metastatic bone tumors: a new and effective approach to a difficult problem. Skeletal Radiol 2006; 35(1):1–15.

67. Hynynen K, Jolesz FA. Demonstration of potential noninvasive ultrasound brain therapy through an intact skull. Ultrasound Med Biol 1998; 24(2):275–283.

68. Hynynen K, Clement GT, McDannold N, et al. 500-element ultrasound phased array system for noninvasive focal surgery of the brain: a preliminary rabbit study with ex vivo human skulls. Magn Reson Med 2004; 52(1):100–107.

69. Hynynen K, McDannold N, Clement G, et al. Pre-clinical testing of a phased array ultrasound system for MRI-guided noninvasive surgery of the brain-A primate study. Eur J Radiol 2006; 59:149–156.

70. Morocz IA, Hynynen K, Cudbjartsson H, et al. Brain edema development after MRI-guided focused ultrasound treatment. J Magn Reson Imag 1998; 8(1):136–142.

71. McDannold N, Moss M, Killiany R, et al. MRI-guided focused ultrasound surgery in the brain: tests in a primate model. Magn Reson Med 2003; 49(6):1188–1191.

72. Foldes K, Hynynen K, Shortkroff S, et al. Magnetic resonance imaging-guided focused ultrasound synovectomy. Scand J Rheumatol 1999; 28(4):233–237.

73. Wu F, Chen WZ, Bai J, et al. Tumor vessel destruction resulting from high-intensity focused ultrasound in patients with solid malignancies. Ultrasound Med Biol 2002; 28(4):535–542.

74. Hynynen K, Colucci V, Chung A, et al. Noninvasive arterial occlusion using MRI-guided focused ultrasound. Ultrasound Med Biol 1996; 22(8):1071–1077.

75. Hynynen K, Damianou CA, Colucci V, et al. MR monitoring of focused ultrasonic surgery of renal cortex: experimental and simulation studies. J Magn Reson Imag 1995; 5(3): 259–266.

76. Hynynen K, Chung AH, Colucci V, et al. Potential adverse effects of high-intensity focused ultrasound exposure on blood vessels in vivo. Ultrasound Med Biol 1996; 22(2):193–201.

77. Vaezy S, Martin R, Schmiedl U, et al. Liver hemostasis using high-intensity focused ultrasound. Ultrasound Med Biol 1997; 23(9):1413–1420.

78. Vaezy S, Martin R, Yaziji H, et al. Hemostasis of punctured blood vessels using high-intensity focused ultrasound. Ultrasound Med Biol 1998; 24(6):903–910.

79. Otsuka R, Fujikura K, Hirata K, et al. In vitro ablation of cardiac valves using high-intensity focused ultrasound. Ultrasound Med Biol 2005; 31(1):109–114.

80. Vykhodtseva NI, Hynynen K, Damianou C. Histologic effects of high intensity pulsed ultrasound exposure with subharmonic emission in rabbit brain in vivo. Ultrasound Med Biol 1995; 21(7):969–979.

81. Hynynen K, Vykhodtseva NI, Chung AH, et al. Thermal effects of focused ultrasound on the brain: determination with MR imaging. Radiology 1997; 204(1):247–253.

82. Vykhodtseva N, Sorrentino V, Jolesz FA, et al. MRI detection of the thermal effects of focused ultrasound on the brain. Ultrasound Med Biol 2000; 26(5):871–880.

83. Hynynen K. The threshold for thermally significant cavitation in dog's thigh muscle in vivo. Ultrasound Med Biol 1991; 17(2):157–169.

84. Xie F, Tsutsui JM, Lof J, et al. Effectiveness of lipid microbubbles and ultrasound in declotting thrombosis. Ultrasound Med Biol 2005; 31(7):979–985.

85. McCreery TP, Sweitzer RH, Unger EC, et al. DNA delivery to cells in vivo by ultrasound. Methods Mol Biol 2004; 245:293–298.

86. Unger EC, Hersh E, Vannan M, et al. Local drug and gene delivery through microbubbles. Prog Cardiovasc Dis 2001; 44(1):45–54.

87. Unger EC, Hersh E, Vannan M, et al. Gene delivery using ultrasound contrast agents. Echocardiography 2001; 18(4):355–361.

88. Unger EC, Matsunaga TO, McCreery T, et al. Therapeutic applications of microbubbles. Eur J Radiol 2002; 42(2):160–168.

89. Vannan M, McCreery T, Li P, et al. Ultrasound-mediated transfection of canine myocardium by intravenous administration of cationic microbubble-linked plasmid DNA. J Am Soc Echocardiogr 2002; 15(3):214–218.

90. Unger EC, Porter T, Culp W, et al. Therapeutic applications of lipid-coated microbubbles. Adv Drug Deliv Rev 2004; 56(9):1291–1314.

91. Siegel RJ, Cumberland DC, Myler RK, et al. Percutaneous peripheral ultrasonic angioplasty. Herz 1990; 15(5):329–334.

92. Kim HJ, Greenleaf JF, Kinnick RR, et al. Ultrasound-mediated transfection of mammalian cells. Hum Gene Ther 1996; 7(11):1339–1346.

93. Kinoshita M, Hynynen K. A novel method for the intracellular delivery of siRNA using microbubble-enhanced focused ultrasound. Biochem Biophys Res Commun 2005; 335(2): 393–399.

94. Huber PE, Pfisterer P. In vitro and in vivo transfection of plasmid DNA in the Dunning prostate tumor R3327–AT1 is enhanced by focused ultrasound. Gene Ther 2000; 7(17): 1516–1525.

95. Madio DP, van Gelderen P, DesPres D, et al. On the feasibility of MRI-guided focused ultrasound for local induction of gene expression. J Magn Reson Imag 1998; 8(1):101–104.

96. Guilhon E, Quesson B, Moraud-Gaudry F, et al. Image-guided control of transgene expression based on local hyperthermia. Mol Imag 2003; 2(1):11–17.

97. Hynynen K, McDannold N, Vykhodtseva N, et al. Non-invasive opening of BBB by focused ultrasound. Acta Neurochir Suppl 2003; 86:555–558.

98. McDannold N, Vykhodtseva N, Raymond S, et al. MRI-guided targeted blood-brain barrier disruption with focused ultrasound: histological findings in rabbits. Ultrasound Med Biol 2005; 31(11):1527–1537.

99. Sheikov N, McDannold N, Hynynen K, et al. Cellular mechanisms of the blood-brain barrier opening induced by ultrasound in presence of microbubbles. Ultrasound Med Biol 2004; 30 (7):979–989.

100. Kinoshita M, McDannold N, Jolesz FA, et al. Noninvasive localized delivery of Herceptin to the mouse brain by MRI-guided focused ultrasound-induced blood-brain barrier disruption. Proc Natl Acad Sci USA 2006; 103(31):11719–11723.

101. Kinoshita M, McDannold N, Jolesz FA, et al. Targeted delivery of antibodies through the blood-brain barrier by MRI-guided focused ultrasound. Biochem Biophys Res Commun 2006; 340(4):1085–1090.

8

Magnetic Resonance Imaging–Guided Breast Focused Ultrasound Surgery

Eva C. Gombos and Daniel F. Kacher
Department of Radiology, Brigham and Women's Hospital and Harvard Medical School, Boston, Massachusetts, U.S.A.

INTRODUCTION

One of the most important potential applications of focused ultrasound surgery (FUS) ablation is the treatment of breast tumors. Breast cancer is the most commonly diagnosed cancer in women in the United States. In 2006, breast cancer is expected to account for 212,920 new cases (31% of all new cancer cases among women) and 40,970 deaths (1). Between 1991 and 2001, a 2.3% annual decrease in the age-adjusted breast cancer death rate was documented, mainly due to earlier diagnosis as well as advances in treatment.

A shift to limited treatment from mastectomy to breast-conservation treatment (BCT) with lumpectomy and radiation therapy has occurred in patients with early stage tumors. The standard treatment for women with breast cancer desiring breast conservation is lumpectomy followed by external beam radiation therapy. Several randomized trials showed that women who undergo a lumpectomy alone and do not receive breast radiation therapy have at least a three-fold increase in local recurrence compared with those who received adjuvant radiation therapy following surgery (2–5). Lumpectomy alone without radiation results in local failure up to 39%. These data imply that surgical removal is an approximate removal of the bulk of the cancer and a more complete eradication of the microscopic residual tumor is achieved primarily by radiation therapy. Magnetic resonance imaging–guided focused ultrasound surgery (MRIgFUS) may offer an alternative to conventional surgical lumpectomy if the majority of the cancer cells are destroyed during MRIgFUS treatment.

The cosmetic results and side effects after conventional BCT are acceptable to most patients; however, the noninvasive ablation method with FUS is thought to be psychologically and cosmetically more satisfactory. MRIgFUS is also suitable for treating patients who are at high risk for surgery; the nonsurgical procedures require less anesthesia and are associated with reduced in-hospital recovery time and therefore cost, less risk of infections, and less scar formation.

PATIENT SELECTION CRITERIA FOR BREAST MRIgFUS

Selection of appropriate patients is of paramount importance for determination of the success of MRIgFUS. If a definitive treatment is planned, this method can be applied only in a limited group of women. Candidate patients should have limited disease with good prognostic factors and the tumor should not be adjacent to the skin nor the chest wall. Exclusion criteria in most studies include the following: large or multifocal tumors, large ductal carcinoma in situ, cancers with extensive intraductal component or lymphovascular invasion, tumors with irregular margins, history of radiation or local thermal therapy, significant background illness or underlying medical condition, contraindications for magnetic resonance imaging (MRI), or an inability to lie still for up to 150 minutes. The ultrasound (US) beam can potentially heat scars on the skin. Patients with scarring should be excluded if the treatment plan requires that the scar lie in the path of the beam. Pregnant or lactating patients and those receiving anticoagulation therapy are also obviously excluded. There are not enough data on treatment of invasive lobular cancer or other special types of cancer (mucinous, medullary, papillary, etc.) and patients with these diagnoses may not be ideal candidates for MRIgFUS. Lesion location is also an important criterion. For superficial targets, there are risks for skin burn and undertreatment, leaving residual tumor cells close to the skin. Also patients with cancers in close proximity to the nipple may not be suitable candidates.

Criteria can be relaxed for patients who are not candidates for open surgery for medical reasons and MRIgFUS would be utilized as a palliative therapy. The noninvasive treatment of fibroadenomata with MRIgFUS is a promising alternative for patients who are uncomfortable with palpable lumps and prefer noninvasive therapy to avoid surgical scars.

TECHNIQUES FOR BREAST MRIgFUS

Patient preparation for MRIgFUS is similar to that for MRI-guided diagnostic procedures (e.g., core needle biopsy or wire localization) regarding imaging, contraindications, anesthesia, and approach. Core biopsy is always obtained prior to treatment to establish histological diagnosis as well as attain status of receptors and prognostic factors. Local anesthetic is typically used and deeper planes of anesthesia and analgesia (e.g., conscious sedation) may be used for MRIgFUS due to potentially intense pain and longer procedure duration.

Prerequisites for MRIgFUS of breast tumors include ability to localize tumor and its surrounding anatomic structure allowing clear definition of targeted tissue volume. The tumor location has to be favorable to be able to target it within the FUS focal volume. Lesions should be between 1 and 20 cm from the skin and not adjacent to the chest wall. The ability to monitor temperature or thermal effects during energy deposition in real time is also required as well as controlling amount of energy deposited and spatial extent of ablation. Low field open scanners have limited signal-to-noise ratio and limited temperature resolution; breast MRIgFUS is best done at higher field strengths (1.5 T and higher).

In FUS ablation, the patient lies prone with the breast positioned on water pillow on a specialized table that fits inside of an MRI scanner. The transducer is acoustically coupled with the water bath and embedded in magnetic resonance (MR) table (Figs. 1–3).

Before the start of the procedure, an anxiolytic is given to reduce movement and an analgesic is administered to counter the associated discomfort. The transducer is then positioned so that the US beam is focused directly on specific positions within the tumor, outlining its margins as accurately as possible. At these focal points within the cancer, the beam produces temperature elevations that result in coagulation necrosis. FUS treatment

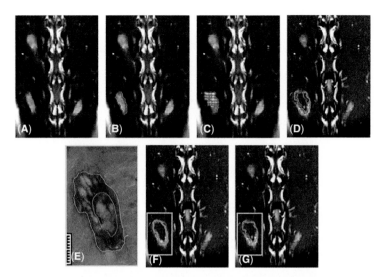

Figure 3.1 Demonstration of MR guidance for treatment planning, monitoring, and verification of focused ultrasound treatment delivery from a prototype system used to ablate a canine transmissible venereal tumor inoculated in the paraspinal muscle. (*For full caption, see page 26.*)

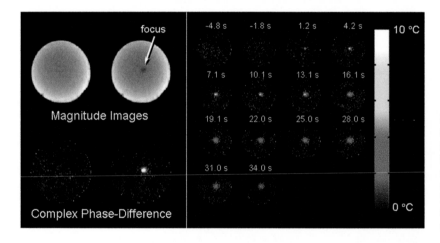

Figure 3.4 Example output of typical fast gradient-echo MRTI images during focused ultrasound heating of an agar phantom (3 sec per image, 0.7×0.7×3 mm resolution). (*For full caption, see page 32.*)

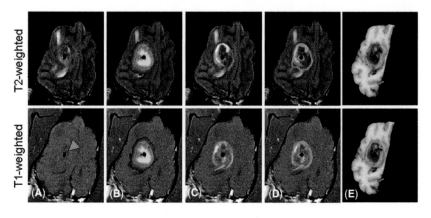

Figure 3.5 Demonstration of MR-guided ablation of canine transmissible venereal tumors in the brain using a multi-element ultrasound applicator. (*For full caption, see page 34.*)

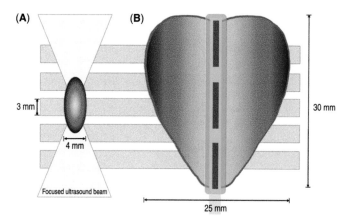

Figure 3.6 A challenge in temperature monitoring thermal therapies utilizing ultrasound is conforming the MRTI technique to the geometry and timing. (*For full caption, see page 35.*)

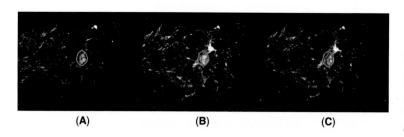

Figure 3.9 MR-guided focused ultrasound ablation of breast cancer at The University of Texas M. D. Anderson Cancer Center. (*For full caption, see page 37.*)

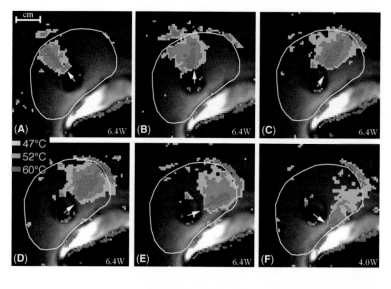

Figure 4.1 Three transverse MRI-based temperature images showing sonications in canine prostate using an interstitial ultra-sound probe. (*For full caption, see page 45.*)

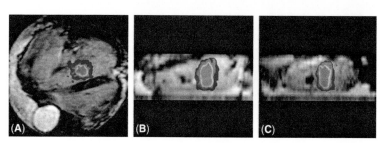

Figure 4.3 Temperature maps in rabbit thigh muscle in vivo obtained at the end of a spiral trajectory with closed-loop MR thermometry-based control. (*For full caption, see page 47.*)

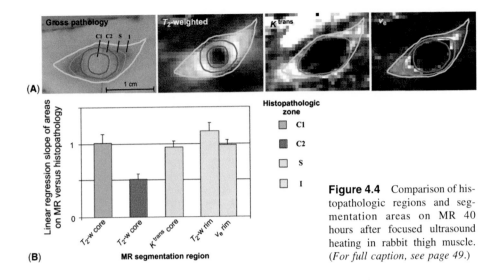

(A)

(B)

Figure 4.4 Comparison of histopathologic regions and segmentation areas on MR 40 hours after focused ultrasound heating in rabbit thigh muscle. (*For full caption, see page 49.*)

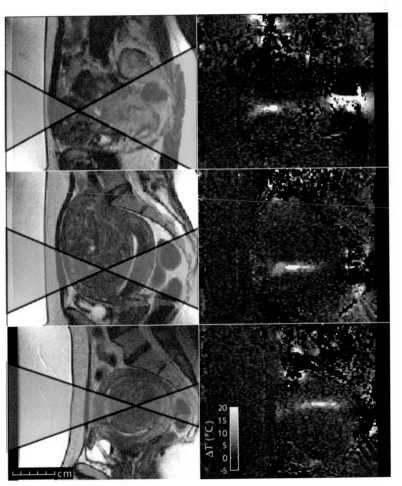

Figure 5.1 Anatomical T_2-weighted MR images (*left*) and MRI-derived temperature maps of three sonications delivered at different depths into uterine fibroids (*right*). (*For full caption, see page 57.*)

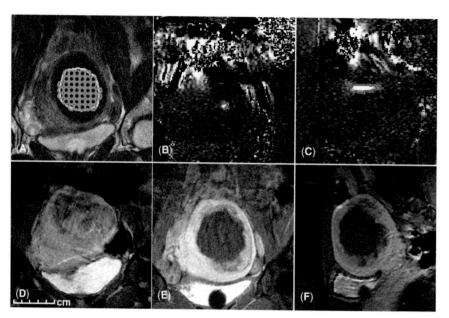

Figure 5.4 MR images of a uterine fibroid acquired before, during, and after focused ultrasound surgery. (*For full caption, see page 60.*)

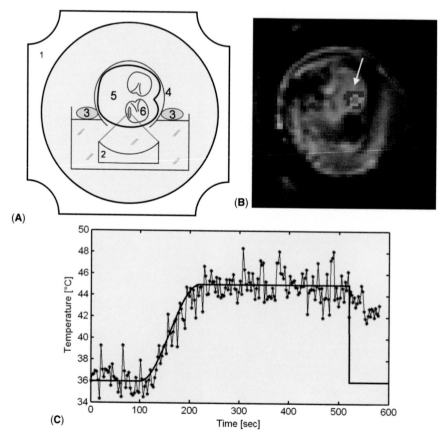

Figure 14.1 Noninvasive local hyperthermia with MRI-controlled focused ultrasound in the kidney. (*For full caption, see page 174.*)

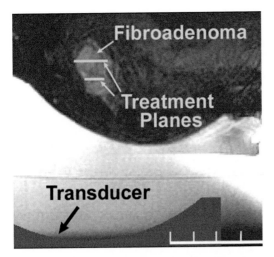

Figure 1   FUS treatment of a fibroadenoma. FS T2WI FSE MR. The patient is prone, with the breast positioned on the water pillow. The transducer is outlined at the bottom. *Abbreviations*: FSE, fast spin-echo; MR, magnetic resonance. *Source*: From Ref. 6.

consists of a series of sonications inside of the prescribed region of treatment comprising the tumor itself plus a surrounding margin.

Many focal points within prescribed region of treatment are individually heated to sculpt the ablation zone. As with all MRIgFUS, in breast treatment, the heat builds and dissipates quickly, and the desired rapid temperature elevation to 60°C to 90°C is produced.

CLINICAL APPLICATION OF BREAST MRIgFUS

The first clinical protocol to test the feasibility of MRIgFUS for management of benign fibroadenomata was reported by Hynynen et al. using an early commercial delivery system (General Electric Medical Systems, Milwaukee, Wisconsin, U.S.A.) with a single channel US transducer (6). From the 11 lesions treated, eight treatments were partially or nearly completely successful. Temperature-sensitive phase-difference-based MRI was performed during each sonication to monitor focus localization and tissue temperature elevation (from 12.8°C to 49.9°C) from these treatments. Success was established on the basis of postcontrast T_1-weighted images showing a partial or complete lack of contrast material uptake as well as clinical examination, revealing that the treated fibroadenomata were smaller and softer. One patient experienced treatment failure due to the placement of excess local anesthetic anterior to the fibroadenoma. Unavoidable microscopic bubbles in the local anesthetic caused scattering of the US beam and thus limited the power delivered to the target. The authors recommended that if local anesthetic is used, it should be placed not in front rather beyond the lesion. Moreover, they recommended that the tumor location be monitored throughout therapy. No adverse effects were detected, except for one case of transient edema in the pectoralis muscle two days after therapy. The authors suggested that the best time for follow-up MRI may be approximately one week following FUS, when edema has resolved in the treated area. With this single-channel prototype, sonication times were each approximately 10 seconds to treat a focal size of 4 × 6 mm. Lesions up to 10 cm from the surface of the skin could be treated with this generation of the technology.

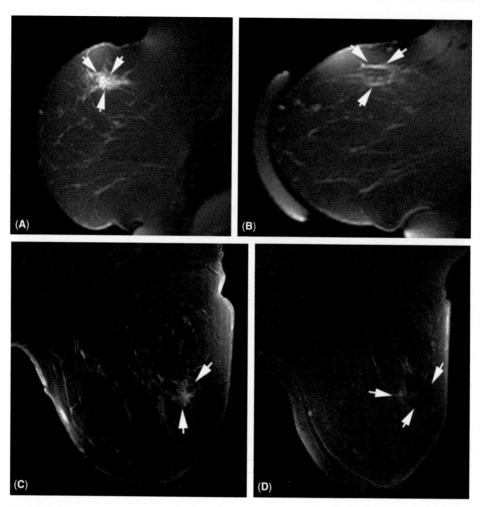

Figure 2 MRI images of a 1.8 cm poorly differentiated invasive ductal carcinoma MRIgFUS in a 44-year-old woman. Pretreatment sagittal (**A**) and axial (**C**) images: an irregular enhancing mass is seen in the upper outer quadrant of the right breast in the pretreatment CE T_1-weighted fat saturated images (*arrow heads*). Posttreatment sagittal (**B**) and axial (**D**) images: three days after MRIgFUS, minimal strikes of enhancement are seen without mass-like enhancement (*arrow heads*) (CE T_1-weighted fat saturated images). This may represent hyperemia due to reactive inflammation or residual tumor. On the axial image, dark signal void area is seen at the site of the prior enhancing mass. At histopathology, about 50% of the carcinoma and adjacent normal tissue showed thermal effects. The remaining portion of the carcinoma appeared viable. *Abbreviations*: CE, contrast enhanced; MRI, magnetic resonance imaging. *Source*: Courtesy of Drs. K. Hynynen, D. Smith, C. Kaelin, and N. McDannold.

A subsequent feasibility test for breast cancer treatment by MRIgFUS was performed in 2001 at the Brigham and Women's Hospital on two breast cancers (unpublished), using the original General Electric (GE) prototype system, and one additional patient was treated with a prototype therapy system (InSightec-TxSonics, Haifa, Israel and Dallas, Texas, U.S.A.) with a 1.5 T MRI scanner (Magnetom Vision Plus, Siemens, Erlangen, Germany) (7). All three patients underwent lumpectomy revealing partial thermal effects and residual viable carcinoma cells.

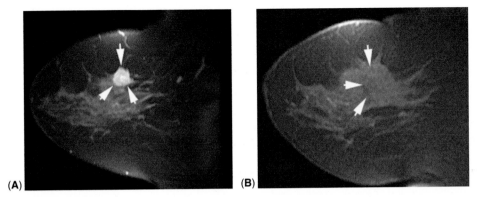

Figure 3 MRI images of a 1.4 cm Grade II invasive ductal carcinoma MRIgFUS in a 57-year-old woman. (**A**) A rapidly enhancing mass is seen in the upper outer quadrant of the right breast in the pretreatment sagittal CE T_1-weighted fat saturated images (*arrows*). (**B**) Six days after MRIgFUS, no enhancement is seen at the site of the tumor (*arrows*) (sagittal CE T_1-weighted fat saturated images). At histopathology, about 25% of the carcinoma and adjacent normal tissue showed thermal effects. The remaining portion of the carcinoma appeared viable. *Abbreviations*: CE, contrast enhanced; MRI, magnetic resonance imaging. *Source*: Courtesy of Drs. K. Hynynen, D. Smith, C. Kaelin, and N. McDannold.

The collaborating studies concluded that MRI-guided FUS of breast cancer is feasible and effective in selected breast cancer patients. Gianfelice et al. conducted the first Phase I trial of MRIgFUS (8) with a next-generation treatment system that evolved from the GE technology (InSightec-TxSonics), used in conjunction with a 1.5 T MRI scanner (Signa Horizon, GE Medical Systems, Milwaukee, Wisconsin, U.S.A.). Histopathologic analysis of the resected specimen showed that residual cancer was predominantly identified at the periphery of the tumor mass. This shortcoming indicated the need to increase the total targeted area at the periphery. FUS ablation was well tolerated by the patients, and with the exception of minor skin burns in two patients, no complications occurred. In a later study by the same authors, with the use of improved technology, 24 patients were treated by MRIgFUS followed by adjuvant hormonal treatment with tamoxifen (9). Percutaneous biopsy was performed after six-month follow-up, and if residual tumor was present, a second MRIgFUS treatment session was initiated, followed by repeat biopsy one month later. Nineteen of 24 patients (79%) had negative biopsy results after one or two treatment sessions. In a subsequent report by Gianfelice et al., dynamic contrast-enhanced (CE) MRI was used both to identify the target volume and to assess residual tumor following MRIgFUS treatment. Twelve women with invasive breast cancers measuring less than 3.5 cm (10) were treated. The ablated region was identified as a dark nonenhancing area, surrounded by enhancing edematous regions. The treatment system evolved over the course of this study. Graduation from a single channel transducer to a phased array transducer, used in the later treatments, enabled focal depths of up to 20 cm from the skin surface. Moreover, the necessary number of sonications to treat a volume was reduced. Flexibility in directing energy to the target was facilitated with the addition of the ability to angle the transducer.

Zippel and Papa conducted another Phase I clinical trial between 2002 and 2004 to examine the possibility of ablating breast carcinoma using MRIgFUS (11). Ten patients underwent the procedure at the Chaim Sheba Medical Center in Israel, using the ExAblate® 2000 (InSightec, Ltd., Haifa, Israel.). On average, 20 to 50 sonications were delivered over a one- to two-hour period to complete a treatment. All patients underwent standard lumpectomy and axillary sampling to complete standard treatment. Histopathology showed no viable tumor cells in two patients. The remaining eight patients had varying amounts of residual tumor up to 30%.

In the most recent Phase II MRIgFUS trial, a cohort of 29 patients was treated with the ExAblate 2000 by Furusawa et al., correlative pathology revealed 97% ± 4% tumor destruction (12). The treatment was well tolerated, with a minimum of adverse effects, especially when performed under local anesthesia. One patient, however, experienced a third-degree burn to the skin below the transducer array, which was attributed to user error. Pathology specimens from lumpectomy showed that residual tumor in two patients was located on the anterior or posterior margins of the treatment. These outcomes emphasized the need to include a 5 mm safety margin in the prescribed region of treatment.

Feasibility of guiding FUS with US has been shown by Wu et al. (13,14). Without MRI guidance, no temperature mapping was possible, and the delineation of the treated volume was less accurate. However, there were no severe side effects, and histo-pathologic analysis supported the prior trials revealing homogeneous coagulative necrosis, including the tumor and normal breast tissue within the target region (14,15).

Past studies have provided data about treatment accuracy, efficiency, and safety. Many questions regarding MRIgFUS and generally about nonsurgical ablation can only be answered through well-conducted prospective studies. To date, the ExAblate 2000 System has been used to treat approximately 150 breast cancer patients. In addition, the InSightec, Ltd. is currently conducting an Food and Drug Administration (FDA) investigational device exemption (IDE)-approved Phase II protocol in breast cancer. This protocol will include treatment by MRIgFUS, follow-up MRI to assess treatment outcome, lumpectomy, and pathological assessment of the excised tissue.

In November 2001, the FDA cleared InSightec for a Phase III IDE for breast fibroadenomata. In Phase III, patients will not undergo subsequent surgery. Studies evaluating MRIgFUS safety and efficiency in treating breast lesions, both benign and malignant, have been conducted at independent sites worldwide. During this trail, a definitive study on the frequency of local recurrence will be conducted.

Furusawa et al. have treated 16 patients to date, as part of a 100-patient Phase III trial (16). In this trial, patients will receive adjuvant radiation therapy instead of lumpectomy and rate of recurrence will be closely monitored. Additional 22 patients, who did not meet criteria for enrollment into the clinical trial, were treated with MRIgFUS. One case of local recurrence of pure type mucinous carcinoma was noted (16).

The American College of Radiology Imaging Network is planning to start a trial to determine the effectiveness of MRIgFUS, with the goal to ablate 95% of the volume of an invasive breast cancer in at least 70% of appropriately selected patients. In this proposed study, patients with histologically proven breast cancer will be treated with MRIgFUS prior to their surgery. The potential effect of treatment on lymphatic drainage as well as the sensitivity of post-treatment MRI in identifying residual cancer will be investigated.

HISTOPATHOLOGY OF BREAST MRIgFUS

Macroscopic examination of breast specimens that are excised after FUS typically shows treatment-induced complete coagulative necrosis as a yellow-white area of central necrosis surrounded by a red hemorrhagic ring (Fig. 4) (7,12–15,18–20).

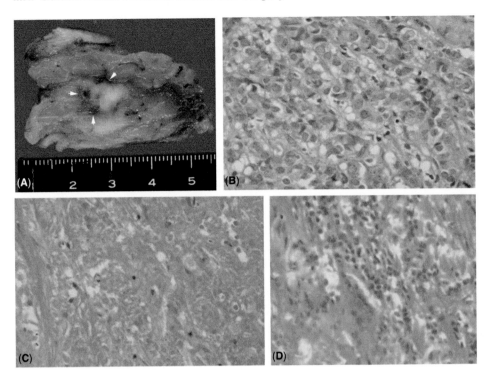

Figure 4 Pathological changes following MRIgFUS of breast cancer. (**A**) Macroscopic specimen shows the target as white area with a hyperemic rim (*arrows*). (**B**) Pretreatment histology shows invasive carcinoma with lobular features (H&E). (**C**) Posttreatment histology shows almost coagulative necrosis in the treated area (H&E). (**D**) Posttreatment histology on other areas shows thermal fixation with preserved tissue architecture and microscopic cellular details in the treated area (H&E). *Abbreviation*: H&E, hematoxylin and eosin. *Source*: From Ref. 17.

At the margin between the treated and untreated regions, there is typically a rim of congestion that represents an inflammatory reaction to thermal ablation. Corresponding histopathology of resected specimens characteristically reveals coagulative necrosis and thermal fixation of the treated tissue, which should include the tumor and margin of an obviously normal breast tissue surrounding the tumor (Fig. 4). The marginal rim of congestion is composed of inflammatory cells, including histiocytes, lymphocytes, macrophages, and giant cells. Normal fatty breast tissue frequently shows histologically signs of fat necrosis.

Pathologic evaluation to assess treatment response postablation is comparable to assessment after neoadjuvant treatment of breast cancer. There are several evaluation systems for breast cancer treatment response (B-18 by Fisher, Miller-Payne, Symmans, AJCC, Chevallier, Sataloff, Rouzier, MNPI) differing mainly in number of categories (21–23). Most of these systems define complete pathologic response as the absence of invasive breast cancer in the breast; a prerequisite is that the tumor site must be identified. Residual tumor is often found at histology in scattered nests within the tumor bed; therefore, extensive pathological examination of the specimen is needed to establish a correct correlation with treatment effectiveness.

MRI may accurately predict the pathologic response; however, there is possibly a high false-negative rate with decreased or no enhancement detected by MRI despite viable tumor cells. Non–tumor-related enhancement might also increase after treatment secondary to reactive inflammation and fat necrosis, leading to potentially false-positive MRI exams.

ADVANTAGES OF BREAST MRIgFUS

From the patient perspective, MRIgFUS produces minimum of adverse effects and is well-tolerated especially when performed under local anesthesia. Moreover, the procedure does not compromise cosmesis or result in scarring or disfigurement of the breast.

The two main technical advantages of MRIgFUS over the other minimally invasive ablation techniques are its noninvasiveness and its real-time, closed-loop MR feedback. MRIgFUS can precisely deliver energy to a given point in soft tissue, accurate within 1 mm, without interrupting skin integrity. High sensitivity of MRI for breast cancer allows accurate treatment planning and later examination for residual tumor. In addition, during MRIgFUS, there is ongoing feedback detailing temperature changes at and around the treated region, which allows the operator to be fully in control of the induced thermal effect (24,25).

The experience so far shows that MRIgFUS can be used for complete ablation of breast tumors in a safe and reliable way. Safety results are measured by the adverse event reports that were captured by the treating physicians. Hardly any severe [third-degree skin burn (12)] and a few minor adverse events were reported. Proximity to the skin should be avoided and it is important to keep safety margins during the MRIgFUS treatment of breast carcinomas.

Disadvantages of Breast Cancer Ablation

The main argument against noninvasive treatments of breast cancer, including MRIgFUS, is that the margin status cannot be assessed due to lack of pathologic specimen. Radiologic assessment, mainly postprocedure CE MRI, must replace histopathology. As no additional tissue is obtained, the histological diagnosis and tumor markers (estrogen and progesterone receptor status and HER2 status) must be determined from the pretreatment core biopsy. Additional tissue can be taken at core biopsy for molecular profiling, which is increasingly becoming part of standard practice.

Nonsurgical ablation also relies on imaging for an accurate determination of tumor extent. CE MRI is very sensitive for detection of invasive breast cancer and may improve the determination of the invasive tumor size (26–28). For small node negative breast cancers, size remains the major determinant of the need for adjuvant systemic therapy. Although MRI is shown to be more accurate than mammography or US in size assessment, even MRI currently cannot exclude small amount of residual invasive cancer.

Axillary lymph node sampling is standard for breast cancer staging. Sentinel lymph node (SLN) surgery is increasingly utilized in early breast cancer. No data are collected to date on FUS therapy effect on lymphatic drainage. Vargas et al. studied the success rate of SLN biopsy in patients enrolled in a clinical trial of preoperative focused microwave phased-array tumor ablation (19). Sentinel nodes were found with an overall success rate of 91% of patients treated with antecedent breast tumor ablation, which is comparable with other reports on success rate of SLN biopsy in the literature. These results imply that there is no impairment in the ability to perform sentinel node biopsy after thermal ablative treatment.

In the breast, medium-sized vessels (2–5 mm in diameter or larger) are frequently encountered. In vicinity of prominent vessels, local heat may be insufficiently delivered to the target volume, because the blood vessels may act as heat sink. As a result, islands of tumor cells in the presence of a larger vessel may survive.

A potential cause for insufficient local heating is generation of microscopic bubbles by local analgesic injection. These may cause scattering of the US beam and limited the power delivery to the tumor (6).

MR thermal monitoring may be challenging in a breast that is of predominantly fatty composition (25). Proton resonance frequency shift techniques work in aqueous tissue, but not in fatty tissue. Moreover, subtraction-based temperature-sensitive sequences are very sensitive for motion. Misregistration due to breathing or bulk patient movement may be problematic.

CONCLUSIONS

MRIgFUS of breast tumors is feasible and safe, without marked adverse effects. The published studies have shown that MRI is suitable for both FUS treatment planning and delineation of FUS therapy-induced changes.

There is a possibility of residual viable cancer cells with MRIgFUS; however, residual tumor is a frequent finding with surgical removal and re-excision: In 50% or more of lumpectomies, the margins are inadequate, involved, or close. Histopathological studies also demonstrated that histologically negative or close biopsy margins do not guarantee complete excision (29,30).

The desired result of MRIgFUS is a total coagulation of the tumor, which would be equivalent to surgical removal at lumpectomy. MRIgFUS has the potential to become an important modality for the local treatment of malignant breast tumors in combination with radiation therapy. Additional studies are needed to prove that this noninvasive method is equivalent to conventional surgery in safety and total ablation of the target and further follow-up is desired to compare long-term local control of the disease.

REFERENCES

1. Jemal A, Siegel R, Ward E, et al. Cancer statistics, 2006. CA Cancer J Clin 2006; 56: 106–130.
2. Fisher B, Anderson S, Bryant J, et al. Twenty-year follow-up of a randomized trial comparing total mastectomy, lumpectomy, and lumpectomy plus irradiation for the treatment of invasive breast cancer. N Engl J Med 2002; 347:1233–1241.
3. Veronesi U, Cascinelli N, Mariani L, et al. Twenty-year follow-up of a randomized study comparing breast-conserving surgery with radical mastectomy for early breast cancer. N Engl J Med 2002; 347:1227–1232.
4. Bartelink H, Horiot JC, Poortmans P, et al. Recurrence rates after treatment of breast cancer with standard radiotherapy with or without additional radiation. N Engl J Med 2001; 345: 1378–1387.
5. Liljegren G, Holmberg L, Bergh J, et al. 10-Year results after sector resection with or without postoperative radiotherapy for stage I breast cancer: a randomized trial. J Clin Oncol 1999; 17: 2326–2333.
6. Hynynen K, Pomeroy O, Smith DN, et al. MR imaging-guided focused ultrasound surgery of fibroadenomas in the breast: a feasibility study. Radiology 2001; 219:176–185.
7. Huber PE, Jenne JW, Rastert R, et al. A new noninvasive approach in breast cancer therapy using magnetic resonance imaging-guided focused ultrasound surgery. Cancer Res 2001; 61: 8441–8447.

8. Gianfelice D, Khiat A, Amara M, et al. MR imaging-guided focused US ablation of breast cancer: histopathologic assessment of effectiveness—initial experience. Radiology 2003; 227: 849–855.

9. Gianfelice D, Khiat A, Boulanger Y, et al. Feasibility of magnetic resonance imaging-guided focused ultrasound surgery as an adjunct to tamoxifen therapy in high-risk surgical patients with breast carcinoma. J Vasc Interv Radiol 2003; 14:1275–1282.

10. Gianfelice D, Khiat A, Amara M, et al. MR imaging-guided focused ultrasound surgery of breast cancer: correlation of dynamic contrast-enhanced MRI with histopathologic findings. Breast Cancer Res Treat 2003; 82:93–101.

11. Zippel DB, Papa MZ. The use of MR imaging guided focused ultrasound in breast cancer patients; a preliminary phase one study and review. Breast Cancer 2005; 12:32–38.

12. Furusawa H, Namba K, Thomsen S, et al. Magnetic resonance-guided focused ultrasound surgery of breast cancer: reliability and effectiveness. J Am Coll Surg 2006; 203:54–63.

13. Wu F, Wang ZB, Zhu H, et al. Extracorporeal high intensity focused ultrasound treatment for patients with breast cancer. Breast Cancer Res Treat 2005; 92:51–60.

14. Wu F, Wang ZB, Cao YD, et al. A randomised clinical trial of high-intensity focused ultrasound ablation for the treatment of patients with localised breast cancer. Br J Cancer 2003; 89:2227–2233.

15. Wu F, Wang ZB, Cao YD, et al. Heat fixation of cancer cells ablated with high-intensity-focused ultrasound in patients with breast cancer. Am J Surg 2006; 192:179–184.

16. Gombos EC, Kacher DF, Furusawa H, et al. Breast focused ultrasound surgery with magnetic resonance guidance. Top Magn Reson Imag 2006; 17(3):181–8.

17. Topics in Magnetic Resonance Imaging. Philadelphia, PA: Lippincott Williams and Wilkins, 2007. In press.

18. Wu F, Chen WZ, Bai J, et al. Pathological changes in human malignant carcinoma treated with high-intensity focused ultrasound. Ultrasound Med Biol 2001; 27:1099–1106.

19. Vargas HI, Dooley WC, Gardner RA, et al. Success of sentinel lymph node mapping after breast cancer ablation with focused microwave phased array thermotherapy. Am J Surg 2003; 186:330–332.

20. Coad JE, Kosari K, Humar A, et al. Radiofrequency ablation causes 'thermal fixation' of hepatocellular carcinoma: a post-liver transplant histopathologic study. Clin Transplant 2003; 17:377–384.

21. Rajan R, Poniecka A, Smith TL, et al. Change in tumor cellularity of breast carcinoma after neoadjuvant chemotherapy as a variable in the pathologic assessment of response. Cancer 2004; 100:1365–1373.

22. Mamounas EP, Fisher B. Preoperative (neoadjuvant) chemotherapy in patients with breast cancer. Semin Oncol 2001; 28:389–399.

23. Abrial C, Mouret–Reynier MA, Amat S, et al. Tumor parameters, clinical and pathological responses, medical management, and survival through time on 710 operable breast cancers. Med Oncol 2005; 22:233–240.

24. Bohris C, Jenne JW, Rastert R, et al. MR monitoring of focused ultrasound surgery in a breast tissue model in vivo. Magn Reson Imag 2001; 19:167–175.

25. Hynynen K, McDannold N, Mulkern RV, et al. Temperature monitoring in fat with MRI. Magn Reson Med 2000; 43:901–904.

26. Morris EA, Liberman L, Ballon DJ, et al. MRI of occult breast carcinoma in a high-risk population. AJR Am J Roentgenol 2003; 181:619–626.

27. Morris EA. Breast cancer imaging with MRI. Radiol Clin North Am 2002; 40:443–466.

28. Schnall MD, Blume J, Bluemke DA, et al. Diagnostic architectural and dynamic features at breast MR imaging: multicenter study. Radiology 2006; 238:42–53.

29. Dillon MF, Hill AD, Quinn CM, et al. A pathologic assessment of adequate margin status in breast-conserving therapy. Ann Surg Oncol 2006; 13:333–339.

30. Silverstein MJ, Gierson ED, Colburn WJ, et al. Can intraductal breast carcinoma be excised completely by local excision? Clinical and pathologic predictors. Cancer 1994; 73: 2985–2989.

9

Uterine Fibroids and MRI-Guided Focused Ultrasound Surgery

Miriam M.F. Hanstede
*Departments of Obstetrics, Gynecology, and Reproductive Biology and Radiology,
Brigham and Women's Hospital and Harvard Medical School, Boston, Massachusetts,
and Mayo Clinic, Rochester, Minnesota, U.S.A.*

Elizabeth A. Stewart
Department of Obstetrics and Gynecology, Mayo Clinic, Rochester, Minnesota, U.S.A.

Clare M.C. Tempany
*Division of MRI, Department of Radiology, Brigham and Women's Hospital and
Harvard Medical School, Boston, Massachusetts, U.S.A.*

UTERINE FIBROIDS

Definition and Introduction

Leiomyomata uteri are the most frequent myometrial disorders and the most common
pelvic tumor in women. Although they are commonly referred to as fibroids, the tumor
consists of uterine smooth-muscle tissue and is enriched in fibrous extracellular matrix
(1). In some cases, fibroids appear to originate from smooth-muscle cells of the uterine
blood vessels (2).

Macroscopically, these clonal tumors are firm, round, or oval-shaped. Microscopic-
ally, they are composed of smooth-muscle bundles in a whirl-like pattern, well circumscribed but not encapsulated. Of importance in therapy, they are often highly vascular.
They can be singular, but generally, there are multiple fibroids in the same uterus varying
in dimensions and location. In extremely rare cases, approximately 0.1%, a uterine
sarcoma is identified on pathology instead of a fibroid and thus malignant transformation
of myomas into sarcoma is rare.

Incidence

The prevalence of clinically significant fibroids peaks toward the end of a woman's
reproductive cycle, in her perimenopausal years, and declines after menopause
(3). Although most women with uterine leiomyomas do not seek therapy, 20% to 25%
of women in the reproductive age do have significant enough symptoms caused by these
fibroids to cause the woman to seek and warrant therapy (2). Genetic predisposition
seems to contribute. Fibroids are particularly common in the black populations with a

three-fold increase compared to Caucasian populations. Also, the clinical disease of black women is more severe (4). Parity reduces risk, and a familial tendency to develop fibroids reduces the risk significantly (5), as does obesity and early age at menarche. Depending on the method of the diagnosis, the incidence of women having these lesions varies from 5.4% to 77% (6).

Etiology and Pathogenesis

The etiology and pathogenesis of fibroids remain largely unknown. Fibroids decrease in size during menopause and under other hypoestrogenic conditions and also after downregulation treatment with gonadotrophin-releasing hormone (GnRH) agonists (7). This supports the fact that fibroids are steroid-dependant tumors. Although estrogen has been implicated as the important hormone, evidence has been found on the role that progesterone also plays on the growth of fibroids. It is controversial whether estrogen or progesterone is the more important influence (8).

Classification

Fibroids are classified by their location, which affects the symptoms they may cause and how they can be treated. Leiomyomas may be subserosal, submucosal, or intramural; however, most fibroids are combinations. Subserosal myomas are on the external surface of the uterus the uterine serosa, and they can be can be sessile or pedunculated. This type of fibroid is the easiest to remove by laparoscopy. Submucous myomas are in the inner aspect of the myometrium, in the endometrial cavity, and some of these can also be removed by hysteroscopic resection. Intramural leiomyomas predominantly occur within the thick myometrial layer (intramural) of the uterus. They may distort the uterine cavity or cause an irregular external uterine contour. Many of these do not cause symptoms unless they become quite large.

Symptoms

Fibroids can present with a variety of symptoms depending on their size, location, and the reproductive status of the woman. Uterine fibroids can cause abnormal uterine bleeding, pain, and pelvic pressure symptoms (9). The impact of uterine leiomyomas on reproduction is more controversial.

　　　The most common kind of abnormal bleeding associated with leiomyomas is menorrhagia or hypermenorrhoea, prolonged or excessively heavy menstruation (10). The heavy bleeding can cause medical problems and frequently results in iron deficiency anemia. The frequent change of tampons or pads may cause a significant interruption in women's productivity.

　　　Pelvic pressure is due to mass effects from the fibroid and enlarging of the uterus. The pelvic and abdominal discomfort is analogous often to the discomfort women experience during pregnancy. Neighboring structures can be pressed on by the fibroid and may lead to difficulty with urination when there is an anterior myoma or defecation and/ or dyspareunia when there is a myoma located posterior.

　　　Acute pain is rare but can occur in situations with degeneration of the fibroid due to insufficient blood supply, for example, torsion of a pedunculated fibroid. Even so, acute abdominal pain can occur in situations of cervical dilatation where a submucous fibroid is protruding through the lower uterine segment.

Diagnosis

Physical Examination

When there is a suspicion of leiomyomas, a regular pelvic examination is the first step. The myomatous uterus produces an enlarged irregular uterine contour, but many times submucosal or deeply intramural myomas can be missed if the examiner relies just on the examination. Also, other conditions such as adenomyosis, ovarian cysts, or ovarian neoplasm may be mistaken for fibroids. Office hysteroscopy is an additional diagnostic tool using a hysteroscope, which is a thin telescope that is inserted through the cervix into the uterus. The uterine cavity is filled with either saline or carbon dioxide in order to distend and better visualize the uterine cavity.

Imaging Examination

Pelvic or transvaginal ultrasonography (TVUS) is often used to confirm the diagnosis of uterine fibroids (Fig. 1) and exclude other conditions and assists in documenting finer levels of discrimination of myomas growth than that obtained by pelvic examination. Some fibroids are too large for TVUS and thus transabdominal ultrasound (US) can be done. For smaller central ones, saline infusion sonohysterography, a TVUS with sterile saline instillation into the endometrial cavity is used when a clear view of the uterine cavity is required (11,12). It is a significant advance in TVUS evaluation of the endometrial cavity because it has an accurate sensitivity for the detection of structural endometrial pathology affecting the uterine cavity including submucous fibroids. In addition, US enables accurate measurement of the size of the uterine fibroids. Three-dimensional (3D) TVUS, although not widely available, allows detailed evaluation of uterine cavity with an additional dimension. Unfortunately, neither of these two advances in US are routinely available and both require sonologists with special expertise to both perform and interpret these studies. Thus, US, although very sensitive for the detection of enlarged bulky uteri, is not very specific for the diagnosis or precise location of fibroids (Fig. 1). Problems also arise when faced with differentiating adnexal or subserosal or

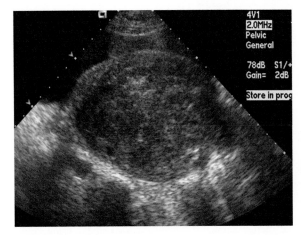

Figure 1 Transvaginal ultrasound exam of the uterus reveals an enlarged uterus with a hyperechoic texture, compatible with a fibroid uterus. Note that the number, size, or volume of individual fibroids is not easily discernable.

pedunculated masses. In this situation, multiplanar magnetic resonance imaging (MRI) with intravenous contrast can be very useful.

Computed axial tomography (CAT) scan or computed tomography (CT) scan is too nonspecific to be of routine use for the imaging evaluation of uterine pathology or fibroids. It does have the unique advantage of detecting calcium, which is relatively common in degenerated fibroids. Also, in the instance where differentiation of a pedunculated fibroid from pelvic mass may be arising from the uterus or the bowel, CT with rectal contrast can be useful. But, it is not helpful in characterizing adnexal masses in general. One situation where it is helpful is in assessing disseminated leiomyomatosis and for mapping the extent of disease.

MRI has gained widespread use and popularity for use in pelvic imaging and in gynecology. It is noninvasive and safe, with no radiation effects, especially important for younger women. The multiplanar sequences allow differentiation of the substructure of the uterus, cervix, vagina, and ovaries (Fig. 2). It allows the radiologist to differentiate uterine anatomy and reliably localizes precisely pelvic pathology. The routine use of both T1- and T2-weighted (T1W and T2W) sequences, before and after the injection of i.v. gadolinium, allows for optimization of the inherent tissue contrast available with MRI. It is uniquely able to characterize soft tissues with these sequences and can provide precise diagnoses for many forms of abnormalities.

It has special advantages for imaging of fibroids. The first and foremost one is to confirm the diagnosis. There are many different types of fibroids, clinically, and pathologically, they have a broad range of features. So, not surprisingly, there are variations in their location and appearance on MRI (Figs. 3–5). Magnetic resonance (MR) allows characterization of the fibroids; with accurate size and volume measurement, the tissue can be characterized such as fibrotic or hypercellular (Fig. 5) and by using i.v. contrast, the perfusion, vascularity, and presence of necrosis can be determined (Fig. 6).

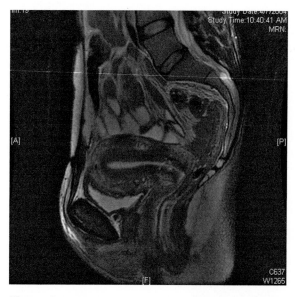

Figure 2 MR appearance of a normal uterus. Sagittal T2-weighted MRI image using eight-channel external multicoil array. This image shows the uterus and its substructures—the myometrium, junctional zone, and endometrium—are all clearly visualized. *Abbreviations*: MR, magnetic resonance; MRI, magnetic resonance imaging.

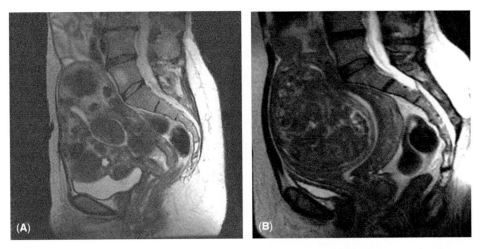

Figure 3 MR appearance of uterine fibroids. (**A**) Sagittal T2W image showing multiple well-defined low (*dark*) signal intensity masses. These are typical of fibroids with very well-defined borders. (**B**) Sagittal T2W image of single large fibroid with heterogeneous mixed T2W signal throughout. *Abbreviations*: MR, magnetic resonance; T2W, T2 weighted.

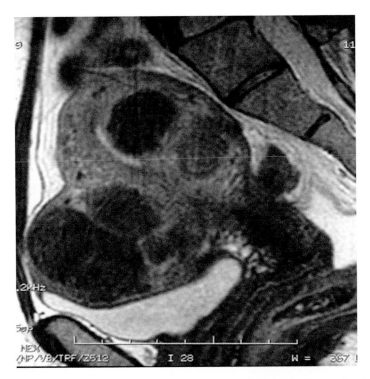

Figure 4 MR appearance of uterine fibroids. Sagittal T2W image showing multiple fibroids; the MR defines the locations that may be correlated with clinical symptoms. Most of these are in the myometrium and one is a submucosal fibroid with extension into the cavity. Note the locations—above and compressing the bladder and one just above and stretching the endometrial cavity. *Abbreviations*: MR, magnetic resonance; T2W, T2 weighted.

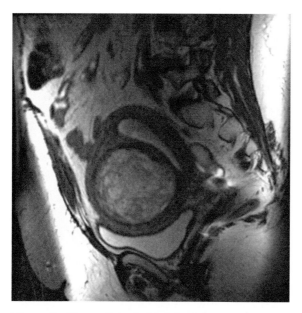

Figure 5 Hypercellular "white" fibroid. MR appearance of a hypercellular "white" fibroid. Note the focal anterior uterine mass, which has high T2 signal throughout. *Abbreviation*: MR, magnetic resonance.

MR Appearance of Fibroids

The ability to classify tissue on MRI is based upon a multiparametric analysis of all the sequences with T1, T2, T1 fat-suppressed, and i.v. contrast-enhanced sequences all playing critical roles. The T2W images first allow location and diagnosis of fibroids as described above. The MR signal on any of the sequences can be isointense and higher or lower than skeletal muscle. The i.v. gadolinium can determine the solid or cystic/necrotic nature of the tissue and if done in rapid bolus fashion can help with perfusion analysis. The gradient echo technique used for gadolinium imaging can also be used to detect fat or calcium. The "classic" fibroid is a well-circumscribed mass with low signal intensity

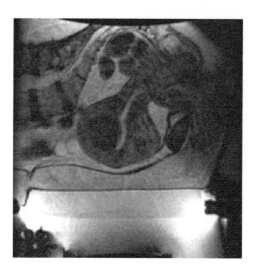

Figure 6 Overview of the MRIgFUS ExAblate 2000 system—an image of a patient in set-up position. *Abbreviation*: MRIgFUS, magnetic resonance–guided focused ultrasound surgery.

on all pulse sequences. On T2W MRI exams, uterine fibroids are usually easily identifiable (Figs. 3–5). These will normally enhance with i.v. contrast or gadolinium. As is well known, in older perimenopausal women, adenomyosis and fibroids may have very similar clinical presentations (Fig. 6).

Treatment

Assessing Outcome in Uterine Fibroid Studies

There are many ways to assess the efficacy of fibroid therapy. Clearly, the simplest is complete resolution of symptoms after definitive surgical removal of the entire uterus and all fibroids, as in a hysterectomy. In other less invasive therapies, the patient's subjective response along with physical and imaging findings can be evaluated in total. The classic way to assess outcome has been to assess the size and volume of the uterus. The very early studies often did this with unblinded examiners by pelvic exam, which clearly made understanding the real treatment effects difficult. However, as GnRH agonists were developed and tested in the 1980s and 1990s, the use of US volumetric measurements was introduced. This is a powerful technique since a relatively small change in a measure diameter can result in a significant difference in the volume. However, for this reason, it is also prone to error again, because small differences in measurement can appear to produce significant differences in volumetric analysis.

Moreover, the volumetric analysis typically derived from the formula for the volume of a prolate ellipsoid. While this is an accurate measure of a concentrically enlarged uterus without subserosal fibroids, it is again prone to error as the shape of the uterus becomes more irregular.

Additionally, volume reduction was not always necessary or helpful in terms of reducing symptoms. Some women with uterine fibroids have only symptoms of heavy menstrual bleeding, and a volume reduction does not predict clinical success. Therefore, newer studies often assess both the endpoints of menorrhagia and impairment of quality-of-life (QOL) through validated questionnaires or instruments.

The classic measurements of QOL are general questionnaires, such as the short form (SF)-36 and the SF-12 developed by the medical outcome trust. These measure general QOL and can be used across procedures and disease states. They are especially useful in terms of looking at postoperative recovery and disease related impairment.

In addition, there is a validated uterine fibroid-specific QOL instrument. This is called the uterine fibroid symptoms quality of life (UFS-QOL) (13). This has two major sections. The symptom severity score (SSS) assesses in a single measurement, both symptoms related to bleeding and those related to bulk or volume-related complaints. The scale runs from 0 to 100. Normal women typically score approximately 20 on the SSS and women with uterine fibroids indicate their increased symptomatology with the mean score of 40. The symptom severity score has eight questions on it and is scored via a five-point Likert scale.

There is also a health-related quality of life (HRQL) component to the UFS-QOL. With this, there is a total HRQL score as well as subscores regarding the following domains: concern, activities, energy/mood, control, self-consciousness, and sexual function. The direction of scoring on these tests is opposite that of the symptom severity score. A woman with no impairment in these domains would score 100 points. The main score for a subset of normal women placed normal women at a mean of approximately 86, and women with uterine leiomyomas at a mean of 62. Both the HRQL total score and all of the subscores showed a significant difference between women with uterine leiomyomas and normal women.

There are also a series of instruments used to discriminate between normal menstrual flow and abnormal menstrual flow. The most commonly used instrument is the pictorial blood loss assessment chart. This uses standard sanitary products as well as a pictorial diary to quantitate the amount of staining of each sanitary product as well as the amount of clots. There are also several other bleeding diaries that are used. A combination of these two endpoints is often used for assessing the efficacy of fibroid therapy.

Uterine myomas can generally be managed expectantly unless they cause symptoms. But, when treatment is indicated, there are several choices. For many years, hysterectomy or less radical surgery such as myomectomy has been the primary choice of treatment. The traditional treatment for fibroids cause symptoms and because the vast majority of fibroids are intramural they are also difficult to treat in nonsurgical, minimally invasive fashion. Eventually size, location, presenting symptoms, age, reproductive desires, and the skills of the surgeon all factor in determining the mode of treatment. Women desiring future fertility or women who want to maintain their uterus for several reasons carry an obvious appeal for effective nonsurgical therapies for uterine fibroids and minimally invasive technology for reducing symptoms from uterine leiomyomas.

Because fibroids are nonmalignant and, therefore, cause morbidity not mortality and because leiomyoma research is underfunded as compared with that for other benign diseases, there has been a historical tendency of little innovation in treatments of fibroids.

Treatment

Uterine myomas can generally be managed expectantly unless they cause symptoms. But, when treatment is wanted, surgery has been the mainstay. Size, location, presenting symptoms, age, reproductive desires, and the skill of the surgeon factor in the mode of treatment.

Surgical Therapy

Hysterectomy is the second most common surgical procedure performed worldwide, exceeded only by cesarean section. Nearly 20% of women will have had a hysterectomy by the age of 40 and one-third by age 65. Hysterectomy has an approximately 3% incidence of major complications. Traditionally, total abdominal hysterectomy has been the surgical approach for gynecological malignancy but in fibroid treatment, there is seldom a need for total hysterectomy, with removal of cervix and ovaries. Vaginal hysterectomy can only be performed when the uterus has a fairly normal size, because the operation is done through the vagina and therefore considered less invasive. Laparoscopic hysterectomy requires a greater surgical expertise than the vaginal and abdominal methods but is increasingly used for fibroids.

Myomectomy conserves the uterus and is offered to women who wish to retain their fertility. The site and size of the fibroids determines the surgical route employed and only the visible and accessible leiomyomas can be removed. Myomectomy is associated with long-term problems such as fibroid recurrence and adhesion formation. Laparoscopy and hysteroscopy also provide minimally invasive options for myomectomy.

Hysteroscopy is associated with lowest morbidity and can be performed without any surgical incisions. The problem with both techniques is that not all leiomyomas can be treated this way. Besides many fibroids that can be easily removed laparoscopically may not require surgical intervention (14).

Endometrial destruction techniques of removing or destroying the full thickness of the endometrium were introduced halfway through the 1980s. This tissue may be removed under direct hysteroscopic view by transcervical resection of endometrium technique using an electrosurgical loop, laser, or a roller ball to ablate the endometrium using thermal energy of sufficient power to produce necrosis of the endometrium. Other techniques developed to destroy the endometrium are cryoablation (15), hot saline solution irrigation (16), diode laser hyperthermia (17), microwave ablation (18), heated balloon system (19), and photodynamic therapy (intrauterine light delivery) (17,20).

These techniques have also been applied to fibroid treatments. Myolysis is a technique where there is an in situ destruction, coagulation, and devascularization of the myoma by electrical, thermal, and US energy sources or carbon dioxide laser (21) or cryotherapy (22). Current methods of myolysis have achieved success in relieving symptoms relating to myoma volume. This can be performed by laparotomy or laparoscopy.

Image-Guided Therapy

Angiographic imaging of the uterus and fibroids can be performed with intra-arterial catheters placed into the uterine arteries via a groin approach. This technique combined with injection of embolic materials, such as beads or gel foam, is know as uterine fibroid embolization (UFE) or uterine artery embolization (UAE) and was originally devised to reduce pelvic bleeding due to postpartum hemorrhage (23). Since 1995, it has been introduced as a treatment for symptomatic uterine myomas sparing the uterus (24,25). It completely occludes both uterine arteries and subbranches, with particulate emboli to cause ischemic necrosis of the uterine fibroids but has no gross permanent adverse effect on the otherwise normal uterus. Without a good blood supply, it has been shown fibroids will decrease in size between 30% and 50% and decrease in symptomatology (26,27). The normal myometrium rapidly establishes a new blood supply through collateral vessels from the ovarian and the vaginal circulations.

This procedure is not without complications (27,28). Complications include postprocedure pain and postembolization syndrome possibly related to the release of cytokines and toxins from the ischemic tissue. Due to acute degenerative procedure, there is also concern of premature ovarian failure due to interference with the ovarian blood supply and infection leading to fallopian tube damage with subsequent infertility. Other complications that may occur are secondary amenorrhea due to endometrial atrophy or intrauterine adhesions and the unknown effect on conception and pregnancy (27). Many advances have been made more recently to avoid some of these complications with for example more highly selective catheterizations to avoid ovarian artery embolization. A recent randomized controlled study from 27 hospitals in the United Kingdom comparing embolization and surgery showed that patients recover faster, but it was associated with 9% rate of patients seeking an alternative treatment after UAE because of inadequate symptom control (29).

Medical Therapy

Medical therapy, conservative therapy for fibroids is limited because the biology of leiomyomas is not well understood. Combined oral contraceptives, nonsteroidal anti-inflammatory drugs, and progestogens (including the Mirena intrauterine device) are used but are not always effective in the presence of uterine fibroids.

GnRH analogs have been used successfully to achieve hypoestrogenism in uterine myomas, resulting in a uterine shrinkage generally by 35% to 65%, amenorrhea, and a reduction in vascularity and therefore is widely used as a preoperative adjuvant in hysterectomies as myomectomy (30). In addition, this same hypoestrogenism is the limit for this form of therapy, because it induces significant menopausal side effects and the risk of osteoporosis with long-term use. Furthermore, after discontinuation of the medication, there is resumption of menses and the tumor will rapidly regrow.

MRI-Guided Focused Ultrasound Surgery

Magnetic resonance imaging–guided focused ultrasound surgery (MRIgFUS) is a ground-breaking minimally invasive alternative to surgery for fibroids (31–35). This novel therapy with MR guidance and control is unique and has three critical advantages, which are (*i*) it uses MRI to define the pelvic anatomy and pathology, (*ii*) it uses MR thermometry, which allows for immediate feedback on the location and tissue temperature changes of the sonication, and (*iii*) it uses MR with i.v. contrast to show the necrotic tissue immediately after the treatment. Focused ultrasound causes local tissue thermal coagulation, ablates the target fibroid, and allows preservation of uterine function. It is a feasible and safe outpatient procedure that does not require hospitalization (36). Also appealing is that the procedure is preformed as an outpatient procedure, day surgery, and it does not require general anesthesia, which greatly reduces recovery time and the risks of side effects. This has an economical impact also, given the decreased time of return to work following therapy.

Fibroids, an Ideal Application of MRIgFUS

There are a number of reasons why uterine fibroids are well suited to treatment with MRIgFUS. Fibroids are generally quite large, well defined, clearly seen on MR, and, importantly, they are nearly always benign. Therefore, the consequences of partial or incomplete treatment have less of an impact than they would for a malignant tumor. Fibroids are rich in extracellular matrix, which makes them relatively easy to treat with thermoablative energy and fibroids are relatively large and therefore easy to target. Also, the fibroid has the ability to dissipate heat via blood perfusion due to the peripheral blood supply. This cooling mechanism prevents significant heat buildup that could potentially cause thermal injury to adjacent structures. As discussed previously, there has been a history of prior thermoablative techniques used for this lesion. Fibroids are also very common in women, which makes clinical trial recruitment easier.

The MRI that is necessary before, during, and after this therapy also helps in screening and patient selection as well as in making evaluation more straightforward. An objective measurement of volume reduction can be made easily. Likewise, the fact that studies suggest that the nonperfused volume (NPV) following treatment correlates with outcome gives a surrogate marker for treatment outcome. Because of the uterine fibroid symptoms quality-of-life questionnaire (UFS-QFOL), which is the only validated measure of leiomyoma symptomatology (13), evaluating the endpoints of successful management such as change in abnormal uterine bleeding, disappearance of pelvic pressure symptoms, and improvement in QOL can be made fairly easy.

Overview of MRIgFUS Procedure

Patient Selection. Patients with symptomatic fibroids present to their doctors and often self-seek this therapy. MRI of the pelvis with standard imaging (multiplanar T2W and T1W sequences before and after i.v. gadolinium) is obtained in all cases presenting for screening at our institution. The clinical history, physical exam, and MRI findings are all used to determine suitability.

Clearly, the usual exclusion criteria for MR scanning apply to MRIgFUS; thus, women with pacemakers or other major contraindications are not considered. We like to scan all our patients in the prone position during screening and thus emulate the treatment position as much as possible. This allows the patient to understand what she may undergo and we can determine the position of the uterus and fibroids. The fibroids and uterus should be directly below the anterior abdominal wall, with no bowel loops intervening. We also mark all lower abdominal wall scars with markers such as vitamin E capsule, to allow visualization on the MR images. We ask our technologists to be sure to cover the entire anterior wall, all the way through the skin surface. This allows us to determine if there will be significant beam passage through scar tissue. This must be avoided if at all possible as it can lead to problems with skin heating and possible skin burns. The T2W images as shown above allow planning and selection of key targets for therapy. The i.v. contrast images determine perfusion, and it is our contention that the fibroid should not have significant necrosis within it, before therapy to allow for optimal treatment effect. The only way to document this is by doing the pretreatment MR with i.v. contrast.

So, in summary, the ideal patient with fibroids for treatment is one with a fibroid of size of 12 weeks' gestation or between 5 and 10 cm, located anteriorly, with no bowel loops in front, and is well perfused (enhance with gadolinium) and the patient is "family complete" and clearly symptomatic.

Procedure Day.   The procedure is done as a day surgery or outpatient treatment; the patient comes to the MR suite, fasting from midnight the night before, and is prepared before entering the magnet. The preparation involves assessment by the treating physician and nurse. An i.v. line and Foley catheter are placed. It is routine to use intravenous conscious sedation (IVCS) for this procedure. This is a combination of a sedative and pain medication that allows the patient to be relatively pain-free, comfortable, awake, and responsive all through the procedure. This form of anesthesia requires the full-time presence of a nurse and a doctor to ensure no complications or adverse events.

As the US beam can cause skin heating, and internal thermal necrosis and distal beam passage through the back can cause nerve heating, the patient must be closely monitored for any of these sensations. Prior to the procedure, the patient is told what may be expected and that she should immediately report any skin heating, internal pain, sciatic nerve stimulation, or back pain. Thus, it is very important for the treating physician to establish regular and clear lines of communication with the patient all through the treatment.

Skin preparation: Prior to entering the magnet, the patients skin is inspected for hair removal and to ensure no scars or focal lesions are present before starting the procedure.

Skin injuries can occur due to defocusing of the US beam, which is most commonly due to superficial scars. A recent case where this occurred and lead to skin burn illustrates this problem (37).

In the magnet, the patient is positioned prone on the ExAblate 2000 table containing the transducer (Fig. 6). This position is confirmed with fast imaging to ensure the transducer is aligned with the fibroid to allow direct US beam passage.

For the duration of the entire procedure, which is over three hours, the patients lie prone on the table with the transducer. This position can be uncomfortable for some and can lead to neck and back pain. For this reason, we use supportive pillows and pain medications.

One very important aspect of this procedure is the continuous communication between the treating physician and the patient. She must understand that the feedback regarding what she feels during each sonication is very important. Her reports of burning in the skin and sciatic nerve pain/stimulation are both critical clues to the treating doctor to change the sonication parameters.

The procedure begins with the delivery of low-power (50–100 watt) sonication, with real-time thermometry acquired simultaneously. The resultant images will provide feedback on location, allowing the operator to determine the correct placement of the focal spot. Any alterations in location can be made at this point and after any individual sonication in the procedure. If the sonication location is correct and the phase map shows it clearly, then the procedure continues with increases in the power gradually up to therapeutic dose.

Once therapeutic dose is achieved, the procedure continues with delivery of all planned sonication. After each one, the operator confirms the patient's comfort and then proceeds. The treatment monitor will display all sonications delivered that have achieved the threshold dose, usually over 60°C. In fact, it is more usual to try to reach 70°C to 80°C, as this will ensure real tissue necrosis. At the end of the procedure, the patient receives 20 cc of i.v. gadolinium and then post gadolinium images are acquired. These will demonstrate the necrotic tissue in the fibroid as a nonperfused area (Fig. 7A and 7B). The patient is then escorted out of the MR suite and recovers for about 30 to 60 minutes and her skin is examined carefully to ensure that there is no damage. There has been one case report of a significant skin burn received during an FUS treatment, which serves to illustrate the real importance of understanding this procedure and taking all possible steps to avoid such events (37). Then, if all is well, the patient can be discharged home and because she has received IVCS, is discharged into the care of an adult family member.

Overview of Clinical Trials and Results

At this time, there have been several large multicenter trials conducted, some in part of the pre-FDA assessment and these are summarized here. Basically, the first trial was a

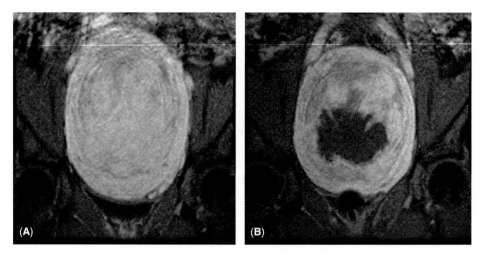

Figure 7 MR assessment of treatment effect. Coronal T1W post-i.v. gadolinium image (**A**) before and (**B**) after MRIgFUS. The pretreatment image shows homogeneous enhancement of the entire fibroid with gadolinium, and the posttreatment image shows the focal area of non-enhancement or necrosis after MRIgFUS. *Abbreviations*: MRIgFUS, magnetic resonance imaging–guided focused ultrasound surgery; i.v., intravenous; T1W, T1 weighted.

safety and feasibility one, treating symptomatic women who then went on to hysterectomy, with pathology evaluation of treatment effect. Several others followed this where the treatment effect was followed by responses to the uterine fibroid quality of life (UF-QOL) and MRI appearance.

The Feasibility Study

The goals of the initial trial treating uterine fibroids were to assess feasibility, safety, and adverse events and confirm correct targeting of MRIgFUS for myomas (36). Furthermore, the relationship between NPV and tissue necrosis was evaluated, as was the completeness of necrosis. The design of the study enrolled women who underwent MRIgFUS treatment within 30 days prior to hysterectomy. However, some sites were required by national authorities to allow women to consider hysterectomy optional (38).

This trial produced some lessons that can be useful for treatment for all indications. First, a wide variety of patients can undergo treatment. Women with body mass indexes (BMIs) from 21 to 41 could all successfully undergo treatment. There was a learning curve in which there were initial issues visualizing low-energy sonication. Also, using gel pads to avoid having sonication pass through the bowel is a learned skill. In patients with anterior abdominal wall scars, there is increased absorption of the treatment beam at that point, which can result in skin burn. The focussed ultrasound beam can be safely angled to avoid this problem. Most patients tolerate the procedure very well with the given medication, which is titrated and administered according to the individual patient's needs. Therefore, procedure-related pain is not a major component in coagulative necrosis caused by MRIgFUS, in contrast to the pain after the procedure due to ischemic necrosis in UAE.

The MR-based volume and pathologic volumes were greater than the planned treatment area; in some patients, this might suggest that coagulation of blood vessels occurred, caused by the focused ultrasound beam, which results in necrosis of the tissue periphery (36). A good correlation was found between the NPV and necrosis. Using focused ultrasound prior to surgery led to increased febrile morbidity in three of the early patients. Using prophylactic antibiotics prior to MRIgFUS when followed by surgery appeared to eliminate this risk. In later trials where surgery was no longer a part of the design, the antibiotics were no longer indicated.

The Clinical Outcome Study

The goal of this study was to achieve effective treatment at 6 to 12 months after MRIgFUS while maintaining a low risk of adverse effects. Fibroid volume, fibroid symptoms, and QOL scores were measured before treatment and six months after treatment. In this study, almost 80% of women who had been treated reported a significant improvement in their uterine fibroid symptoms on follow-up HRQL questionnaires. The mean reduction in fibroid volume at six months was 13.5%, but nonenhancing volume remained within the treated fibroid at six months. This early description of MRIgFUS therapy treatment of fibroids includes follow-up data and shows that although the volume reduction is moderate, it correlates with treatment volume and the symptomatic response to this treatment is encouraging.

In this multicenter clinical trial setting, women were interviewed at six months with an extension of followup to one year, using a 10-point improvement in the transformed SSS of the UFS-QOL as the primary endpoint (13). Secondary endpoints included the HRQOL scores, a second UFS-QOL scale that measured six dimensions of HRQL and

SF-36 (Medical Outcomes Trust) scores, an additional method of assessment of HRQOL. Furthermore, a strict reporting of adverse events was in conformity with the Standard Code of Federal Regulations.

In a study by Stewart et al., 109 women were enrolled and screened, and 62% underwent treatment (39). The remaining 67 were screen failures. Of these, 40% did not meet all the inclusion and exclusion criteria. The remaining 60% of the exclusions occurred after review of MRI images prior to treatment screening. Typical reasons were that the fibroid was not safely accessible to the FUS beam, the fibroid was already necrotic, or that there was adenomyosis present. All included patients had significant fibroid symptoms as measured by the SSS. A significant improvement of QOL parameters in women undergoing MRIgFUS was shown with a volume reduction relative to treatment reduction [77%, respectively 51.2% (38) SSS]. The baseline SSS is the only covariate of efficacy. The SSS discriminates between women with symptomatic fibroids and normal women (27). MRIgFUS appeared to be a safe intervention for uterine fibroids and showed no complications as seen in other new investigational devices for fibroids or UAE. The study design did not maximize efficacy because of the strict treatment guidelines (only 10% of the fibroid volume was treated). The volume reduction was small but could support the fact that volume reduction is not essential for symptoms' resolution. The mean time of return to work after MRIgFUS is significantly lower compared with UAE and abdominal myomectomy or hysterectomy, which has an important economical impact.

There are now multiple studies reporting the growing clinical experience with MRIgFUS in the treatment of uterine fibroids (36,38,40,41). Initial studies were confined to smaller volumes in targeted fibroids and these have shown highly effective symptom relief. The original treatment guidelines determined by the FDA and used in the early clinical trials were restricted by volume to be ablated and, more importantly, by the length of the procedure. The technology, as it was first developed, was relatively slow as there was a required cool-down period between sonications and the time allowed by the FDA was limited to two to three hours in total. In an attempt to overcome this problem, the group at St Mary's hospital in London developed a way of potentiating the results of FUS within large fibroids by the pretreatment of uterine fibroids with GNRH agonists. This regulatory neuropeptide causes a hypoestrogenic state by interfering with the hypothalamic–pituitary–ovarian axis. They decrease the vascularity of the fibroids and make the operation much less risky by lowering blood loss to produce a much more avascular field and can help optimize FUS treatment in large vascular fibroids. The results have been published by Smart et al. who found that by utilizing GNRH agonists given intramuscularly once a month for three months prior to FUS treatment, we can reduce the size of the target fibroid uterus by approximately 30% to 40% and this fibroid can then be readily treated with FUS at the end of this time when it is in a much smaller state (42).

The MRIgFUS technology is improving and more effective sonications are now available and the ExAblate device has recently been approved by the FDA for use on 3 T MRI. These advances will lead to shorter treatment times, more effective tissue necrosis, and with the higher signal-to-noise ratio afforded by 3 T will allow greater accuracy and smaller lesions to be treated. An example of improved efficacy with changing protocols is demonstrated in the most recent study to be published in *Radiology* in June 2007, by Fennessy et al. (43). Under the original study protocol, A, 96 patients were treated; and 64 patients were treated under an optimized protocol, B. Protocol A allowed a maximum treatment time of 120 minutes and a maximum fibroid treatment volume of 100 cc (roughly 6 cm in diameter) or up to 33% of total fibroid volume. Protocol B allowed a maximum treatment time of 180 minutes and maximum fibroid treatment volume of 150 cc (about 7 cm in diameter) or up to 33% of total volume in subserosal fibroids (those on the outer wall of the uterus). The findings showed significant symptom relief in three and six months and sustained relief in one year. Women treated with the optimized protocol reported greater symptom relief and QOL improvement than those treated with the original protocol. No serious adverse effects were reported.

As more results are studied and published, there will be several key features to look for; these include the continuing safety of the procedure, especially as we tend toward larger volume treatments. There is now a registry being established for tracking all treatments that will lead to similar methods of analysis as the UFE or fibroid registry has been able to provide. The other important aspect is to evaluate the durability of the response to the treatment and the rate of alternative treatments sought after MRIgFUS. We are currently awaiting the completion of the three-year follow-up studies that should provide important results to address these issues.

CONCLUSIONS

MRIgFUS is an excellent noninvasive method of treating uterine fibroids. It represents a major change in the clinical approach to this disease as truly disruptive technology is forcing new challenges upon the health-care system and its delivery. It will remain to be seen how fast this becomes integrated into routine clinical care, but there is no doubt it will eventually become a major treatment option not just for uterine fibroids but for many solid tumors throughout the body.

REFERENCES

1. Stewart E. Uterine fibroids. Lancet 2001; 357:293–298.
2. Cramer SF, Patel A. The frequency of uterine leiomyomas. Am J Clin Pathol 1990; 94: 435–438.
3. Flake GP, Anderson J, Dixon D. Environ Health Perspect 2003; 111:1037.
4. Kjerulff KH et al. Uterine leiomyomas: racial differences in severity, symptoms and age at diagnosis. J Reprod Med 2004; 41:483–490.
5. Luoto R, Kaprio J, Rutanen EM, Taipale P, Perola M, Koskenvuo M, et al. Heritability and risk factors of uterine fibroids: the Finnish Twin Cohort study. Maturitas 2000; 37:15–26.
6. Lethaby A, Vollenhoven B, Sowter M. Fibroids. Clin Evid 2002; 8:666–678.
7. West C. GnRH analogues in the treatment of fibroids. Reprod Med Rev 1993; 2:1–97.
8. Reinsch RC, Morales AJ Yen, et al. The effect of RU486 and leuprolide acetate on uterine blood flow in the fibroid uterus: a prospective randomised study. Am J Obstet Gynecol 1994; 170:1623–1628.
9. Buttram VC, Reiter RC. Uterine leiomyomata: etiology, symptomatology and management. Fertil Steril 1981; 36:433–445.
10. Rybo G, Leman J, Tibblin R. Epidemiology of Menstrual Blood Flow. New York: Raven Press, 1985:181–193.
11. Cicinelli E et al. Transabdominal sonohysterography, transvaginal sonography, and hysteroscopy in the evaluation of submucous myomas. Obstet Gynecol 1995; 85:42–47.
12. de Kroon CD, Jansen FW, Trimbos JB. Saline contrast hysterosonography in abnormal uterine bleeding: a systematic review and meta-analysis. BJOG 2003; 110:938–947.
13. Spies JB, Coyne K, Guaou N. UFS-QOL, a new disease-specific symptom and health related quality of life questionnaire for leiomyomata. Obstet Gynecol 2002; 99(2):290–300.

14. Hurst BS. Laparoscopic Myomectomy. 2nd ed. New York: Springer-Verlang, 1997:163–172.
15. Pittrof R, Majid S, Murray A. Initial experience with transcervical cryoablation using saline as a uterine distension medium. Minim Invasive Ther 1993; 2:69–73.
16. Baggish M, Paraiso M, Breznock EM, Griffey S. A computer-controlled, continuously circulating hot irrigating system for endometrial ablation. Am J Obstet Gynecol 1995; 173: 1842–1848.
17. Donnez J, Polet R, Mathieu PE, Konwitz E, Nisolle M, Casanas-Roux F. Endometrial laser interstitial hyperthermia: a potential modality for endometrial ablation. Obstet Gynecol 1996; 87:459–464.
18. Sharp NC, Cronin N, Evans M, Hodgson D, Ellis S, Feldberg I. Microwaves for menorrhagia: a new fast technique for endometrial ablation. Lancet 1995; 346:1003–1004.
19. Singer A, Almanza R, Haber G, Gutierrez A. Preliminary clinical experience with thermal balloon endometrial ablation method to treat menorrhagia. Obstet Gynecol 1994; 83:732–737.
20. Fehr MK, Madsen SJ, Tromberg BJ, Eusebio J, Berns MW, Tadiry Y, Svaasand LO. Intrauterine light delivery for photodynamic therapy of the human endometrium. Hum Reprod 1995; 10:3067–3072.
21. Hindley J, Law P, Hickey M, et al. Clinical outcomes following percutaneous magnetic resonance image guided laser ablation of symptomatic uterine fibroids. Hum Reprod 2002; 17:2737–2741.
22. Sewell PE, Arriola RM, Robinette L, Cowan BD. Real-time I-MR-imaging—guided cryoablation of uterine fibroids. J Vasc Interv Radiol 2001; 12:891–893.
23. Greenwood LH, Glickman MG, Schwartz SS, Morse SS, Denny DF. Obstetric and non malignant gynecologic bleeding: treatment with angiographic embolization radiology. Radiology 1987; 164:155–159.
24. Goodwin SC, Vedantham S, McLucas B, Forno AE, Perrella R. Preliminary experience with uterine fibroid embolization for uterine fibroids. J Vasc Interv Radiol 1997; 8:517–526.
25. Ravina JH, Bouret JM, Ciraru-Vigneron N, et al. Recourse to particular arterial embolization in the treatment of some uterine leiomyoma. Bull Acad Natl Med 1997; 181:233–243.
26. Lumsden M. Embolization versus myomectomy versus hysterectomy: which is the best, when? Hum Reprod 2002; 17:253–259.
27. Spies JB, Warren EH, Mathias SD, Walsh SM, Roth AR, Pentecost MJ. Uterine fibroid embolization: measurement of health-related quality of life before and after therapy. J Vasc Interv Radiol 1999; 10:1293–1303.
28. Godfrey CD, Zbella EA. Uterine necrosis after uterine artery embolization for leiomyoma. Obstet Gynecol 2001; 98:950–952.
29. The Rest Investigators. Uterine-artery embolization versus surgery for symptomatic uterine fibroids. N Engl J Med 2007; 356:360–370.
30. Friedman AJ, Barbieri RL, Benacerraf BR, Schiff I. Treatment of leiomyomata with intranasal or subcutaneous leuprolide, a gonadotropin-releasing hormone agonist. Fertil Steril 1987; 48: 560–564.
31. Cline HE, Schenck JF, Hynynen K, Watkins RD, Souza SP, Jolesz FA. MR-guided focused ultrasound surgery. J Comput Assist Tomogr 1992; 16:956–965.
32. Jolesz FA, Hynynen K. Magnetic resonance image-guided focused ultrasound surgery. Cancer J 2002; 8(suppl 1):S100–S112.
33. Hynynen K, Freund WR, Cline HE, et al. A clinical, noninvasive, MR imaging-monitored ultrasound surgery method. Radiographics 1996; 16:185–195.
34. Hynynen K, Darkazanli A, Unger E, Schenck JF. MRI-guided noninvasive ultrasound surgery. Med Phys 1993; 20:107–115.
35. Lele PP. A simple method for production of trackless focal lesions with focused ultrasound: physical factors. J Physiol 1962; 160:494–512.
36. Tempany CM, Stewart EA, McDannold N, Quade BJ, Jolesz FA, Hynynen K. MR imaging-guided focused ultrasound surgery of uterine leiomyomas: a feasibility study. Radiology 2003; 226:897–905.

37. Leon-Villapalos J, Kaniorou-Larai M, Dziewulski P. Full thickness abdominal burn following magnetic resonance guided focused ultrasound therapy. Burns 2005; 31:1054–1055.
38. Stewart EA, Gedroyc W, Tempany C. Focused ultrasound treatment of uterine fibroids: safety and feasibility of a noninvasive thermoablative technique. Am J Obstet Gynecol 2003; 189: 48–54.
39. Stewart ERJ, Tempany CMC, Inbar Y, Regan L, Gastout B, Hesley G. Clinical outcomes of focused ultrasound surgery for the treatment of uterine fibroids. Fertil Steril 2006; 85:22–29.
40. Hindley J, Gedroyc WM, Regan L, et al. MRI guidance of focused ultrasound therapy of uterine fibroids: early results. AJR Am J Roentgenol 2004; 183.
41. McDannold N, Tempany CM, Fennessy FM, et al. Uterine leiomyomas: MR imaging-based thermometry and thermal dosimetry during focused ultrasound thermal ablation. Radiology 2006; 240:263–272.
42. Smart O, Hindley J, Regan L, Gedroyc WM. Gonadotrophin-releasing hormone and magnetic-resonance-guided ultrasound surgery for uterine leiomyomata. Obstet Gynecol 2006; 108:49–54.
43. Fennessy F, Tempany C, McDannold N, et al. MRI-guided focused ultrasound surgery of uterine leiomyomas; results of different treatment guideline protocols. Acad Radiol 2005; 12(9):1158–1166.

10

MRI-Guided Focused Ultrasound Treatment of the Brain

Kullervo H. Hynynen
*Department of Medical Biophysics, University of Toronto and Department
of Imaging Research, Sunnybrook Health Sciences Centre, Toronto,
Ontario, Canada*

Ferenc A. Jolesz
*Department of Radiology, Brigham and Women's Hospital and Harvard Medical
School, Boston, Massachusetts, U.S.A.*

INTRODUCTION

Magnetic resonance imaging (MRI)-guided noninvasive ultrasound treatment of the brain has substantial advantage over invasive neurosurgery in which unavoidable disruption of anatomic structures results in functional disturbances. Since the early 1940s, the potential of focused ultrasound to produce focal, targeted deep destruction within the brain has been researched extensively. Early on, animal and clinical results were encouraging, showing well-defined tissue coagulation at the focal zone (1–5). However, the experiments of Lynn et al. (6) demonstrated that ultrasound is strongly attenuated by bone, and the energy loss increases bone temperature, resulting in brain-tissue coagulation close to the skull. Another problem is related to the variable thickness and density of the skull bone, which results in distortion of the ultrasound wave front propagating through the bone. Because of these two problems, it is difficult to focus ultrasound beams through the cranium. As a result, most scientists accepted that therapeutic ultrasound could not be delivered through an intact skull.

After craniotomy, when the bony flap is removed through an acoustic window, the brain can be sonicated. There are a few clinical studies that have explored ultrasound surgery after craniotomy. In the first clinical trial, ultrasound was used to ablate small tissue volumes for the treatment of Parkinson's disease (7). The ultrasound beams were delivered into the brain through the intact dura with the aid of X ray–identified bony landmarks. After the sonications, the skull bone and the skin were replaced. Thus, the whole procedure was performed under sterile conditions. The lesion-inducing method was relatively successful in a series of over 100 patients (7). In later clinical trials, the skull bone was removed and the skin was placed over the bony defect. Then, after the wound healed, the sonications were performed through the intact skin. This allowed multiple sonication sessions, and there was no need for a sterile operating room setting. This method was also used in the ablative treatment of a small series of glioma patients demonstrating feasibility (8). In another study with glioma patients, focused ultrasound beams were used only to induce mild temperature elevations (5–7°C for 30 minutes, hyperthermia) to sensitize the tumor for subsequent radiation therapy (9). More recently, the feasibility of both ultrasound (10) and MRI (11)-guided thermal ablation of brain tissue and tumors has been demonstrated through a surgically created bony window. The requirement for the removal of a piece of the skull prior to the sonication makes the procedure that is potentially noninvasive quite invasive and expensive and adds to the risk of complications.

ULTRASOUND PROPAGATION THROUGH THE SKULL

Although ultrasound attenuation in the human skull is high (12), some ultrasound does propagate through the bone. This was shown by early clinical studies that used transskull transmission of ultrasound pulses for detecting the midline shift of the brain (13). This method was commercialized and clinically used to diagnose intracranial mass effect due to bleeding or tumors. The propagation of ultrasound through the skull for therapeutic purposes was demonstrated by Fry and Barger (12) who investigated the insertion losses caused by pieces of human skull. More recently, the density dependence of speed of sound (14,15) has been demonstrated. These measurements indicated that frequencies below 1 MHz may provide an adequate transmission through skull for tissue-destruction purposes. Later, computer simulations (16,17) and experiments with ex vivo human skulls (18) have demonstrated that the optimal frequency is dependent on the skull thick-ness but is, on average, approximately 700 kHz. The optimal frequency is a compromise between the absorption that decreases and the diameter of the focus (inversely proportional to the focusing gain) that increases with decreasing frequency. Simulation studies have shown that thermal coagulation of the deep brain structures should be possible with large arrays that propagate the ultrasound beam through most of the available and relatively large skull surface (16).

FOCUSING THROUGH HUMAN SKULL

Fry (19) produced thermal lesions in cat brains through a piece of human skull immersed in water. These studies showed that in favorable conditions, a low-frequency (around 0.5 MHz) beam could be focused through some parts of the skull and adequate energy for thermal ablation could be transmitted through the skull bone. However, the results showed that the location of the focus is shifted by several millimeters from its geometric focus. In addition, only very limited exposures were done without investigations of the location-to-location or skull-to-skull variations. Most importantly, the thermal exposure on the skull (in water at room temperature) was not investigated (19).

Later studies have shown that when large aperture applicators that are needed to overcome the skull-heating problem are used, the variable thickness of the skull bone causes enough wave propagation variations to completely destroy the focal spot (20). This distortion can be eliminated using phased arrays, as was first demonstrated by experiments investigating the feasibility of transskull diagnostic imaging of the brain (20,21). Later Thomas and Fink (22) used a linear imaging array to show that phase and amplitude compensation can be used to refocus the beam through the skull, based on hydrophone measurements inside of the skull. The first experiments using two-dimensional arrays, practical for therapy delivery, demonstrated the feasibility of focusing through the skull by using a hydrophone at the focus to determine the phase corrections (23). That study evaluated the beam area gain requirements for focal therapy delivery and concluded that thermal therapy was marginally feasible if surface cooling was utilized for most of the skull area. In addition, the study investigated the potential for cavitation-enhanced focal tissue destruction and demonstrated its advantage over the utilization of linear ultrasound absorption to increase the tissue temperature. The main advantage in using cavitation-enhanced tissue destruction is that the time average power can be reduced, due to either the bubble-enhanced energy absorption (24,25) or direct tissue damage of the tissue (23,26). Also, it has been shown that intravenously injected ultrasound contrast agents can reduce the required power and even the temperature threshold for tissue ablation (27). Furthermore, that study gave the first indication that through-skull focusing is possible with very low frequencies (250 kHz) without any distortion correction. This observation was studied in detail with simulations (28) and it was shown that the method may simplify the device requirements for cavitation base therapies that do not require high time average powers and sharp focusing [such as the disruption of the blood-brain barrier (BBB)].

The first demonstrations of through-skull focusing were done with small hydrophones (22,29), but the goal of noninvasive, model-based focusing was quickly achieved. The first experiments showed that it was possible to achieve good quality focusing by deriving the skull shape and thickness from magnetic resonance (MR) images and using them in an acoustic model, together with the average skull properties measured by Fry and Barger (12), to calculate the phase shifts required to compensate for the skull-induced distortions (30). However, this information was not adequate when multiple skulls were tested and it became clear that the speed of sound dependency on the skull density needs to be taken into account (14). The first reliable transskull focusing with multiple skulls was achieved by determining the skull density along the beam path from computed tomography scans and then modeling the beam propagation through the skull to determine the phase shifts required (31). Similar results were later reported by others (32). Further simulation studies have investigated optimal methods for intensity compensation (33) and multifrequency sonications, where each transducer element is operating at the frequency that provides the maximum power transmission through the local skull bone traversed by the beam (34).

DEVELOPMENT OF LARGE GAIN THERAPEUTIC ULTRASOUND ARRAYS

Based on simulation studies (16,17), the first large-scale array able to deliver adequate ultrasound gain and power for thermal or cavitation-based ablation of tissues was developed in-house at the focused ultrasound lab at the Brigham and Women's Hospital (18). The 64-element array was hemispherical in shape with a diameter of 30 cm. The next array had 500 elements (custom manufactured by Imasonic, Inc., France), and it was made MRI-compatible and tested by coagulating in vivo rabbit brains through ex vivo human skulls (35). The driving system of the array was developed by InSightec, Inc., Haifa, Israel.

The group, lead by Mathius Fink, developed an ultrasound-guided 300-element system and used it to ablate sheep brains with the aid of an implanted needle hydrophone (36). Recently the group reported successful ablation in monkey brain with noninvasive beam focusing. This series of experiments provided independent verification that transskull ultrasound surgery is feasible.

CLINICAL MRI-GUIDED FOCUSED ULTRASOUND SYSTEM

Based on the early experience, InSightec Inc., in collaboration with the scientists at Brigham and Women's Hospital, developed a clinical prototype device. The hemispherical array with 500 elements (later 512 elements) had similar dimensions and shape as the original 64-element array. The array was coupled to the patient's head with the aid of a rubber membrane that allowed water to be circulated between the head and the array. This water space allows coupling of the ultrasound beams to the head and provides skin cooling. The details of the system are described elsewhere (35). The system was tested first with monkeys (37), then with an initial series of three patients, and demonstrated feasibility. The plan is to continue this initial trial at the Brigham and Women's Hospital in Boston.

CLINICAL POTENTIAL

The potential of focused ultrasound to treat brain tumors was recognized in the early 1940s. Most direct neurosurgical approaches cause damage to cortical areas immediately surrounding a lesion, as well as to the white matter at the depths of the lesion and to brain tissue involved in the surgical trajectory. Therefore, a noninvasive tumor destruction method is particularly useful for tumors positioned deep in the brain. Focused ultrasound is an "ideal" surgical tool with maximal destructive effect within the target and with minimal permanent injury to surrounding normal brain tissue and, more importantly, no resultant neurological deficit. The early trials to treat brain tumors were aborted because of the inability to achieve good focusing through the intact skull bone and the heating of the skull bone during sonication. In addition, there was no imaging method to delineate the targeted brain tumors, and it was impossible to identify or monitor the focal spot by temperature-sensitive imaging.

With the introduction of MRI as a localizing, targeting, and monitoring method for thermal therapies, a novel mechanism for controlling energy deposition became available. By combining focused ultrasound with MRI-based guidance and control, it may be possible to achieve complete tumor ablation without any associated structural injury or functional deficit. Many MRI parameters (T_1, diffusion, proton resonance frequency) are sensitive to temperature changes, which makes MRI appropriate for providing image guidance or image-based control for thermal ablations.

The role of MRI during thermal ablations is twofold: to monitor temperature changes and to detect tissue coagulation. Both information types can be used to establish a closed-loop feedback mechanism. In the brain, physiologic effects such as perfusion or metabolic response to elevated temperature can also be used for monitoring the ablation. The integrity of the nontargeted surrounding tissue can also be monitored by imaging sequences, which are sensitive to biophysical, vascular, metabolic, or functional parameters. Both flow and tissue perfusion can affect the rate and extent of energy delivery and the size of the treated tissue volumes. Diffusion imaging, functional MRI, and MR spectroscopy all can be utilized to detect changes in adjacent normal brain parenchyma.

Since the original description of MRI monitoring and control of laser-tissue interactions (38), MRI-guided laser ablation of brain tumors has become a clinically tested and accepted minimally invasive treatment option. It is a relatively simple straight-forward method, which can be well adapted to the interventional MRI environment (39,40). Overall, early results suggest that interstitial laser therapy (ILT) is a safe and effective therapy method. During and after ILT, the induced edema is clinically tolerable and relatively large tumors can be treated without craniotomy.

The positive results and feasibility of MRI-guided ILT treatments are encouraging for any other thermal therapy methods including focused ultrasound. The most important comparison for MRI-guided focused ultrasound surgery (FUS), however, is not ILT but stereotactic radiotherapy and radiosurgery. Advantages of FUS over radiation therapy and radiosurgery are multiple. Primarily because of the lack of radiation toxicity, which is an unavoidable side effect of radiation therapy. Radiosurgery of lesions >4 cm is associated either with an unacceptable level of radiation toxicity or an ineffectual radiation dose. Radiosurgery also causes cranial nerve neuropathy. Radiation sensitivity of the optic nerve is especially problematic. Focused ultrasound has no radiotoxicity, the treatments are repeatable without limit, and online temperature monitoring can assure that critical structures, like nerves, will not be damaged by heat.

FUS will be particularly successful in the treatment of benign brain tumors like meningiomas. It will be extremely helpful for the ablation of meningiomas located in regions where complete surgical resection cannot be safely achieved (for example, meningiomas of the cavernous sinus or other skull base locations), It remain to be seen how FUS measure up to traditional neurosurgery for surgically accessible meningiomas in the areas of the convexity, falx, and parasagittal region, where today complete resection is the treatment of choice. In the case of acoustic neurinoma radiosurgery, the surgical paradigm has already been challenged. If MRI-guided FUS can achieve hearing preservation, it could be the method of choice over traditional or radiosurgery. Given the prevalence and the benign nature of the pituitary adenomas, a noninvasive treatment option can replace microsurgery. If the microadenoma can be targeted and coagulated without the heating of the hypothalamus, optic nerve and the cavernous sinus FUS can be an exceptionally simple and effective therapy solution.

As far as the primary malignant brain tumors are concerned, FUS will not radically change the field. FUS is a surgical method and as such it requires a well-defined target. Most of the gliomas are diffuse and infiltrative and cannot be fully excised or ablated. MRI-guided FUS may be valuable in treating low-grade thalamus gliomas. Their deep location makes them difficult to access and surgery is rarely feasible. FUS may also be applicable as a palliative solution for recurrent glioma when the regrowth is relatively well circumscribed. Brain metastases are the most common intracranial tumors in adults. The lesions are usually well circumscribed and marginated, therefore targeting is relatively straightforward. FUS can be the choice over surgery for single metastasis. Unfortunately, multiple metastatic lesions are seen in 60% to 75% of all cases and in patients who were initially thought to have a single brain metastasis by MRI. Although, FUS has a great potential to treat well-marginated single brain metastasis, in the case of multiplicity, it will not be applicable as the only treatment. However in combination with chemotherapy (especially after the FUS-induced opening of the BBB), FUS may be the future primary treatment of brain metastasis.

Beyond thermal coagulation of tissue, FUS has various other effects that can be therapeutically useful. The capability of occluding vessels could make FUS a therapeutic tool for the treatment of vascular malformation (41). Lesions can be induced using MRI targeting to treat movement disorders (Parkinson's) or epilepsy. FUS can be used not only as a functional neurosurgical method, but also as a way to achieve targeted drug delivery. FUS can be used to selectively open the BBB and introduced large molecular drugs into targeted brain regions (42–45). These large molecules can be used for chemotherapy or can act as functional neuropharmacological agents (46,47). MRI-guided focal opening of the BBB, combined with ultrasound technology that permits sonications through the intact skull, will open the way for new, noninvasive, targeted therapies.

REFERENCES

1. Fry FJ, Kossoff G, Eggleton RC, Dunn F. Threshold ultrasound dosages for structural changes in the mammalian brain. J Acoust Soc Am 1970; 48:1413–1417.

2. Fry WJ, Barnard JW, Fry FJ. Ultrasonically produced localized selective lesions in the central nervous system. Am J Phys Med 1955; 34:413–423.

3. Fry WJ, Mosberg W, Barnard JW, Fry FJ. Production of focal destructive lesions in the central nervous system with ultrasound. J Neurosurg 1954; 11:471–478.

4. Fry WJ, Barnar JW, Fry FJ, Krumins RF, Brennan JF, Fry WJ. Ultrasonic lesions in the mammalian central nervous system. Science 1955; 122:517–518.

5. Lele PP. Production of deep focal lesions by focused ultrasound—current status. Ultrasonics 1967; 5:105–122.

6. Lynn JG, Zwemer RL, Chick AJ, Miller AE. A new method for the generation and use of focused ultrasound in experimental biology. J Gen Physiol 1942; 26:179–193.

7. Fry WJ, Fry FJ. Fundamental neurological research and human neurosurgery using intense ultrasound. IRE Trans Med Electron 1960; ME-7:166–181.

8. Heimburger RF. Ultrasound augmentation of central nervous system tumor therapy. Indiana Med 1985; 78:469–476.

9. Guthkelch AN, Carter LP, Cassady JR, et al. Treatment of malignant brain tumors with focused ultrasound hyperthermia and radiation: results of a phase I trial. J Neuro Oncol 1991; 10:271–284.

10. Park J-W, Jung S, Junt TY, Lee M-C. Focused ultrasound surgery for the treatment of recurrent anaplastic astrocytoma: a preliminary report. In: Clement GT, McDannold NJ, Hynynen K, eds. Therapeutic Ultrasound: 5th International Symposium on Therapeutic Ultrasound. New York: American Institute of Physics, 2006:238–240.

11. Ram Z, Cohen ZR, Harnof S, et al. Magnetic resonance imaging-guided, high-intensity focused ultrasound for brain tumor therapy. Neurosurgery 2006; 59(5):949–955.

12. Fry FJ, Barger JE. Acoustical properties of the human skull. J Acoust Soc Am 1978; 63(5): 1576–1590.

13. White DN. Neurosonology pioneers. Ultrasound Med Biol 1988; 14(7):541–561.

14. Clement GT, Hynynen K. Correlation of ultrasound phase with physical skull properties. Ultrasound Med Biol 2002; 28(5):617–624.

15. Connor CW, Clement GT, Hynynen K. A unified model for the speed of sound in cranial bone based on genetic algorithm optimization. Phys Med Biol 2002; 47(22):3925–3944.

16. Sun J, Hynynen K. The potential of transskull ultrasound therapy and surgery using the maximum available skull surface area. J Acoust Soc Am 1998; 104(4):2519–2527.

17. Sun J, Hynynen K. Focusing of ultrasound through a human skull: a numerical study. J Acoust Soc Am 1998; 104(3):1705–1715.

18. Clement GT, Sun J, Giesecke T, Hynynen K. A hemisphere array for non-invasive ultrasound brain therapy and surgery. Phys Med Biol 2000; 45(12):3707–3719.

19. Fry FJ, Goss SA. Further studies of the transskull transmission of an intense focused ultrasound beam: lesion production at 500 KHz. Ultrasound Med Biol 1980; 6(1):33–38.

20. Smith SW, Phillips DJ, von Ramm OT, Thurstone FL. Some advances in acoustic imaging through skull. In: Hazzard DG, Litz ML, eds. Symposium on Biological Effects and Characterizations of Ultrasound Sources. Rockville, MA: HEW, FDA, 1977:37–52.

21. Smith SW, Trahey GE, von Ramm OT. Phased array ultrasound imaging through planar tissue layers. Ultrasound Med Biol 1986; 12(3):229–243.

22. Thomas JL, Fink MA. Ultrasonic beam focusing through tissue inhomogeneities with a time reversal mirror: application to transskull therapy. IEEE Trans Ultrason Ferroelectr Freq Contr 1996; 43(6):1122–1129.

23. Hynynen K, Jolesz FA. Demonstration of potential noninvasive ultrasound brain therapy through intact skull. Ultrasound Med Biol 1998; 24(2):275–283.

24. Hynynen K. The threshold for thermally significant cavitation in dog's thigh muscle in vivo. Ultrasound Med Biol 1991; 17:157–169.

25. Sokka SD, Hynynen KH. The feasibility of MRI-guided whole prostate ablation with a linear aperiodic intracavitary ultrasound phased array [In Process Citation]. Phys Med Biol 2000; 45(11):3373–3383.

26. Xu Z, Ludomirsky A, Eun LY, et al. Controlled ultrasound tissue erosion. IEEE Trans Ultrason Ferroelectr Freq Control 2004; 51(6):726–736.

27. McDannold NJ, Vykhodtseva NI, Hynynen K. Microbubble contrast agent with focused ultrasound to create brain lesions at low power levels: MR imaging and histologic study in rabbits. Radiology 2006; 241(1):95–106.

28. Yin X, Hynynen K. A numerical study of transcranial focused ultrasound beam propagation at low frequency. Phys Med Biol 2005; 50(8):1821–1836.

29. Clement GT, Hynynen K. Micro-receiver guided transcranial beam steering. IEEE Trans Ultrason Ferroelectr Freq Control 2002; 49(4):447–453.

30. Hynynen K, Sun J. Transskull ultrasound therapy: the feasibility of using image derived skull thickness information to correct the phase distortion. IEEE Trans Ultrason Ferroelectr Freq Contr 1998; 46(3):752–755.

31. Clement GT, Hynynen K. A non-invasive method for focusing ultrasound through the human skull. Phys Med Biol 2002; 47(8):1219–1236.

32. Aubry JF, Tanter M, Pernot M, Thomas JL, Fink M. Experimental demonstration of noninvasive transskull adaptive focusing based on prior computed tomography scans. J Acoust Soc Am 2003; 113(1):84–93.

33. White J, Clement GT, Hynynen K. Transcranial ultrasound focus reconstruction with phase and amplitude correction. IEEE Trans Ultrason Ferroelectr Freq Control 2005; 52(9):1518–1522.

34. White PJ, Clement GT, Hynynen K. Local frequency dependence in transcranial ultrasound transmission. Phys Med Biol 2006; 51(9):2293–2305.

35. Hynynen K, Clement GT, et al. 500-element ultrasound phased array system for noninvasive focal surgery of the brain: a preliminary rabbit study with ex vivo human skulls. Magn Reson Med 2004; 52(1):100–107.

36. Pernot M, Aubry JF, Tanter M, Boch AL, Kujas M, Fink M. Adaptive focusing for ultrasonic transcranial brain therapy: first in vivo investigation on 22 sheep. AIP Conf Proc 2005; 754(1):174–177.

37. Hynynen K, McDannold N, Clement G, et al. Pre-clinical testing of a phased array ultrasound system for MRI-guided noninvasive surgery of the brain-A primate study. Eur J Radiol 2006; 59(2):149–156.

38. Jolesz FA, Bleier AR, Jakab P, Ruenzel PW, Huttl K, Jako GJ. MR imaging of laser tissue interactions. Radiology 1988; 168:249–253.

39. Kettenbach J, Silverman SG, Hata N, et al. Monitoring and visualization techniques for MR-guided laser ablations in an open MR system. J Magn Reson Imag 1998; 8(4):933–943.

40. Schwarzmaier HJ, Eickmeyer F, von Tempelhoff W, et al. MR-guided laser-induced interstitial thermotherapy of recurrent glioblastoma multiforme: preliminary results in 16 patients. Eur J Radiol 2006; 59(2):208–215.

41. Hynynen K, Colucci V, Chung A, Jolesz FA. Noninvasive artery occlusion using MRI guided focused ultrasound. Ultrasound Med Biol 1996; 22(8):1071–1077.

42. Hynynen K, McDannold N, Vykhodtseva N, Jolesz FA. Noninvasive MR imaging-guided focal opening of the blood-brain barrier in rabbits. Radiology 2001; 220(3):640–646.

43. Hynynen K, McDannold N, Sheikov NA, Jolesz FA, Vykhodtseva N. Local and reversible blood-brain barrier disruption by noninvasive focused ultrasound at frequencies suitable for trans-skull sonications. NeuroImage 2005; 24(1):12–20.

44. Hynynen K, McDannold N, Vykhodtseva N, et al. Focal disruption of the blood-brain barrier due to 260-kHz ultrasound bursts: a method for molecular imaging and targeted drug delivery. J Neurosurg 2006; 105(3):445–454.

45. McDannold N, Vykhodtseva N, Hynynen K. Targeted disruption of the blood-brain barrier with focused ultrasound: association with cavitation activity. Phys Med Biol 2006; 51(4): 793–807.

46. Kinoshita M, McDannold N, Jolesz FA, Hynynen K. Noninvasive localized delivery of Herceptin to the mouse brain by MRI-guided focused ultrasound-induced blood-brain barrier disruption. Proc Natl Acad Sci USA 2006; 103(31):11719–11723.

47. Kinoshita M, McDannold N, Jolesz FA, Hynynen K. Targeted delivery of antibodies through the blood-brain barrier by MRI-guided focused ultrasound. Biochem Biophys Res Commun 2006; 340(4):1085–1090.

11

New Clinical Applications of Magnetic Resonance–Guided Focused Ultrasound

Wladyslaw M.W. Gedroyc
St. Mary's Hospital, Imperial College London, London, U.K.

INTRODUCTION

The ability to use magnetic resonance (MR) for the accurate targeting of delivery of high-intensity focused ultrasound, together with the easy depiction of tissue thermals results, means that focused ultrasound surgery (FUS) can potentially be used in a wide variety of applications in the body. Different inherent tissue responses to heating and variable heating responses due to alterations in vascularity can be easily appreciated using online thermal mapping carried out with MR in response to focused ultrasound heating. As a result, it is relatively easy to take steps to overcome different tissue responses either between individuals or within an individual so that a consistent and accurately placed lesion can be produced with each sonication. Multiple alterations in the parameters of the ultrasound deposition can be carried out such as power, spot site, cooling durations, frequency of transducer, etc. to interact with tissue variations and keep the response visualized in the tissues constant. Similarly, areas of subtle tissue abnormality that may not be visualized on other modalities, such as ultrasound or computed tomography, are frequently easily appreciated on MR and therefore complex targeting of such abnormalities can be quite readily achieved using online MR imaging.

These qualities allow MRIgFUS to potentially be used as a destructive noninvasive tool in many different body areas with great accuracy of delivery and substantial safety in its application since adjacent organs and the path of the ultrasound beam are particularly well visualized with MR, so that possible involvement of tissues that could be inadvertently damaged can be appreciated very rapidly at an early stage and avoided (1).

Despite this potential, many individual problems in the widespread application of MRIgFUS remain. Motion, predominately due to respiration, is problematic because it is often inconsistent and the movement of the upper abdominal organs in response to respiration for instance is usually not entirely consistent making exact targeting difficult. Ribs overlying the path of the focused ultrasound would disrupt the beam, preventing accurate application of destructive energy and marked vascularity of a target in the tissue may prevent an easy visualizable tissue response.

TREATING LARGE FIBROIDS

The largest experience to date in terms of patient numbers with MRIgFUS has been in the treatment of uterine fibroids (2). Initial studies were confined to smaller fibroids and these have shown highly effective symptom relief. The problem of how to treat much larger fibroids, however, remains. Conventional sonications require a long procedure time to cover a large fibroid, which may be anywhere between 10 and 20 cm in diameter. Frequently the time required to cover this whole area is inappropriate for patients since they would have to be on the machine for probably several sessions lasting more than four hours each, and, similarly, the time it takes out of the MR scanning schedule may also be highly problematic. In an attempt to overcome this problem, our group has developed a way of potentiating the results of focused ultrasound within these large fibroids by the pretreatment of uterine fibroids with gonadotrophin-releasing hormone (GNRH) agonists. This regulatory neuropeptide causes a hypoestrogenic state by interfering with the hypothalamic-pituitary-ovarian axis. Fibroids, which are highly estrogen dependant, will shrink when GNRH agonists are given over a period of time. This effect is well known in gynecological surgery where GNRH agonists are frequently used as a pretreatment in patients who are going to have myomectomies. Surgeons utilize this effect to decrease the vascularity of the fibroids and make the operation much less risky by lowering blood loss to produce a much more avascular field. We have found that by utilizing GNRH agonists given intramuscularly once a month for three months prior to focused ultrasound treatment, we can reduce the size of the target fibroid uterus by approximately 30% to 40%, and this fibroid can then be readily treated (2) with focused ultrasound at the end of this time, when it is in a much smaller state (Fig. 1).

In addition, at this time, the vascularity has been reduced, and the response to each individual sonication is much greater (3). On average, there is a 50% larger response in terms of tissue destruction per unit joule applied after GNRH pretreatment. In a series of consecutive patients with fibroids greater than 10 cm, who all had three months of GNRH pretreatment, we found that our symptomatic responses were completely comparable to those of a group of patients who had fibroids smaller than 10 cm. Overall, our results showed that 83% of patients treated in this way had a greater than 10-point improvement in symptom severity scores [considered to be highly significant (see Chapter 8)] when treatment was applied in this manner, which is similar to the results of the group of patients with fibroids that were all smaller than 10 cm. In addition, the median symptomatic responses showed a highly significant fall in these large fibroids at three and six months, and this was prolonged to 12 months posttreatment. All of these patients had procedure times broadly similar to those of patients with the much smaller fibroids. The results of this work with GNRH is that we have developed a way of potentiating the effect of heat within fibroids by a simple medical pretreatment, which we believe alters the vascularity of the fibroids and, as a result, influences the thermal response of this tissue to focused ultrasound. This technique therefore allows us to much more easily treat the larger fibroids found in many women, which may be symptomatic and difficult to control conservatively or with other more invasive therapies. The elegance of this approach has highlighted the potential for finding similar methods for the treatment of other solid viscera with this paradigm. If we can find hormonal or other potentiators, which influence vascularity in tissue for organs such as liver, kidney, prostate, etc., we may be able to potentiate the treatment of such abnormalities in these organs in a totally noninvasive fashion.

LIVER MR-GUIDED FOCUSED ULTRASOUND

There is very extensive work available in the field of liver thermal ablation indicating great promise in destroying local liver disease (4). Multiple modalities of heat application have been used and all achieved broadly promising outcomes. The largest experience in

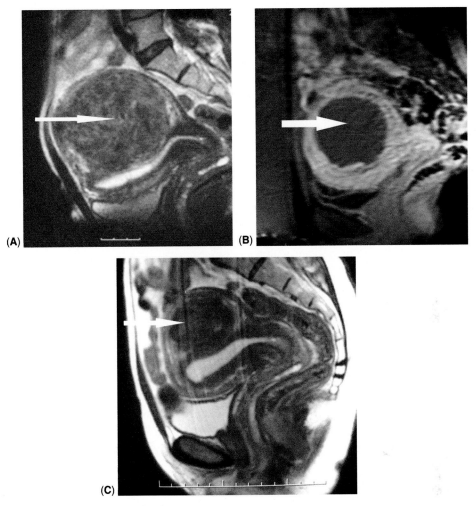

Figure 1 (**A**) Patient with 10-cm diameter posterior-wall fibroid (*arrow*) pre-GNRH treatment. (**B**) Same patient post-GNRH treatment and postfocused ultrasound. Note that the overall size of the posterior-wall fibroid has shrunk very substantially and that postfocused ultrasound, almost the entirety of the fibroid has been treated with a large nonperfused area (*arrow*) induced in the previously large fibroid when it was in a smaller state. (**C**) Same patient as above three months following FUS and GNRH treatment. At this stage, the patient's symptomatology is much improved, and the overall size of the previously large fibroid is now a maximum of 5 cm diameter, with a very substantial overall reduction in volume. *Abbreviations*: FUS, focused ultrasound surgery; GNRH, gonadotrophin-releasing hormone.

any one center has been from Vogl et al. (5) with more than 1500 patients treated with approximately 35% to 40% five-year survival in patients who are otherwise unsuitable for surgery after thermal ablation and up to a 56% five-year survival in groups of patients who would otherwise be suitable for surgery but simply refused it. The majority of this series is concerned with treatment of metastatic disease but similar, very promising results have been achieved with hepatocellular carcinomas from a variety of groups, predominately using radiofrequency ablations (6).

Percutaneous radiofrequency, microwave, laser ablation, and cryotherapy have all been utilized to treat livers masses successfully. Several papers have also emerged using ultrasound guidance for high-intensity focused ultrasound procedures used to treat liver lesions (7,8), and these papers also suggest that this type of application is extremely promising. It is clear from all of this body of work that excellent results may be achieved in the liver relatively easily, without substantial complications, and that excellent improvements in patient survival and symptomatology may be achieved with this type of approach, in contradistinction to the much larger, more invasive surgeries that are required to achieve this type of response in this field. Liver metastases and increasingly hepatocellular carcinomas, in conjunction with the worldwide pandemic of hepatitis c, are now important and common causes of death, which otherwise have relatively poor treatments available for them, ranging from the quite toxic in terms of chemotherapy to the very invasive with surgery. The potential therefore of minimally invasive work in this field is highly desirable and could help a great many patients. Nevertheless conventional minimally invasive procedures still require a significant invasion with large bore needles passing though the liver, which when there is underlying liver disease as is usually the case with hepatocellular carcinoma can be problematic in terms of bleeding complications, etc. Many of the patients with liver disease have associated coagulation defects, which may or may not be easily treatable and while minimally invasive procedures are a substantial improvement in terms of morbidity in comparison to surgery, they still have their problems. The potential of focused ultrasound is the ability to achieve a completely noninvasive method of treating such local abnormalities requiring any needles to pass through the liver. Clearly this potential must be investigated as the advantages this could bring to the treatment of these patients are immense. It would be very feasible to treat patients before surgery or transplantation without any influence on the surgery and it would be very easy to treat a much larger group of patients with a wide range of tumors if this technology could be applied to all liver lesions.

Currently our application of MRIgFUS cannot reach lesions behind ribs or lung and is confined at the moment to treatment of low liver lesions, which peak out from below the rib line or to left lobe lesions, which can be accessed with conventional application through the epigastrium. It is anticipated that improvements in the transducer technology available will allow access to lesions between ribs in the relatively near future allowing us to treat many more patients but at the moment these are the simple limitations.

Respiratory movement is also currently a problem due to the repeated motion of the liver, which is often inconsistent so that the variability of the liver position may be very problematic for any procedure. To recapture control of the three-dimensional space around the target liver lesion, we perform our liver cases at the moment under general anesthetic. We use MR-compatible ventilators, which are linked to and under the control of the FUS machine. This means that at the time of sonication, the respiratory excursion of the patient is controlled by the ventilator via the FUS machine so that it is always at the same point. This means that the transducer and the target are in constant relationship to one another at the time of the sonication. As a result, we can place lesions with great confidence in a particular target at the exact desired site and subsequent lesions can be placed with confidence in relation to these initial lesions to produce an overlapping confluent area of destruction in the target. Using general anesthesia in this context overcomes the problems of respiratory motion of the liver, although it certainly does nothing for the complexity and duration or the potential invasiveness of the whole process. It is hoped that in the future, we may be able to carry out procedures that can lock onto lesions by scanning so quickly that they may be followed throughout the phases of respiration, no longer requiring general anesthesia. Until these problems are resolved with improvements in technology, general anesthesia allows an achievable, safe, and accurate procedure to be carried out. Despite the anesthesia, the patient can still walk out following the procedure once they have recovered from the general anethesia (GA). We are carrying out pilot work in this area using the above technology. To date we have treated only two patients with this type of approach. The first patient was a purely palliative case where we treated a large tumor, part of which presented below the rib line, that we could reach with focused ultrasound, and we achieved a reasonable palliation with approximately 20% destruction of this tumor. Subsequently, we have successfully and easily treated a 2 cm hepatocellular carcinoma in the left lobe of the patient, which was easily accessible via the epigastrium (Fig. 2).

In both cases, we found that lesions could be readily produced in the targeted liver with no complications and that the general anesthesia system for the control of respiration worked highly effectively without any danger to the patient; accurate, confluent lesions could be placed to encompass the whole lesion plus margins of at least 0.5 cm or more, if required, on all sides. This procedure in the second case took 120 minutes. Interestingly, the patient had virtually no significant pain postprocedure and returned to normal activities the next day.

We are currently trying to recruit more patients with suitable accessible lesions as described above so that we can gain further experience with this type of approach.

Further technological improvements in the speed and targeting of the scanning along with transducer developments should allow us to be able to treat many more patients, hopefully without the use of general anesthesia, within 18 months as technology matures.

KIDNEY

Renal tumors are relatively slow-growing and very frequently asymptomatic for the majority of their time course. They are found increasingly common at quite early stages due to the widespread use of cross-sectional imaging. This has resulted in more patients seeking minimally invasive treatments such as thermal ablations rather than the larger surgical procedures, which are available. Multiple papers are now available describing the use of radiofrequency cryotherapy or laser approaches for the destruction of renal masses using minimally invasive procedures, which show very good early promise when the whole mass of the tumor can be treated (9,10). Long-term results are not yet available, but this is due to the relatively recent evolution of these processes. Many of the same problems that are encountered in MRIgFUS of the liver apply equally to renal procedures. The kidney is an even more mobile organ than the liver and has much greater respiratory excursion than the liver, so control of this motion is absolutely crucial in the undertaking of such a process. We believe that similar procedures to those described in the liver however should be able to treat renal masses particularly the lower pole, which are visible below the liver and we are in the process of recruiting patients to this area but we believe that focused ultrasound should provide an excellent totally noninvasive method for the treatment of appropriate renal tumors in the near future.

MR-GUIDED FOCUSED ULTRASOUND OF BONE

Many patients with bony metastatic deposits have continuing disabling pain despite the use of other conventional therapies such as radiotherapy, chemotherapy, hormonal manipulation, and analgesics. Further palliative therapeutic options for this group of patients are therefore highly desirable to improve the way we treat these patients. The percutaneous delivery of thermal ablative energy directly into skeletal metastases is evolving as a very effective new modality in the palliation of painful deposits. The

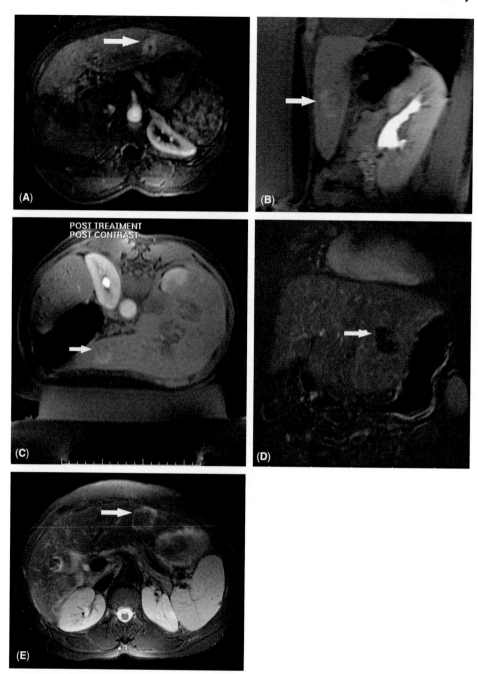

Figure 2 (**A**) A 35-year-old patient with hepatitis C. This is a postcontrast dynamic arterial phase fat saturated echo image. Note the area of arterial blush in the left lobe in the midline, which is a new lesion representing a hepatocellular carcinoma. This patient has previously undergone laser thermal ablation of a right lobe lesion. (**B**) Same patient as above post–focused ultrasound therapy in the sagittal planes. Image obtained still on the focused ultrasound table. Note area of hyperintensity in the left lobe (*arrow*), which represents hemoglobin degradation encompassing the previously noted arterially hyperintense lesion. Contrast in pelvicalyceal system posteriorly is from previous injection of gadolinium. (**C**) Axial view post-focused ultrasound therapy while still on the focused ultrasound table. (*Caption continues on page 143*)

majority of the studies in this area have been carried out using radiofrequency electrodes as the source of heat, although studies using cryotherapy and laser fibers are also in the literature with similar promising overall results (11,12).

Callstrom et al. (11) have reported on a study of 62 patients who had severe pain secondary to bony secondaries. All their patients were treated with percutaneous radio-frequency ablation techniques either with conscious sedation or under general anesthesia. Ninety-five percent of their patients experienced a significant drop in pain scores, which continued to improve over 24 weeks of follow-up. This improvement was associated with a very significant fall in the opiate usage in this group. These types of studies have indicated that there is substantial gain to be achieved in the palliation of difficult metastases with this type of simple approach—using heat sources to destroy areas of tumor tissue within bone. An interesting aspect to emerge from this study is that the tumor interface with normal bone should always be treated for best pain relief, and if the thermal ablation is limited to the center of the tumor, very little gain is achieved in terms of pain improvement.

Bone absorbs ultrasound very avidly, which explains why it disrupts ultrasound beams, making treatment of lesions obscured by bones so problematic as described above. However, this ability of bone can be utilized in thermal ablation treatments by targeting the abnormal areas with focused ultrasound and depositing energy into these areas in order to raise the temperatures sufficiently to cause tissue destruction. This process suggests that we may be able to utilize focused ultrasound as a modality to treat bone lesions palliatively in the first instance in a fashion similar to the type of work that has been so successfully pioneered with percutaneous placement of radiofrequency probes. So far, only a few cases have been attempted on painful deposits; the initial results are promising with relatively quick improvements in pain scores in most patients without the need to undergo any form of interventional procedure. MR is simply used to target the focused ultrasound deposition so a very effective, easy, and accurate way of depositing the heat is achieved. Diagnostic ultrasound cannot be used for this type of targeting in bones for the above mentioned reason that ultrasound is absorbed by bones, preventing visualization.

This particular application is in a very early stage of development with several investigators slowly recruiting patients. The potential for this type of approach is large and there is clearly a need for a further therapy modality in this field to improve our overall treatment of painful metastases, which are refractory to simple treatments. It is hoped that focused ultrasound guided with MR may be able to fulfill this particular role.

NEW POTENTIAL AREAS OF TREATMENT

MR-guided focused ultrasound provides us with a controllable tissue destructive modality, which works on a simple physical principle common to all living tissue. This is the coagulation of cellular proteins by raising the temperature so they become inactive

---

(*Caption continued from page 142*) Area of hyperintensity (*arrow*) represents hemoglobin degradation with no significant enhancement post-i.v. contrast. (**D**) Image obtained immediately post–focused ultrasound therapy while still on the table post–contrast administration. This is a subtraction image indicating that there is an area of decreased perfusion (*arrow*), which represents the treated lesion post–focused ultrasound. (**E**) Same patient as above but one month later. This is a T_2-weighted image with no contrast. Note the area of hyperintensity in a ring around the previously treated portion, representing hemoglobin degradation products (*arrow*); no activity was noted in this lesion at this time. *Abbreviation*: i.v., intravenous.

and the cells die. It is not dependant on the responsiveness of individual histologies or cell receptors, etc. but purely depends on whether enough power can be deposited at the target site. Having said this, multiple other physical factors of course determine whether enough power can be deposited, and tissue vascularity and obscuration by overlying structures are highly important factors to the success of such individual procedure.

By destroying tissue, focused ultrasound can therefore potentially be used to treat a great variety of soft-tissue abnormalities—if a suitable way of applying it to the target tissue can be achieved, which overcomes the problems of suitable acoustic windows and patient motion (Fig. 3).

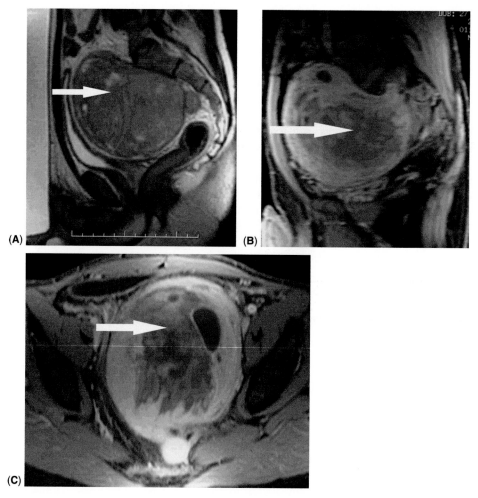

Figure 3 (**A**) Sagittal T_2-weighted images of the pelvis showing a large mass in the center of the pelvis superficially resembling a uterine fibroid (*arrow*). This, however, is a male patient, and this was due to a large pelvic schwannoma. Surgery was considered highly problematic in this young patient and focused ultrasound was carried out to try to debulk the area. (**B**) The same projection as in (**A**) but in a postcontrast fat-saturated T_1-weighted gradient-echo image showing enhancement of the periphery of the mass with no perfusion in the center post—focused ultrasound indicating the areas of destruction here (*arrows*). (**C**) Similar sequence to (**B**) but in the axial plane again showing areas of noncontrast enhancement indicating destroyed portions of the patient's schwannoma post–focused ultrasound (*arrow*).

The more subtle use of focused ultrasound therapy in drug and gene probe delivery systems is not considered in this chapter.

Slow-flow arterial venous malformations are often extremely problematic and long-lasting and cause recurrent problems for patients. Surgery is frequently disfiguring and unsuccessful and embolization procedures have variable success. We have tried to treat some of these slow-flow arteriovenous malformation's (AVM), particularly within the pelvis, with focused ultrasound, with initially very limited success. We anticipate that improvements in technology will allow much greater power deposition to be achieved within individual slow-flow AVMs, which should be able to overcome some of the problems. Much of the vascular flow of these lesions, which is very slow, is responsible for the difficulty with which heat can be deposited within them, but if focused ultrasound could be utilized successfully to treat such abnormalities, it could be a very successful and useful way of taking the treatment of this type of lesion forward.

Other soft-tissue masses, either primary or residual/recurrent malignancies after other forms of therapy, such as surgery and radiotherapy, should also be potentially amenable to focused ultrasound treatment in many instances. The high tissue specificity of MR allows excellent targeting of such areas and this combination of MR guidance and focused ultrasound may provide an excellent adjuvant form of therapy in this and other similar soft-tissue abnormalities. The minimization of treatment-associated morbidity and disfigurement from more radical surgery particularly in recurrent disease under these circumstances would be of great benefit to these patients.

REFERENCES

1. Hindley J, Gedroyc WM, Regan L, et al. MR guidance of focused ultrasound therapy of uterine fibroids: early results. Am J Roentgenol 2004; 183(6):1713–1719.
2. Stuart EA, Gedroyc WM, Temponey CM, et al. Focused ultrasound of uterine fibroid tumours: safety and feasibility of a non-invasive thermo ablative technique. Am J Obstet Gynaecol 2003; 189(1):48–54.
3. Smart O, Regan L, Gedroyc WM. Potentiation of size of uterine fibroid thermal ablation with GNRH pre-treatment. Eur J Radiol 2006; 59(2):163–167.
4. Mack MG, Straub R, Eichler K, et al. Breast cancer metastases in the liver, colon, laser induced interstitial thermo therapy—local tumour control rate and survival data. Radiology 2004; 233(2):400–409.
5. Vogl T, Straub R, Eichler K, et al. Colorectal carcinoma metastases in the liver: laser induced interstitial thermo therapy—local tumour control rate and survival data. Radiology 2004; 230(2):450–458.
6. Livraghi T, Meloni F, Morabito A, et al. Multi modal image guided tailored therapy of early and intermediate hepatocellular carcinoma: long term survival in the experience of a single radiological referral centre. Liver Transbl 2004; 10(2 suppl 1):S98–S106.
7. Wu F, Wang Z, Chen W, et al. Extra corporeal high intensity focused ultrasound ablation in the treatment of patients with large hepatocellular carcinoma. Ann Surgical Oncol 2004; 11 (12):1061–1068.
8. Kennedy J, Wou F, ter Haar G, et al. High intensity focused ultrasound for the treatment of liver tumours. Ultrasonics 2004; 42:931–935.
9. Weld K, Landman J. Comparison of cryoablation, radio frequency ablation and high intensity focused ultrasound for treating small renal tumours. Brit J Urol Int 2005; 96: 1224–1229.
10. Jervis D, Arellano R, Mueller P, et al. Percutaneous ablation of kidney tumours in non surgical candidates. Oncology 2005; 19(11 suppl 4):6–11.

11. Callstrom M, Charboneau J, Goetz M, et al. Image guided ablation of painful metastatic bone tumours: a new and effective approach to a difficult problem. Skeletal Radiol 2006; 35: 1–15.
12. Groenemeyer D, Schrip S, Gevargez A. Image guided percutaneous thermal ablation of bone tumours. Acad Radiol 2002; 9:467–477.

12
Targeted Drug Delivery

Manabu Kinoshita
Department of Radiology, Brigham and Women's Hospital and Harvard Medical School, Boston, Massachusetts, U.S.A.

INTRODUCTION

With the advancement of acoustic technology, ultrasound has become not only a diagnostic but also a therapeutic tool. Among many therapeutic applications of ultrasound, here I would like to focus on its capability for drug delivery both in vivo and in vitro. I will also discuss on the methods and issues for enhancing ultrasound therapeutic capability by using sonosensitizers that accumulate at tumor tissues.

DRUG DELIVERY BY ULTRASOUND IN VITRO

Background of Sonoporation In Vitro

It has been known that ultrasound has the capability of delivering exogenous substances into cells through the cell membrane. The report from Saad and Hahn is one of the early works that has shown that ultrasound can enhance the cell membrane permeability (1). Studies from Fechheimer et al. showed that a large molecule such as a plasmid DNA can be introduced into cells using ultrasound (2). Although ultrasound-induced drug/gene delivery into cells was an interesting and appealing technique, it was not able to become a standard drug/gene delivery method compared to electroporation and lipofection. The low efficiency was one of the main issues that had to be solved to make this method practical.

Recently, however, with the appearance of microbubble-based ultrasound contrast agents, drug/gene delivery into cells by ultrasound is starting to be extensively investigated. This phenomenon is named "sonoporation," which is an analogy of the word "electroporation." Both researches on improving the sonoporation efficiency and also on the mechanism behind it are the most important in this field.

The most widely accepted model and explanation for sonoporation is that the collapse of the microbubble caused by ultrasound produces a transient hole in the cell membrane making exogenous substances enter the cell. Tachibana et al. showed pores created on cell membranes by ultrasound through an electron microscopic examination (3). Moreover, Deng et al. showed physiological evidence that ultrasound with microbubble is triggering transient cell membrane porosity by directly measuring the transmembrane current during ultrasound exposure in *Xenopus oocyte*. They were able to show that ultrasound exposure with microbubble ultrasound contrast agent Optison was indeed creating membrane pores and that this event was reversible in a second order (4). The importance of microbubbles in sonoporation was also evaluated from a different perspective. Guzman et al. evaluated the relationship between the cell-to-bubble ratio and the bioeffects caused by ultrasound. According to their study, it was concluded that cells must have a proper distance to the microbubbles to achieve sonoporation. Cells too close to bubbles will be destroyed by the collapse (blast) of the bubbles caused by ultrasound, while cells located too far away from the bubbles will receive no effect (Fig. 1) (5). They also evaluated whether the molecular size of the exogenous substance will affect the transportation efficiency of those molecules into the cells by sonoporation and showed that the molecular size of the substance does not contribute to the sonoporation and delivery efficiency at least up to 464 kDa (6). This result is one strong evidence that supports the idea that ultrasound-induced drug/gene delivery is caused by transient membrane porosity. If exogenous substances are introduced into cells through these pores, it is reasonable that the size of the substance will not affect the efficiency of delivery up to the size of the pores themselves. Zarnitsyn and Prausnitz have also shown that when cells are sonoporated with plasmid DNAs, gene expression efficiency is lower than the sonoporation efficiency (7). They showed that a substantial amount of plasmid DNA must be delivered into cells to achieve gene expression, and that, as the amount of plasmid DNA delivered into cells differ in each sonoporated cell, only those cells that up took enough amount of plasmid DNA can achieve gene expression.

The major problem of the sonoporation technique in vitro is its low efficiency. Although the efficiency has improved with the use of ultrasound contrast agent, the overall outcome of sonoporation is still inferior to those by electroporation and lipofection. Another problem is its high toxicity. The blast of microbubbles causes destruction of cells, which can be named cell lysis. For example, according to the experiments that we have performed, more than 50% of the whole cell population is destroyed, while only less than 10% of the cells can achieve sonoporation even at the most suitable condition (8). These numbers are in a comparative range with those reported by others (5–7), again addressing the necessity to improve the total sonoporation efficiency. There are reports suggesting that the sequence of ultrasound exposure, such as duty cycle and pulse repetition frequency, can be an important factor for improving sonoporation efficiency. The experimental settings, however, differ from one report to another and the most important factor is not yet determined.

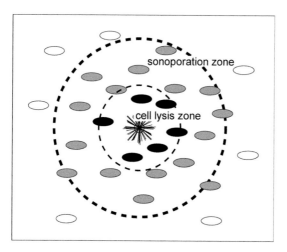

Figure 1 A theoretical model of sonoporation. Cells located too far from the collapse of the microbubbles will not receive any biological effect from the collapsing bubbles. On the other hand, cells located too close will be destroyed and lysed. Cells located between the two ranges will be sonoporated.

Methods to Evaluate Sonoporation

The easiest and most reliable method to evaluate sonoporation of cells is to sonicate cells with a molecule named calcein. Calcein (fluorescein-methylene-iminodiacetic acid) is a fluorescent indicator for calcium with a molecular weight of 622 Da. Once calcein is introduced into cells, it emits green fluorescence excited by blue light, which can be detected by a fluorescent microscope or a flow cytometer. Nonviable cells can be simultaneously stained with propidium iodide, which is a red fluorescent die that stains the nucleus of nonviable cells. Simultaneous detection of these two dies makes it possible to evaluate whether the cells are sonoporated, nonviable, or viable without being sonoporated. Evaluation can be done by using either microscopes or flow cytometers. When using flow cytometers, cell viability can also be evaluated by measuring the size and complexity of the cells using forward and side scatter measurements, as viable cells tend to show larger values of size and complexity. Moreover, flow cytometers allow data collection with a large number of events in a shorter time. The intracellular localization of the fluorescence can be confirmed by confocal laser scanning microscopic examination. The correlation between the molecular size of the exogenous substance and sonoporation efficiency can be investigated by using different fluorescence with various molecular sizes (5,6,8,9).

Materials Tested for Sonoporation In Vitro

Several materials have been tested for intracellular delivery of exogenous substances using sonoporation. As mentioned in section entitled Methods to Evaluate Sonoporation, fluorescent substances, such as calcein (662 kDa), fluorescein isothiocyanate (FITC) conjugated bovine serum albumin (BSA) (66 kDa), 42 kDa-dextran conjugated FITC, and 464 kDa-dextran conjugated FITC, have been used for sonoporation efficacy measurements (5,6). In some experiments, plasmid DNA labeled with YOYO-1™, a fluorescence label, was used to evaluated the sonoporation efficiency with plasmid DNA itself (7).

Other materials tested for investigating the feasibility of using sonoporation as a drug delivery method are plasmid DNAs, peptides, and short interfering RNA (siRNA). For plasmids, different kinds of genes have been tried out. As most of the studies reported have focused on demonstrating gene expression using sonoporation, reporter genes such as green fluorescent protein (GFP), luciferase, and β-galactosidase were mostly used. In the case of peptides, the cell-killing Bak BH3 peptide was tested to enhance cell killing by sonoporation (9). And finally, sonoporating cells with siRNA, a short double-strand RNA that knocks down gene expression, have been shown to be feasible in suppressing target gene expression by using a GFP-targeting siRNA with a GFP-expressing cell line (8).

All of the materials tested so far have proven that sonoporation can be used for intracellular delivery of the molecules. The efficiency, however, has still not caught up with other methods such as electroporation and lipofection, and sonoporation is not yet a standard method for intracellular drug/gene delivery in vitro in the basic biological field.

DRUG DELIVERY BY ULTRASOUND IN VIVO

In this section, two applications of ultrasound as a method for drug delivery will be discussed. The first will be delivering drug/gene intracellularly at the target organ by ultrasound (sonoporation) in vivo. The second will be enhancing the delivery of drugs at target tissues by ultrasound.

The Rational of Using Sonoporation In Vivo

As mentioned in the above in vitro section, the capability of sonoporation for intracellular drug/gene delivery has also been tested in vivo. The most widely used method of in vivo gene delivery is the virus method. The virus method achieves high transfection efficiency and does not require any special devices for transfection. This feature has a great advantage over other gene delivery methods. The safety, however, of using viruses for gene delivery has not been established and this has been a major drawback (10). Electroporation is another conventional but hopeful technique. It enables site-specific transfection of naked plasmid DNAs without using viruses for vector. The necessity of inserting electrodes in the tissue, however, brings up the problem of using this technique in the real clinical setting (11). This method might be useful in transfecting genes into solid organs. It would entail many difficulties, however, to apply this technique to transfect gene into vascular tissues, such as blood vessels.

Ultrasound-induced sonoporation has attracted great attention for gene transfer into the vasculature in vivo, as there is no need to either insert any device into tissue or to use hazardous materials to achieve gene transfection to the target tissue. Theoretically, once the plasmid DNAs and microbubbles are introduced into the vascular system, the exposure of ultrasound to the target vasculature will trigger sonoporation only around the target area and the DNAs will be up taken by the surrounding endothelial cells. Several studies have already shown success in controlling and inhibiting hyperplasia of the endothelial cell in the arterial system in arterial-restenosis models. In these studies, not only plasmid DNAs but also decoy oligonucleotides have been used (12–14) as therapeutic substances. There are also reports suggesting that gene therapy using sonoporation can recover cardiac function or control fibrosis in the kidney (15,16). Most of the studies, however, have focused only on demonstrating gene expression or intracellular drug delivery using sonoporation in vivo.

Demonstration of Intracellular Drug/Gene Delivery In Vivo by Sonoporation

Various tissues have been tested for demonstrating drug/gene delivery by sonoporation. Muscle (17–20), kidney (14,16,21), heart (15,22–24), brain (25), cornea (26), spinal cord (27), and carotid or femoral artery (12,13,28,29) have been reported (Table 1) (30–32). In most of the reports, ultrasound contrast agents are used in conjunction with ultrasound exposure and some reports compare the efficiency of sonoporation between various kinds of contrast agents (17,21). Optison from GE healthcare has been chosen to be the most suitable contrast agent in most reports. For demonstrating in vivo sonoporation, reporter genes such as *GFP*, luciferase, and β-galactosidase have been used. The advantage of using luciferase and β-galactosidase is that the actual quantification of the amount of gene expression is possible. On the other hand, *GFP* makes it possible to visually confirm the number of cells that is expressing the gene in the target area. In the case of demonstrating intracellular delivery of oligonucleotides, FITC-conjugated oligonucleotides were used (31). Recently, Sunoda et al. showed for the first time that delivery of siRNA by sonoporation is possible in vivo (26). This report is significant, as developing the delivery method for siRNA is one major issue today. They have shown that siRNAs delivered into the endothelial cells or the coronary artery knocked down the expression of *GFP* in a *GFP* transgenic mouse.

Drug/Gene Therapy in Animals Models Using Sonoporation

Here, several examples of successful reports on gene therapy via sonoporation will be discussed.

Table 1 Reported Drug/Gene Delivery In Vivo

Organ	Tested material
Muscle	Luciferase and HGF (20), GFP (17,18), luciferase and TFPI (19)
Kidney	Luciferase and GFP (21), Smad-7 (16), NFκB-decoy ODN (14)
Brain	Luciferase and GFP (25)
Spinal cord	Luciferase and GFP (27)
Heart	HGF (15), TNF-α-targeting antisense-ON (23), β-galactosidase and eNOS (22), GFP, β-galactosidase, luciferase, and siRNA (24)
Carotid artery	β-galactosidase (28), E2F-decoy ODN (12), p53 (29)
Femoral artery	NFκB-decoy ODN (13)
Cornea	GFP (26)
Dental pulp stem cells	GFP, β-galactosidase and Gdf11 (30)
Intrauterine fetus	GFP, β-galactosidase and FITC-ODN (31)
Chick embryo	β-galactosidase, GFP and Shh (32)

Abbreviations: FITC, fluorescin isothiocyanate; GFP, green fluorescent protein; HGF, hepatocyte growth factor; NFκB, nuclear factor-kappa-B; ODN, oligodeoxynucleotide; Shh, sonic hedgehog; siRNA, short interfering RNA; TFPI, tissue factor pathway inhibitor; TNF, tumor necrosis factor.

Restenosis of the arterial system after angioplasty is one major issue in the field of cardiovascular treatment (33,34). Angioplasty is a procedure that is performed in the coronary artery of the heart or the carotid artery in the neck. Narrow segments of the artery reduce the blood flow of the perfusion territory of the vessel and can cause ischemic changes leading to myocardial or cerebral infarction (heart attack or stroke). To prevent these events, the narrow segments of the vessel can be widened by using balloon catheters and metallic stents. These procedures have proven to be effective in preventing and treating myocardial or cerebral infarction, and furthermore, have lessened the number of direct surgery performed, such as coronary artery bypass graft surgery and carotid endarterectomy. Although angioplasty and stenting have shown great success, it does have some problems. It is reported that some portion of the patients with these procedures develop restenosis after treatment (33,34), requiring repeated surgery or alternative treatments. In this context, preventing restenosis after angioplasty and stenting is an important issue to be solved.

One of the approaches is to deliver genes that can inhibit proliferation of the endothelial cells to the target vessel. As sonoporation can be performed in vessel organs, this technique has attracted great attention in this field. Taniyama et al. showed that by delivering plasmid DNAs encoding *p53* gene into the carotid artery of a carotid artery-restenosis model, restenosis of the artery was significantly inhibited after injury treatment of the vessel (29). P53 is a protein that has a capability to arrest the cell cycle or kill cells via apoptosis, both of which are favorable features to prevent hyperplasia of the endothelial cells. Their histological study also showed that tissue damage related to the procedure was minimal.

Another approach is to use decoy oligonucleotides instead of genes. In many cases, for the gene to be expressed, transcription factors (proteins that regulate the expression level of each or group of genes) must bind to the genomic DNA and start the transcription of the gene into mRNAs. Nuclear factor-kappa B (NFκB) or E2F is one of these transcription factors that has been suggested to be necessary for neointima formation (35) or cell cycle regulation (36). The concept of using decoy oligonucleotides is to deliver DNA fragments with the binding-site sequences of these transcription factors into cells and capture the active transcription factors with the "decoy" fragments before they actually bind to the genomic DNA for gene expression. Hashiya et al. have shown that intracellular delivery of E2F-decoy oligodeoxynucleotide (ODN) into the carotid artery via sonoporation is possible and that intracellular delivery of E2F-decoy ODN inhibited stenosis of the artery with a carotid artery injury model (12). Similarly, Inagaki et al. showed the effect of intracellular delivery of NFκB-decoy ODN via sonoporation in the femoral artery (13).

Other organs that have been shown that gene therapy via sonoporation is effective include heart and kidney. Kondo et al. showed that delivery of plasmid DNA encoding the hepatocyte growth factor via sonoporation recovered cardiac function in an acute myocardial infarction model (15). On the other hand, Hou et al. showed that delivery of Smad-7 into kidney via sonoporation inhibited renal fibrosis in a remnant kidney (16).

All of these reports hold great promise in using sonoporation as an intracellular drug/gene delivery method in vivo. The simplicity of the whole procedure, compared to electroporation or others, is a great advantage that sonoporation has. One fundamental question, however, remains in order to understand and use this technique in the real clinical setting. In most of the in vivo reports, the transfection efficiency is remarkably higher and tissue damage is less severe than those shown in in vitro experiments (14,16,21). This might be partially explained by the fact that, in the case of in vitro experiments, cells are usually prepared in a solution and that cells are subjected to other forces than sonoporation, such as microstreaming, while this is unlikely to take place in an in vivo setting. A more careful and thorough investigation is necessary to clear out this question.

Target Delivery of Systemic Agents by Ultrasound

In addition to sonoporation, ultrasound has shown another possibility in drug delivery in vivo. It has been reported that ultrasound can enhance the delivery of molecules across tissues, which are usually impermeable to large size molecules. For an excellent example, transdermal delivery of large molecular proteins, including insulin, using ultrasound has been reported (37–39). Skins are impermeable to various substances, and it has been considered that the reorganization of the outer layer of the skin by ultrasound makes it possible for transdermal delivery of these molecules (39). Enhanced delivery of systemic chemotherapeutic agent into solid tumors has also been reported (40). Furthermore, we have demonstrated that focused ultrasound, in conjunction with microbubbles, can disrupt the blood-brain barrier and deliver macromolecular agents through the barrier into the brain parenchyma (41–43). These techniques provide the possibility to deliver drugs to target tissues where drugs cannot be delivered without invasive aids such as direct catheter insertions. As ultrasound is now used for ablation of malignant diseases (44), its capability to enhance delivery of chemotherapeutic agents to the target tissue may become a powerful adjuvant therapy for ultrasound surgery.

ENHANCEMENT OF ULTRASOUND-INDUCED CELL LYSIS BY TUMOR-ACCUMULATING SONOSENSITIZERS (SONODYNAMIC THERAPY)

Sonodynamic effect of ultrasound with porphyrin derivatives was proposed by Umemura et al. (45–49). They showed that porphyrin derivatives such as ATX-70, ATX-S10, and hematoporphyrin can enhance the cell-killing effect of ultrasound both in vitro and in vivo.

Porphyrins are famous for their photosensitizing effect. Various kinds of porphyrins have been tested in the field of photodynamic diagnosis (PDD) and photodynamic therapy (PDT). The key feature of using porphyrins in PDD or PDT is that they selectively accumulate to malignant tissues. The contrast of the porphyrin concentration between normal and malignant tissues enables selective photodiagnosis or phototherapy of the target tissue by exciting the photosensitizers by lights with specific wavelength. This feature has been used in the treatment of skin cancers (50) and lately, many neurosurgical groups have started using porphyrins for PDD of malignant gliomas during surgery (51).

Similar to PDT, the key concept underlying the sonodynamic effect of porphyrin derivatives holds that the cell-killing effect of ultrasound can be concentrated only in tumor tissues that take up porphyrin derivatives. Umemura et al. examined whether it is possible to enhance cell-killing effect of ultrasound using porphyrin derivatives or not in an in vitro setting. They used ATX-S10, ATX-70, and other porphyrin derivatives, and treated sarcoma 180 cells with ultrasound in vitro. They observed an enhanced loss of viability of cells when cells were treated with these porphyrins (46,47,52). During the course of investigating sonodynamic effect, many other molecules than porphyrins showed a similar sonodynamic effect (53). Umemura et al. also showed that this sonodynamic effect can be triggered in an in vivo setting (46). They have shown various studies that porphyrins accumulating at the tumor can enhance the cell-killing effect of ultrasound in a tumor-bearing mouse model (54–56).

Although sonodynamic therapy using tumor-accumulating porphyrins is an appealing concept for enhancing the effect of ultrasound surgery against malignant tumors, the main mechanism of sonodynamic effect is not fully understood and requires careful examination for clinical application. In this section, several models proposed will be reviewed and discussed.

Sonodynamic Effect Via Singlet Oxygen

In the case of PDT, it is widely accepted that the production of reactive oxygen species by excitation of photosensitizers by light is the main mechanism for cell killing (57). Similar to this concept, the role of singlet oxygen in sonodynamic therapy has been addressed (46). As ultrasound exposure condition by Umemura et al. showed the possibility of sonoluminescence production, the fact that porphyrins are photosensitizers brought up a concept that sonodynamic effect of porphyrins was a sonoluminescence-mediated process (58). The excited sonosensitizers by sonoluminescence was considered to produce highly reactive singlet oxygen resulting in loss of viability of cells. One evidence that supports this concept is that histidine, a scavenger for singlet oxygen, but not other free radical scavengers as superoxide dismutase or mannitol, can inhibit the enhanced cell-killing effect of porphyrin by ultrasound (46). Several experiments, however, question this model. One of most important observations is that copper protoporphyrin is showed as an effective sonosensitizer. It is considered that this compound is unable to produce singlet oxygen while showing sonosensitizing effect (59).

Sonodynamic Effect Via Free Radicals

Riesz et al. suggested that porphyrins, or in a broader sense, sonosensitizers, are activated directly by inertial cavitation, to produce peroxyl radicals, enabling them to attack cell membranes (60–62). During inertial cavitation, the violent collapse of the microbubbles produces homolysis of water and leads to the formation of H and OH radicals. In the presence of surfactant molecules (RH) including porphyrins, a large amount of H and OH can be scavenged and produce secondary organic radicals (reaction A) and further lead to the production of organic peroxyl radicals (reaction B).

$$RH + \dot{H}(\dot{O}H) \rightarrow \dot{R} + H_2(H_2O) \quad (A)$$

$$\dot{R} + O_2 \rightarrow RO_2^{\cdot} \quad\quad\quad\quad (B)$$

It is considered that these organic radicals have the capability to diffuse in a distance, making it possible to attack the cell membrane for cell killing (Fig. 2).

As a supporting evidence of this model, when cells were sonicated with porphyrin derivatives with various length of alkyl side chain, there was a good correlation between the length of the *n*-alkyl chain of porphyrins, the amount of CH_3 or CH radicals produced, and the magnitude of the sonodynamic effect in HL-60 and HL-525 leukemia cells (62). As the sonosensitizers must react with inertial cavitation, it has been suggested that the "extracellular" localization of porphyrins is required for the production of the sonodynamic effect. The necessity of extracellular localization of porphyrins for sonodynamic effect has been confirmed by our previous experiments (63). By treating malignant cells with 5-aminolevulinic acid (5-ALA), the intracellular concentration of protoporphyrin IX (PPIX) can be increased. 5-ALA is a precursor for heme synthesis, and, as tumor cells have lower capability for PPIX wash out, PPIX selectively accumulates inside the tumor cells. We have observed in an in vitro setting that not intracellular but extracellular PPIX can trigger sonodynamic effect. Overall, it seems reasonable to consider that this model is one of the most convincing models to explain the mechanism of sonodynamic effect by porphyrins. However, there is one crucial problem in applying this model to explaining sonodynamic effect in vivo, which will be discussed in the next section.

The Difference Between In Vitro and In Vivo Sonodynamic Effect

Although in vitro results for sonodynamic effect by porphyrins seem to be explainable by the above mentioned model, when applying this model to in vivo results, a major problem stands in our way. There are several concepts for the explanation for tumor accumulation of porphyrins. However, one of the mostly accepted is that porphyrins are up taken by

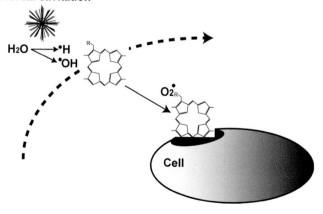

Figure 2 A model for sonodynamic effect by porphyrins. The N-alkyl side chain of the porphyrins will be directly activated by inertial cavitation. These activated porphyrins are much more stable than other free radicals, enabling them to destroy the cell membrane for cell lysis.

tumors and selectively accumulate inside the cells. Involvement of low-density lipoprotein (LDL) receptors, β-glycoprotein, and hyaluronidase in their uptake by tumor cells has been suggested (49,64–69). This "tumor seeking" feature has been used in selective PDT (70) and the development of tumor-specific magnetic resonance (MR) contrast agents (71). In the experiments reported by Sasaki et al. who exposed mice to ultrasound 24 hours after the administration of porphyrins, most of the porphyrins should have been taken up by the tumor mass at the time of ultrasound exposure (49,56). If we should apply the model mentioned above to explain the sonodynamic effect reported in vivo, the main porphyrins that were activated by ultrasound will be the "extracellular" and not the "intracellular" porphyrins that accumulated in the tumor. It seems difficult to explain this discrepancy. One interpretation would be that the enhanced cell killing of ultrasound by porphyrin was achieved by the background concentration of porphyrins. If this is the case, extreme caution should be paid to use this sonodynamic effect in the clinical setting as there would be a possibility that the administered sonosensitizers are lowering the threshold of the whole body for causing cell killing by ultrasound, losing its tumor selectivity. As intracellular porphyrins can enhance thermal toxicity in some conditions (63,72), the sonodynamic effect seen in vivo might be attributable to the thermal effect caused by ultrasound.

The concept of sonodynamic therapy is very appealing. The capability of ultrasound to penetrate deep into tissues, a potential that lights do not possess, brings up a novel use of tumor-accumulating agents as porphyrins. The clinical application of this technique, however, requires caution and a more complete understanding of the underlying mechanism is necessary.

FUTURE DIRECTION IN ULTRASOUND-INDUCED DRUG DELIVERY

Ultrasound-induced drug delivery is thought to be one of the least invasive methods for localized drug delivery to the target lesion. The principle of the concept of ultrasound-induced drug delivery has been well demonstrated in the past studies. The current key question is whether or not the drug delivery efficiency is enough for real therapy of the lesion. For example, when we look into the reported efficiency of sonoporation, it is clear that the current technology is still not enough for clinical application and that ultrasound is not as efficient as other methods such as virus-mediated gene therapy. The direction of research to improve the overall outcome of ultrasound-induced drug delivery will stay unclear unless more detailed studies on the key factors that affect sonoporation or sonodynamic effect is completed.

REFERENCES

1. Saad AH, Hahn GM. Ultrasound enhanced drug toxicity on Chinese-hamster ovary cells-in vitro. Cancer Res 1989; 49(21):5931–5934.
2. Fechheimer M, Boylan JF, Parker S, et al. Transfection of mammalian-cells with plasmid DNA by scrape loading and sonication loading. Proc Natl Acad Sci U S A 1987; 84(23): 8463–8467.
3. Tachibana K, Uchida T, Ogawa K, et al. Induction of cell-membrane porosity by ultrasound. Lancet 1999; 353(9162):1409.
4. Deng CX, Sieling F, Pan H, et al. Ultrasound-induced cell membrane porosity. Ultrasound Med Biol 2004; 30(4):519–526.

5. Guzman HR, McNamara AJ, Nguyen DX, et al. Bioeffects caused by changes in acoustic cavitation bubble density and cell concentration: a unified explanation based on cell-to-bubble ratio and blast radius. Ultrasound Med Biol 2003; 29(8):1211–1222.

6. Guzman HR, Nguyen DX, McNamara AJ, et al. Equilibrium loading of cells with macromolecules by ultrasound: effects of molecular size and acoustic energy. J Pharm Sci 2002; 91(7):1693–1701.

7. Zarnitsyn VG, Prausnitz MR. Physical parameters influencing optimization of ultrasound-mediated DNA transfection. Ultrasound Med Biol 2004; 30(4):527–538.

8. Kinoshita M, Hynynen K. A novel method for the intracellular delivery of siRNA using microbubble-enhanced focused ultrasound. Biochem Biophys Res Commun 2005; 335(2): 393–399.

9. Kinoshita M, Hynynen K. Intracellular delivery of Bak BH3 peptide by microbubble-enhanced ultrasound. Pharm Res 2005; 22(5):716–720.

10. Thomas CE, Ehrhardt A, Kay MA. Progress and problems with the use of viral vectors for gene therapy. Nat Rev Genet 2003; 4(5):346–358.

11. Wells DJ. Gene therapy progress and prospects: electroporation and other physical methods. Gene Ther 2004; 11(18):1363–1369.

12. Hashiya N, Aoki M, Tachibana K, et al. Local delivery of E2F decoy oligodeoxynucleotides using ultrasound with microbubble agent (Optison) inhibits intimal hyperplasia after balloon injury in rat carotid artery model. Biochem Biophys Res Commun 2004; 317(2):508–514.

13. Inagaki H, Suzuki J, Ogawa M, et al. Ultrasound-microbubble-mediated NF-kappa-B decoy transfection attenuates neointimal formation after arterial injury in mice. J Vasc Res 2006; 43(1):12–18.

14. Azuma H, Tomita N, Kaneda Y, et al. Transfection of NF-kappa-B-decoy oligodeoxynucleotides using efficient ultrasound-mediated gene transfer into donor kidneys prolonged survival of rat renal allografts. Gene Ther 2003; 10(5):415–425.

15. Kondo I, Ohmori K, Oshita A, et al. Treatment of acute myocardial infarction by hepatocyte growth factor gene transfer: the first demonstration of myocardial transfer of a "functional" gene using ultrasonic microbubble destruction. J Am Coll Cardiol 2004; 44(3):644–653.

16. Hou CC, Wang W, Huang XR, et al. Ultrasound-microbubble-mediated gene transfer of inducible Smad7 blocks transforming growth factor-beta signaling and fibrosis in rat remnant kidney. Am J Pathol 2005; 166(3):761–771.

17. Li T, Tachibana K, Kuroki M. Gene transfer with echo-enhanced contrast agents: comparison between Albunex, Optison, and Levovist in mice—initial results. Radiology 2003; 229(2): 423–428.

18. Lu QL, Liang HD, Partridge T, et al. Microbubble ultrasound improves the efficiency of gene transduction in skeletal muscle in vivo with reduced tissue damage. Gene Ther 2003; 10(5): 396–405.

19. Pislaru SV, Pislaru C, Kinnick RR, et al. Optimization of ultrasound-mediated gene transfer: comparison of contrast agents and ultrasound modalities. Eur Heart J 2003; 24(18): 1690–1698.

20. Taniyama Y, Tachibana K, Hiraoka K, et al. Development of safe and efficient novel nonviral gene transfer using ultrasound: enhancement of transfection efficiency of naked plasmid DNA in skeletal muscle. Gene Ther 2002; 9(6):372–380.

21. Koike H, Tomita N, Azuma H, et al. An efficient gene transfer method mediated by ultrasound and microbubbles into the kidney. J Gene Med 2005; 7(1):108–116.

22. Teupe C, Richter S, Fisslthaler B, et al. Vascular gene transfer of phosphomimetic endothelial nitric oxide synthase (S1177D) using ultrasound-enhanced destruction of plasmid-loaded microbubbles improves vasoreactivity. Circulation 2002; 105(9):1104–1109.

23. Erikson JM, Freeman GL, Chandrasekar B. Ultrasound-targeted antisense oligonucleotide attenuates ischemia/reperfusion-induced myocardial tumor necrosis factor-alpha. J Mol Cell Cardiol 2003; 35(1):119–130.

24. Tsunoda S, Mazda O, Oda Y, et al. Sonoporation using microbubble BR14 promotes pDNA/ siRNA transduction to murine heart. Biochem Biophys Res Commun 2005; 336(1):118–127.

25. Shimamura M, Sato N, Taniyama Y, et al. Development of efficient plasmid DNA transfer into adult rat central nervous system using microbubble-enhanced ultrasound. Gene Ther 2004; 11(20):1532–1539.

26. Sonoda S, Tachibana K, Uchino E, et al. Gene transfer to corneal epithelium and keratocytes mediated by ultrasound with microbubbles. Invest Ophthalmol Vis Sci 2006; 47(2):558–564.

27. Shimamura M, Sato N, Taniyama Y, et al. Gene transfer into adult rat spinal cord using naked plasmid DNA and ultrasound microbubbles. J Gene Med 2005; 7(11):1468–1474.

28. Huber PE, Mann MJ, Melo LG, et al. Focused ultrasound (HIFU) induces localized enhancement of reporter gene expression in rabbit carotid artery. Gene Ther 2003; 10(18): 1600–1607.

29. Taniyama Y, Tachibana K, Hiraoka K, et al. Local delivery of plasmid DNA into rat carotid artery using ultrasound. Circulation 2002; 105(10):1233–1239.

30. Nakashima M, Tachibana K, Iohara K, et al. Induction of reparative dentin formation by ultrasound-mediated gene delivery of growth/differentiation factor 11. Hum Gene Ther 2003; 14(6):591–597.

31. Endoh M, Koibuchi N, Sato M, et al. Fetal gene transfer by intrauterine injection with microbubble-enhanced ultrasound. Mol Ther 2002; 5(5 Pt 1):501–508.

32. Ohta S, Suzuki K, Tachibana K, et al. Microbubble-enhanced sonoporation: efficient gene transduction technique for chick embryos. Genesis 2003; 37(2):91–101.

33. Mehan VK, Meier B. Conventional coronary angioplasty. Curr Opin Cardiol 1993; 8(4): 645–651.

34. Bult H. Restenosis: a challenge for pharmacology. Trends Pharmacol Sci 2000; 21(7): 274–279.

35. Bourcier T, Sukhova G, Libby P. The nuclear factor kappa-B signaling pathway participates in dysregulation of vascular smooth muscle cells in vitro and in human atherosclerosis. J Biol Chem 1997; 272(25):15817–15824.

36. Weintraub SJ, Prater CA, Dean DC. Retinoblastoma protein switches the E2F site from positive to negative element. Nature 1992; 358(6383):259–261.

37. Tachibana K. Transdermal delivery of insulin to alloxan-diabetic rabbits by ultrasound exposure. Pharm Res 1992; 9(7):952–954.

38. Tachibana K, Tachibana S. Transdermal delivery of insulin by ultrasonic vibration. J Pharm Pharmacol 1991; 43(4):270–271.

39. Mitragotri S, Blankschtein D, Langer R. Ultrasound-mediated transdermal protein delivery. Science 1995; 269(5225):850–853.

40. Yuh EL, Shulman SG, Mehta SA, et al. Delivery of systemic chemotherapeutic agent to tumors by using focused ultrasound: study in a murine model. Radiology 2005; 234(2): 431–437.

41. Kinoshita M, McDannold N, Jolesz FA, et al. Targeted delivery of antibodies through the blood-brain barrier by MRI-guided focused ultrasound. Biochem Biophys Res Commun 2006; 340(4):1085–1090.

42. McDannold N, Vykhodtseva N, Raymond S, et al. MRI-guided targeted blood-brain barrier disruption with focused ultrasound: histological findings in rabbits. Ultrasound Med Biol 2005; 31(11):1527–1537.

43. Hynynen K, McDannold N, Sheikov NA, et al. Local and reversible blood-brain barrier disruption by noninvasive focused ultrasound at frequencies suitable for trans-skull sonications. Neuroimage 2005; 24(1):12–20.

44. Gianfelice D, Khiat A, Amara M, et al. MR imaging-guided focused US ablation of breast cancer: histopathologic assessment of effectiveness—initial experience. Radiology 2003; 227(3):849–855.

45. Yumita N, Sasaki K, Umemura S, et al. Sonodynamically induced antitumor effect of a gallium-porphyrin complex, ATX-70. Jpn J Cancer Res 1996; 87(3):310–316.

46. Yumita N, Nishigaki R, Sakata I, et al. Sonodynamically induced antitumor effect of 4-formyloximethylidene-3-hydroxy-2-vinyl-deuterio-porphynyl (IX)-6,7-dia spartic acid (ATX-S10). Jpn J Cancer Res 2000; 91(2):255–260.

47. Yumita N, Nishigaki R, Umemura K, et al. Hematoporphyrin as a sensitizer of cell-damaging effect of ultrasound. Jpn J Cancer Res 1989; 80(3):219–222.

48. Sasaki K, Kawabata K, Yumita N, et al. Sonodynamic treatment of murine tumor through second-harmonic superimposition. Ultrasound Med Biol 2004; 30(9):1233–1238.

49. Sasaki K, Yumita N, Nishigaki R, et al. Pharmacokinetic study of a gallium-porphyrin photo- and sono-sensitizer, ATX-70, in tumor-bearing mice. Jpn J Cancer Res 2001; 92(9): 989–995.

50. Morton CA. The emerging role of 5-ALA-PDT in dermatology: is PDT superior to standard treatments? J Dermatolog Treat 2002; 13(suppl 1):S25–S29.

51. Stummer W, Novotny A, Stepp H, et al. Fluorescence-guided resection of glioblastoma multiforme by using 5-aminolevulinic acid-induced porphyrins: a prospective study in 52 consecutive patients. J Neurosurg 2000; 93(6):1003–1013.

52. Umemura S, Yumita N, Nishigaki R. Enhancement of ultrasonically induced cell damage by a gallium-porphyrin complex, ATX-70. Jpn J Cancer Res 1993; 84(5):582–588.

53. Rosenthal I, Sostaric JZ, Riesz P. Sonodynamic therapy—a review of the synergistic effects of drugs and ultrasound. Ultrason Sonochem 2004; 11(6):349–363.

54. Yumita N, Umemura S, Nishigaki R. Ultrasonically induced cell damage enhanced by photofrin II: mechanism of sonodynamic activation. In Vivo 2000; 14(3):425–429.

55. Yumita N, Sasaki K, Umemura S, et al. Sonodynamically induced antitumor effect of gallium-porphyrin complex by focused ultrasound on experimental kidney tumor. Cancer Lett 1997; 112(1):79–86.

56. Sasaki K, Yumita N, Nishigaki R, et al. Antitumor effect sonodynamically induced by focused ultrasound in combination with Ga-porphyrin complex. Jpn J Cancer Res 1998; 89(4): 452–456.

57. Fuchs J, Weber S, Kaufmann R. Genotoxic potential of porphyrin type photosensitizers with particular emphasis on 5-aminolevulinic acid: implications for clinical photodynamic therapy. Free Radic Biol Med 2000; 28(4):537–548.

58. Umemura S, Yumita N, Nishigaki R, et al. Mechanism of cell damage by ultrasound in combination with hematoporphyrin. Jpn J Cancer Res 1990; 81(9):962–966.

59. Kessel D, Jeffers R, Fowlkes JB, et al. Porphyrin-induced enhancement of ultrasound cytotoxicity. Int J Radiat Biol 1994; 66(2):221–228.

60. Misik V, Riesz P. Free radical intermediates in sonodynamic therapy. Ann N Y Acad Sci 2000; 899:335–348.

61. Miyoshi N, Misik V, Riesz P. Sonodynamic toxicity of gallium-porphyrin analogue ATX-70 in human leukemia cells. Radiat Res 1997; 148(1):43–47.

62. Miyoshi N, Sostaric JZ, Riesz P. Correlation between sonochemistry of surfactant solutions and human leukemia cell killing by ultrasound and porphyrins. Free Radic Biol Med 2003; 34(6):710–719.

63. Kinoshita M, Hynynen K. Mechanism of porphyrin induced sonodynamic effect: possible role of hyperthermia. Radiat Res 2006; 165(3):299–306.

64. Barel A, Jori G, Perin A, et al. Role of high-, low- and very low-density lipoproteins in the transport and tumor-delivery of hematoporphyrin in vivo. Cancer Lett 1986; 32(2): 145–150.

65. Jori G, Beltramini M, Reddi E, et al. Evidence for a major role of plasma lipoproteins as hematoporphyrin carriers in vivo. Cancer Lett 1984; 24(3):291–297.

66. Kessel D. Porphyrin-lipoprotein association as a factor in porphyrin localization. Cancer Lett 1986; 33(2):183–188.

67. Megnin F, Faustino PJ, Lyon RC, et al. Studies on the mechanism of selective retention of porphyrins and metalloporphyrins by cancer cells. Biochim Biophys Acta 1987; 929(2): 173–181.

68. Mosley ST, Yang YL, Falck JR, et al. Receptor-mediated delivery of photoprotective agents by low-density lipoprotein. Exp Cell Res 1984; 155(2):389–396.

69. Hofmann B, Bogdanov A Jr, Marecos E, et al. Mechanism of gadophrin-2 accumulation in tumor necrosis. J Magn Reson Imaging 1999; 9(2):336–341.

70. Takahashi H, Itoh Y, Nakajima S, et al. A novel ATX-S10(Na) photodynamic therapy for human skin tumors and benign hyperproliferative skin. Photodermatol Photoimmunol Photomed 2004; 20(5):257–265.

71. Takehara Y, Sakahara H, Masunaga H, et al. Assessment of a potential tumor-seeking manganese metalloporphyrin contrast agent in a mouse model. Magn Reson Med 2002; 47(3): 549–553.

72. Saito A, Tanaka R, Takahashi H, et al. Hyperthermic sensitization by hematoporphyrin on glioma cells. Int J Hyperthermia 1998; 14(5):503–511.

13

Blood-Brain Barrier Opening

Nathan McDannold
Department of Radiology, Brigham and Women's Hospital and Harvard Medical School, Boston, Massachusetts, U.S.A.

Kullervo H. Hynynen
Department of Medical Biophysics, University of Toronto and Department of Imaging Research, Sunnybrook Health Sciences Centre, Toronto, Ontario, Canada

INTRODUCTION

The blood-brain barrier (BBB) is a specialized structure of the blood vessel wall that limits transport and diffusion from the vasculature to the central nervous system and is a major limitation for the delivery of many therapeutic and imaging agents into the central nervous system (1–3). It consists of a functional and structural barrier at the level of the basal lamina and intercellular attachments of the endothelial cells known as "tight junctions." The factors that limit passage through the barrier are lipid solubility, molecular size, and charge. The BBB prevents passage of ionized water-soluble molecules with molecular weight greater than 180 Da (2). These limitations exclude many of the available therapeutic and diagnostic agents from being used in the brain.

Major efforts have thus been undertaken to develop pharmaceuticals that circumvent the barrier, such as designing more lipid-soluble drugs, designing water-soluble drugs with high affinities for natural carriers at the BBB, or using vectors such as amino acids and peptide carriers (3–5). Others have diffusely and reversibly disrupted the BBB by introducing a catheter into an arterial branch within the brain and applying an infusion of hyperosmotic solution or other substances (6). The only current method to deliver agents to selected regions of the brain is to directly inject agents (7) or use implanted delivery systems (8). A method to noninvasively and reversibly disrupt the BBB at targeted locations would have a major impact on clinical neuroscience. Indeed, the National Institutes of Health's Brain Tumor Progress Review Group recently recognized the need for such targeted drug delivery (9).

Ultrasound exposure (sonication) has been studied as a method for producing effects in the brain since the 1940s (10–14). Using focused ultrasound, it is possible to produce locally several different effects deep in soft tissue without damage to the surrounding tissue through heating or direct mechanical action. Numerous studies have shown that ultrasound can enhance the delivery of drugs or other agents to skin, soft tissue, tumors, or to cells in culture (15–24). While the exact mechanism for this enhanced delivery is unclear and likely differs among the different applications, it is thought to be related in many cases to the generation of microbubbles and their interaction with the ultrasound field, a phenomenon known as cavitation. Motivated by our work in developing ultrasound phased array systems for focal trans-skull ultrasound delivery (25–29), our group has been interested in using ultrasound via different mechanisms to temporarily disrupt the BBB. In this chapter, ultrasound-induced BBB disruption (BBBD) will be reviewed.

BBBD VIA ULTRASOUND ALONE

Several studies have shown that ultrasound-induced effects can result in localized BBBD, either accompanied with tissue necrosis or, in some cases, without any evident tissue damage at all. In the 1950s, Bakay et al. investigated BBBD associated with lesions produced in the cat brain using Trypan blue and radioactive tracers (30,31). They found that while nonsonicated portions of the brain were not stained with Trypan blue, in large lesions, the area surrounding the lesion was intensely stained, and small, uniformly stained areas could be produced in lesions (with nerve damage) targeted between gray and white matter. Ballantine et al. found that BBBD could be produced on hemorrhagic areas in the cat brain with negligible parenchymal damage using unfocused ultrasound (12). These results led them to conclude that it may be possible to select ultrasound parameters that allow for BBBD without producing discrete lesions. Patrick et al. noted that the BBB is disrupted peripherally in ultrasound-induced lesions in the brain and suggested that this disruption could enhance ultrasound surgery through combination with a therapeutic agent (32). Since the disruption was found at the periphery of the lesion where the temperature was comparatively low, they also suggested that it might be possible to induce the disruption without damage. Disruption without damage was noted later by Vykhodtseva et al., who, in a study of ultrasound-induced bioeffects in rabbit brain produced by short, high-intensity pulses, noted that sometimes BBBD was found at the targeted location without damage to the brain tissue (as detected by the histology staining) beyond the disruption of the BBB (14,33). However, the parameters that produced such disruption sometimes produced neuronal damage, limiting the usefulness of the approach.

More recently, Mesiwala et al. reported a similar finding in rat brain (34). In that work, they too found that they could sometimes produce BBBD alone without damage. Their goal was to provide a method to produce the disruption intraoperatively after surgical resection of brain tumors. They targeted the surface of the brain and suggested that the bubbles in the ultrasound gel that was used for coupling dispersed the beam and aided the procedure. They also examined the brain under electron microscopy, finding that the ultrasound resulted in opening of the tight junctions. However, no evidence was presented that the tight junction widening was responsible for the BBBD. In the case of intraoperative exposure for tumor therapy, it may be acceptable to produce limited damage to the sonicated area, since in that area the brain may already have suffered injury.

BBBD VIA HEAT

The finding that BBBD surrounds of ultrasound-induced lesions (32) as well as findings from hyperthermia studies (35) have led some to suggest that it may be possible to selectively disrupt the BBB with heat without otherwise producing damage (36,37). However, to our knowledge, this has not been demonstrated in vivo.

We have investigated whether ultrasound-induced heating could selectively produce BBBD (38) using the ability of magnetic resonance imaging (MRI) to quantify and map temperature changes (39). In that work, multiple locations were sonicated in rabbit brain while the temperature rise was monitored with MRI. At each location, the acoustic power level was tailored over several sonications to produce a thermal dose (40) near the threshold for damage. BBBD was detected using an MRI contrast agent. We found that while BBBD could be produced in some cases without other changes visible in MRI, histological examination found necrosis in the sonicated region. In our experiments, each sonication was 30 seconds in duration, and the threshold for damage was approximately 48°C (38).

Others are investigating whether longer (20 minutes), lower temperature (~41°C) exposures can result in selective BBBD without damage to the brain. Ng et al. have shown using in vitro models of the BBB that such hyperthermia increases permeability of brain microvessel endothelial cells (36,37). While in vivo results are not yet available for this method, if proven successful, it could provide a means for targeted BBBD via ultrasound.

BBBD VIA ULTRASOUND COMBINED WITH AN ULTRASOUND CONTRAST AGENT

Unfortunately, in all of the studies using ultrasound alone, sonication parameters were not found that could repeatedly and reliably produce BBBD without sometimes producing lesions or necrosis, limiting the usefulness of the method. Because of these findings, we have been investigating the use of ultrasound contrast agents to induce the BBBD. The use of these agents, which consist of preformed microbubbles, limits the interaction of the ultrasound to the endothelial cells, thus reducing the chance of damage to other brain structures. Finally, if the disruption is related to an interaction between the ultrasound field and microbubbles, the acoustic energy needed to produce this interaction is greatly reduced, since there is no need to use the high acoustic intensities necessary to generate the bubbles that will require high intensities in brain (14). This last point also could make the procedure more practical for application through the intact skull, since the cost of the system and risks of overheating the skull would be greatly reduced.

In our initial work, we tested sonications at 1.63 MHz combined with the ultrasound contrast agent Optison (GE Healthcare, Milwaukee, Wisconsin, U.S.A.) (41). We found that 100 msec pulses delivered at a repetition frequency of 1 Hz for 20 seconds could repeatedly produce focal BBBD in rabbit brain without neuronal damage for pressure amplitudes of 0.7 and 1 MPa. Lowering the pulse length from 100 to 10 msec produced similar results. The time average power values used are approximately two orders of magnitude lower than needed to produce thermal brain damage under similar experimental conditions (42). The BBB appeared to be open after approximately two hours for the 1 MPa exposure, and was found to be closed 48 hours after the experiments. Histologically, the effects to the brain appeared to be mostly related to the extravasation of red blood cells in small, isolated regions scattered about the sonicated area.

To investigate the long-term effects of these sonications, a follow-up study was performed using the parameters found earlier that did not produce neuronal damage (43). In that work, more locations were targeted, and effects were examined at one month and 72 hours after sonication. Sections from these experiments and from our initial study were stained to detect ischemia and apoptosis, effects one might expect if severe damage to the blood vessels occurred. We did not observe ischemic or apoptotic regions in the brain, indicating that the effects to the brain were minimal—certainly less than what one would expect from invasive interventions to deliver drugs.

The frequency tested in our initial studies—1.63 MHz—is not optimal for transcranial ultrasound application due to the distorting effects of the skull bone on the ultrasound beam. Thus, in our next studies, we investigated whether the procedure could be performed using the lower frequencies. First, we tested a frequency of 690 kHz, which is being employed in a system designed for thermal ablation (54). Next, we tested the procedure at 260 kHz (44), a frequency at which the ultrasound can be applied through the skull without having to correct for focal distortion (25,45). At both frequencies, we found that we could produce the BBBD reliably and again found no ischemic, apoptosis, or other long-term damages in light microscopy. We also demonstrated that the opening could be achieved through the intact rabbit skull. Also of note was the fact that the number of regions with extravasated erythrocytes was largely reduced at the lower frequencies—with disruption at 260 kHz possible with no extravasations at all. In Figure 1, examples of the focal BBBD in rabbit brain at the three frequencies we have tested to date are shown.

The mechanisms by which focused ultrasound causes BBBD are currently unknown. When microbubbles interact with an ultrasound beam, a range of biological effects have been observed (46). Depending on their size, the bubbles can oscillate within the ultrasound field, growing in size via rectified diffusion. At high enough acoustic pressures, they can collapse during the positive pressure cycle, a phenomenon known as inertial cavitation, producing shock waves and high-velocity jets (47), free radicals (48), and high local temperatures (49,50). In addition, the medium surrounding the bubbles undergoes acoustic streaming (51), which may be associated with large shear stresses. Further, a radiation force on the bubbles is produced along the direction of the ultrasound beam (47). The preformed microbubbles used in ultrasound contrast agents presumably can exhibit these behaviors, either with their shells intact or after being broken apart by the ultrasound beam and their gas contents released. Each of these effects could potentially affect the blood vessels or the blood flow within the microvasculature and be the source of the BBBD. Inertial cavitation, if it exists when the BBBD occurs, would likely be the most significant effect produced by the sonications due to the large energy concentrations in the region of the collapsing bubbles.

We have performed experiments examining the acoustic emission produced over a range of acoustic intensities at 260 kHz (52), and we found that we could produce the disruption without detecting wideband emission, which has been used as a signature for inertial cavitation in vivo (13). This finding, along with the lack of extravasation at these exposure parameters, indicates that inertial cavitation is not necessary for the BBBD, at least at low power levels and at this frequency, and that some other interaction between the ultrasound beam and the contrast agent bubbles is responsible.

When the brain samples have been examined under electron microscopy, it is also not apparent how inertial cavitation is responsible for the disruption. The effect appears to be largely an active transport mechanism (transcellular passage via caveolae and cytoplasmic vacuolar structures), in addition to some paracellular passage via widened tight junctions (44,53,54). It is not clear how inertial cavitation could induce such transcellular transport. In Figure 2, examples of the electron microscopy findings are shown.

One possible mechanism for the disruption was observed in experiments in mice, where a cranial window was attached to the dorsal surface of the skull and various fluorescent tracers were imaged in the vasculature using multiphoton microscopy (55). In those experiments, during the ultrasound pulses, the vasoconstriction was observed

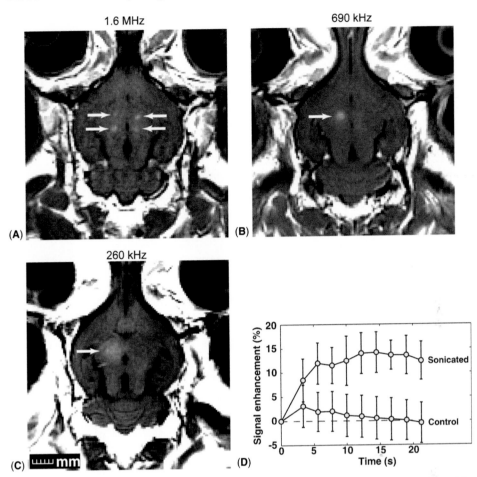

Figure 1 (A–C) Contrast-enhanced T1-weighted MR images showing selective disruption of the BBB at 1.63, 0.69, and 0.26 MHz. The images were acquired perpendicular to the direction of the ultrasound beam. The indicated enhancing spots (*arrows*) show where the MRI contrast agent (Magnevist®) passes through the ultrasound-induced BBB disruption. As the frequency decreases, the diameter of the focal spot increases. The lower frequencies were investigated to facilitate sonication through the skull bone. (**D**) Plot showing contrast enhancement as a function of time for the spot sonicated at 260 kHz and for a control location. *Abbreviations*: BBB, blood-brain barrier; MR, magnetic resonance; MRI, magnetic resonance imaging.

followed shortly after by leakage of the tracer. Such vasoconstriction was observed earlier in high-intensity pulses in rabbit femoral artery (56). These results suggest that the vasoconstriction is related to the BBBD. Perhaps this constriction results in temporary ischemia, which can cause BBBD.

A range of particle sizes have been shown to cross the BBB in the focal zone after sonication. In our studies of this technique, we have shown that MRI contrast agents [(molecular weight: 938 (Magnevist®, Berlex Laboratories Inc., Wayne, New Jersey, U.S.A.) and 10,000 (monocrystalline iron oxide nanoparticles)] (44,57), Trypan blue (molecular weight: 961, larger when bound to albumin) (54), horseradish peroxidase (molecular weight: 40,000) (54), and antibodies (molecular weight 150,000) (58) can pass through the BBB in targeted locations. Immunohistochemistry demonstrating successful

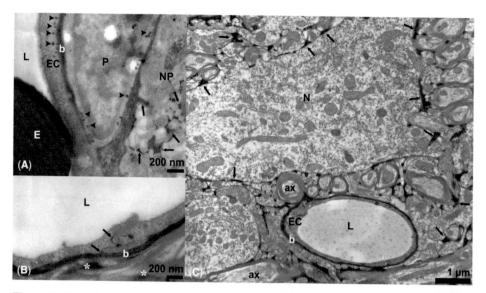

Figure 2 Vessel and perivascular neuropil 19 minutes after sonication at 690 kHz in the presence of HRP. (**A**) Numerous caveolae containing peroxidase (*arrowheads*) have moved to abluminal front of the endothelial cell and into the pericyte. The tracer has infiltrated the basement membrane and the interstitium of the neuropil (*arrows*). (**B**) Passage of HRP through interendothelial clefts with evidently opened tight junctions is shown with arrows. Peroxidase has reached the middle and abluminal part of the cleft and has penetrated the basement membrane. Staining for HRP also is seen outside the vessel's wall in the neuropil (*asterisks*). (**C**) Another microvessel profile in a specimen taken from location sonicated at 260 kHz (60 minutes after ultrasound exposure). HRP is seen in endothelial cell vacuoles again, but also outside the endothelium, in the basement membrane, which looks heavily infiltrated with HRP, and everywhere in the interstitial spaces of neuropil (the dark zones, some of which are pointed to with *arrows*). *Abbreviations*: b, basement membrane; HRP, horseradish peroxidase; P, pericyte; EC, endothelial cell; N, cytoplasm of an adjacent neuron; ax, cross and longitudinal sections of myelinated axons; L, lumen; E, red blood cell in the lumen; NP, neuropil.

delivery of antibodies in the mouse brain is shown in Figure 3. We also have evidence that clinically relevant concentrations of liposomal doxorubicin (Doxil, Ben Venue Laboratories, Bedford, Ohio, U.S.A.) can be delivered to the normal rat brain (59), and have demonstrated that the antibody-based agent Herceptin (trastuzumab; Genentech) can be delivered in mice (60). This agent is effective in treating breast cancer for a certain population of patients, and the ability to deliver it to the brain via BBBD could allow for more effective treatments for breast cancer metastases.

FUTURE WORK

This technique shows great promise, and if proven successful, could offer the possibility of delivering agents that are currently limited by the BBB. Furthermore, the delivery can be targeted to the desired region in the brain, perhaps avoiding dose-limiting side effects. Our research to date has been successful, but significant work remains before this method can be applied clinically.

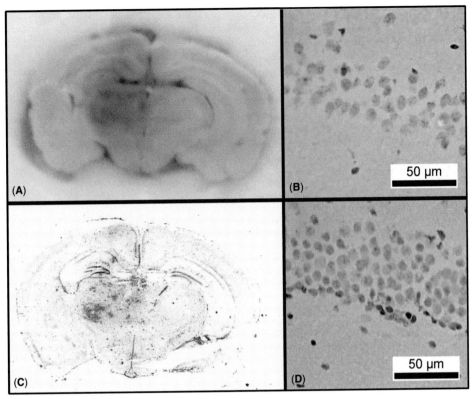

Figure 3 Delivery of intravenously administered dopamine D4 receptor-targeting antibody to the mouse brain using focused ultrasound exposure at 0.69 MHz. (**A**) After removing the brain, the location of the BBB disruption was visualized using Trypan blue. (**B**) Immunohistochemistry showing corresponding delivery of antibodies. (**C** and **D**) Positive signals from the anti-dopamine D4 receptor antibody can be detected at the entire hippocampus, but are weakly stained or absent in control locations. *Abbreviation*: BBB, blood-brain barrier.

Future work needs to be performed to optimize the BBBD, demonstrate that therapeutics delivered across the barrier are effective in a disease model, and to develop a clinical system. Tests should also be performed to determine whether repeated opening of the barrier is safe, as would likely be necessary in many applications, and to look for subtle damage to the brain, including functional changes. Methods to monitor the procedure online, such as the use of contrast agents or monitoring of acoustic emission signatures (52), would also be desirable in making this technique practical.

REFERENCES

1. Abbott NJ, Romero IA. Transporting therapeutics across the blood-brain barrier. Mol Med Today 1996; 2:106–113.
2. Kroll RA, Neuwelt EA. Outwitting the blood-brain barrier for therapeutic purposes: osmotic opening and other means. Neurosurgery 1998; 42:1083–1099.
3. Pardridge WM. Drug and gene delivery to the brain: the vascular route. Neuron 2002; 36: 555–558.
4. Pardridge WM. Drug and gene targeting to the brain with molecular Trojan horses. Nat Rev Drug Discov 2002; 1:131–139.

5. Pardridge WM. Blood-brain barrier genomics and the use of endogenous transporters to cause drug penetration into the brain. Curr Opin Drug Discov Devel 2003; 6:683–691.
6. Doolittle ND, Miner ME, Hall WA, et al. Safety and efficacy of a multicenter study using intraarterial chemotherapy in conjunction with osmotic opening of the blood-brain barrier for the treatment of patients with malignant brain tumors. Cancer 2000; 88:637–647.
7. Bobo RH, Laske DW, Akbasak A, Morrison PF, Dedrick RL, Oldfield EH. Convection-enhanced delivery of macromolecules in the brain. Proc Natl Acad Sci U S A 1994; 91: 2076–2080.
8. Guerin C, Olivi A, Weingart JD, Lawson HC, Brem H. Recent advances in brain tumor therapy: local intracerebral drug delivery by polymers. Invest New Drugs 2004; 22:27–37.
9. NIHR. National institute of neurological disorders and stroke, and National Cancer Institute, report of the brain tumor progress review group. NIH Publication Number 01-4902, November 2000.
10. Lynn JG, Zwemer RL, Chick AJ, Miller AE. A new method for the generation and use of focused ultrasound in experimental biology. J Gen Physiol 1942; 26:179–193.
11. Fry WJ. Intense ultrasound in investigations of the central nervous system. Adv Biol Med Phys 1958; 6:281–348.
12. Ballantine HT, Bell E, Manlapaz J. Progress and problems in the neurological applications of focused ultrasound. J Neurosurg 1960; 17:858–876.
13. Lele PP. Effects of ultrasound on "solid" mammalian tissues and tumors in vivo. In: Repacholi MH, Grondolfo M, Rindi A, eds. Ultrasound: Medical Applications, Biological Effects and Hazard Potential. New York: Plenum Publication Corp., 1987.
14. Vykhodtseva NI, Hynynen K, Damianou C. Histologic effects of high intensity pulsed ultrasound exposure with subharmonic emission in rabbit brain in vivo. Ultrasound Med Biol 1995; 21:969–979.
15. Pitt WG, Husseini GA, Staples BJ. Ultrasonic drug delivery—a general review. Expert Opin Drug Deliv 2004; 1:37–56.
16. Sivakumar M, Tachibana K, Pandit AB, et al. Transdermal drug delivery using ultrasound-theory, understanding and critical analysis. Cell Mol Biol (Noisy-le-grand) 2005; 51(suppl): OL767–OL784.
17. Mitragotri S. Healing sound: the use of ultrasound in drug delivery and other therapeutic applications. Nat Rev Drug Discov 2005; 4:255–260.
18. Tsutsui JM, Xie F, Porter RT. The use of microbubbles to target drug delivery. Cardiovasc Ultrasound 2004; 2:23.
19. Lavon I, Kost J. Ultrasound and transdermal drug delivery. Drug Discov Today 2004; 9: 670–676.
20. Rapoport N. Combined cancer therapy by micellar-encapsulated drug and ultrasound. Int J Pharm 2004; 277:155–162.
21. Miller DL, Pislaru SV, Greenleaf JE. Sonoporation: mechanical DNA delivery by ultrasonic cavitation. Somat Cell Mol Genet 2002; 27:115–134.
22. Unger EC, Matsunaga TO, McCreery T, Schumann P, Sweitzer R, Quigley R. Therapeutic applications of microbubbles. Eur J Radiol 2002; 42:160–168.
23. Ng KY, Liu Y. Therapeutic ultrasound: its application in drug delivery. Med Res Rev 2002; 22:204–223.
24. Tachibana K, Tachibana S. The use of ultrasound for drug delivery. Echocardiography 2001; 18:323–328.
25. Hynynen K, Jolesz FA. Demonstration of potential noninvasive ultrasound brain therapy through an intact skull. Ultrasound Med Biol 1998; 24:275–283.
26. Clement GT, White J, Hynynen K. Investigation of a large-area phased array for focused ultrasound surgery through the skull. Phys Med Biol 2000; 45:1071–1083.
27. Clement GT, Sun J, Giesecke T, Hynynen K. A hemisphere array for non-invasive ultrasound brain therapy and surgery. Phys Med Biol 2000; 45:3707–3719.
28. Clement GT, Hynynen K. A non-invasive method for focusing ultrasound through the human skull. Phys Med Biol 2002; 47:1219–1236.

29. Hynynen K, Clement GT, McDannold N, et al. 500-Element ultrasound phased array system for noninvasive focal surgery of the brain: a preliminary rabbit study with ex vivo human skulls. Magn Reson Med 2004; 52:100–107.

30. Bakay L, Hueter TF, Ballantine HT, Sosa D. Ultrasonically produced changes in the blood-brain barrier. Arch Neurol 1956; 76:457–467.

31. Bakay L, Ballantine HT, Bell E. P32 uptake by normal and ultrasonically irradiated brain tissue from cerebrospinal fluid. Arch Neurol 1959; 1:59–67.

32. Patrick JT, Nolting MN, Goss SA, et al. Ultrasound and the blood-brain barrier. Adv Exp Med Biol 1990; 267:369–381.

33. Vykhodtseva N. Effects of high intensity pulsed ultrasound on brain tissues. The Fifth International Symposium on Ultrasound in Biol Med, Puschino, Russia 1981; 95–97.

34. Mesiwala AH, Farrell L, Wenzel HJ, et al. High-intensity focused ultrasound selectively disrupts the blood-brain barrier in vivo. Ultrasound Med Biol 2002; 28:389–400.

35. Shivers RR, Wijsman JA. Blood-brain barrier permeability during hyperthermia. Prog Brain Res 1998; 115:413–424.

36. Cho CW, Liu Y, Cobb WN, et al. Ultrasound-induced mild hyperthermia as a novel approach to increase drug uptake in brain microvessel endothelial cells. Pharm Res 2002; 19: 1123–1129.

37. Ng KY, Cho CW, Henthorn TK, Tanguay RL. Effect of heat preconditioning on the uptake and permeability of R123 in brain microvessel endothelial cells during mild heat treatment. J Pharm Sci 2004; 93:896–907.

38. McDannold N, Vykhodtseva N, Jolesz FA, Hynynen K. MRI investigation of the threshold for thermally induced blood-brain barrier disruption and brain tissue damage in the rabbit brain. Magn Reson Med 2004; 51:913–923.

39. Ishihara Y, Calderon A, Watanabe H, Okamoto K, Suzuki Y, Kuroda K. A precise and fast temperature mapping using water proton chemical shift. Magn Reson Med 1995; 34: 814–823.

40. Sapareto SA, Dewey WC. Thermal dose determination in cancer therapy. Int J Radiat Oncol Biol Phys 1984; 10:787–800.

41. Hynynen K, McDannold N, Vykhodtseva N, Jolesz FA. Noninvasive MR imaging-guided focal opening of the blood-brain barrier in rabbits. Radiology 2001; 220:640–646.

42. Vykhodtseva NI, Sorrentino V, Jolesz FA, Bronson RT, Hynynen K. MRI detection of the thermal effects of focused ultrasound on the brain. Ultrasound Med Biol 2000; 26: 871–880.

43. McDannold N, Vykhodtseva N, Raymond S, Jolesz FA, Hynynen K. MRI-guided targeted blood-brain barrier disruption with focused ultrasound: histological findings in rabbits. Ultrasound Med Biol 2005; 31:1527–1537.

44. Hynynen K, McDannold N, Vykhodtseva N, et al. Focal disruption of the blood-brain barrier due to 260-KHz ultrasound bursts: a method for molecular imaging and targeted drug delivery. J Neurosurgery 2006; 105:445–454.

45. Yin X, Hynynen K. A numerical study of transcranial focused ultrasound beam propagation at low frequency. Phys Med Biol 2005; 50:1821–1836.

46. Nyborg WL, Carson PL, Carstensen EL, et al. Exposure Criteria for Medical Diagnostic Ultrasound: ii. Criteria Based on all Known Mechanisms (NCRP Report No. 140). Bethesda, MD: National Council on Radiation Protection and Measurements, 2002.

47. Leighton TG. The Acoustic Bubble. San Diego, CA: Academic Press Limited, 1994.

48. Edmonds PD, Sancier KM. Evidence for free radical production by ultrasonic cavitation in biological media. Ultrasound Med Biol 1983; 9:635–639.

49. Flynn HG. Generation of transient cavities in liquids by microsecond pulses of ultrasound. J Acoust Soc Am 1982; 72:1926–1932.

50. Apfel RE. Acoustic cavitation: a possible consequence of biomedical uses of ultrasound. Br J Cancer Suppl 1982; 45:140–146.

51. Miller DL. Particle gathering and microstreaming near ultrasonically activated gas-filled micropores. J Acoust Soc Am 1988; 84:1378–1387.

52. McDannold N, Vykhodtseva N, Hynynen K. Targeted disruption of the blood-brain barrier with focused ultrasound: association with cavitation activity. Phys Med Biol 2006; 51: 793–807.

53. Sheikov N, McDannold N, Vykhodtseva N, Jolesz F, Hynynen K. Cellular mechanisms of the blood-brain barrier opening induced by ultrasound in presence of microbubbles. Ultrasound Med Biol 2004; 30:979–989.

54. Hynynen K, McDannold N, Sheikov NA, Jolesz FA, Vykhodtseva N. Local and reversible blood-brain barrier disruption by noninvasive focused ultrasound at frequencies suitable for trans-skull sonications. Neuroimage 2005; 24:12–20.

55. Raymond SB, Skoch J, Hynynen K, Backsai BJ. Multiphoton imaging of ultrasound/Optison medicated cerebrovasular effects in vivo. J Cereb Blood Flow Metab 2006.

56. Hynynen K, Chung AH, Colucci V, Jolesz FA. Potential adverse effects of high-intensity focused ultrasound exposure on blood vessels in vivo. Ultrasound Med Biol 1996; 22: 193–201.

57. Hynynen K, McDannold N, Josphson L, Vykhodtseva N, Weisleder R, Jolesz FA. Noninvasive MRI-guided focal opening of the blood brain barrier: Demonstration of large particle penetration. In: Proceedings of the 10th Meeting of the International Society for Magnetic Resonance in Medicine, Honolulu, HI, U.S.A. 2002:332.

58. Kinoshita M, McDannold N, Jolesz FA, Hynynen K. Targeted delivery of antibodies through the blood-brain barrier by MRI-guided focused ultrasound. Biochem Biophys Res Commun 2006; 340:1085–1090.

59. Treat LH, McDannold N, Zhang Y, Vykhodtseva N, Hynynen K. Targeted delivery of doxorubicin to the rat brain at therapeutic levels using MRI-guided focused ultrasound. Int J Cancer 2007; 121(4):901–907.

60. Kinoshita M, McDannold N, Jolesz FA, Hynynen K. Noninvasive localized delivery of Herceptin to the mouse brain by MRI-guided focused ultrasound-induced blood-brain barrier disruption. Proc Natl Acad Sci USA. 2006; 103(31):11719–11723.

14

Ultrasound-Induced Expression of a Heat Shock Promoter-Driven Transgene Delivered in the Kidney by Genetically Modified Mesenchymal Stem Cells: A Feasibility Study

Béatrice Letavernier
INSERM, E362 and Université Victor Segalen Bordeaux 2, Bordeaux, France

Rares Salomir
INSERM, U 386, Lyon, France

Yahsou Delmas
INSERM, E362 and Université Victor Segalen Bordeaux 2 and Département de Néphrologie, Hôpital Bordeaux, Bordeaux, France

Claire Rome and Franck Couillaud
CNRS, ERT Imagerie Moléculaire et Fonctionnelle and Université Victor Segalen Bordeaux 2, Bordeaux, France

Alexis Desmoulière and Isabelle Dubus
INSERM, E362 and Université Victor Segalen Bordeaux 2, Bordeaux, France

François Moreau-Gaudry
INSERM, E217 and Université Victor Segalen Bordeaux 2, Bordeaux, France

Christophe Grosset
INSERM, E362 and Université Victor Segalen Bordeaux 2, Bordeaux, France

Olivier Hauger
CNRS, UMR5231 Imagerie Moléculaire et Fonctionnelle, Université Victor Segalen Bordeaux 2, CHRU Bordeaux and Département de Radiologie, Hôpital Bordeaux, Bordeaux, France

Jean Rosenbaum
INSERM, E362 and Université Victor Segalen Bordeaux 2, Bordeaux, France

Nicolas Grenier
CNRS, UMR5231 Imagerie Moléculaire et Fonctionnelle, Université Victor Segalen Bordeaux 2, CHRU Bordeaux and Département de Radiologie, Hôpital Bordeaux, Bordeaux, France

Christian Combe
INSERM, E362, Université Victor Segalen Bordeaux 2, CHRU Bordeaux and Département de Néphrologie, Hôpital Bordeaux, Bordeaux, France

Jean Ripoche
INSERM, E362 and Université Victor Segalen Bordeaux 2, Bordeaux, France

Chrit Moonen
*CNRS, UMR5231 Imagerie Moléculaire et Fonctionnelle and Université Victor Segalen
Bordeaux 2, Bordeaux, France*

INTRODUCTION

Genetically modified stem and progenitor cells have been shown to be potentially useful tools for cell therapy. They can be modified to express a transgene of interest and they offer the possibility of transgene expression at the site where the stem cells are grafted. This has been achieved either by direct administration in tissues or after systemic injection of the modified stem cells. More importantly, because of their ability to differentiate into various cell lineages, they offer the additional potential of repairing and regenerating tissues in response to disease or injury. Mesenchymal stem cells (MSCs) represent some of the most promising stem cells. They are easily available from the bone marrow, need relatively simple requirements for in vitro expansion, self-renew at high proliferation rate, and can be easily transduced with stable long-term gene transfer expression, properties that make them easier to use than hematopoietic stem cells. Genetically, MSCs can repair damaged tissues (1–3). They also have per se potential therapeutic effects as was shown for the degradation of the extracellular matrix in experimental models of fibrosis (4,5) or the facilitation of the grafting of transplanted bone marrow progenitor cells by providing a competent stroma (6). They have a well-established ability to differentiate into the mesoderm lineage, which makes them potentially useful in strategies aiming at targeting the kidney mesangium for instance.

Systemic injection of MSCs results in a wide distribution of the grafted MSCs that can be found in most organs (7). Local injection either directly in the organ or via vascular injection is a potential interesting means to increase the number of grafted MSCs (8). However, even when grafted locally, there is a low but detectable distribution of the grafted MSCs outside the targeted organ. Therefore, in experiments aiming at expressing an MSC-borne transgene specifically to the desired organ, it is necessary to have a means to turn-on the expression of the transgene at the chosen location. Heat-shock promoters (HSPs) have proven to be good candidates as inducible promoters allowing a noninvasive spatial and temporal control of gene expression when combined with the recent development of noninvasive controlled heating of tissues, for instance by focused ultrasound (FUS) (9,10). In this report, we show the feasibility to activate an HSP-driven transgene that has been delivered in the kidney by genetically modified MSCs, using magnetic resonance imaging (MRI)-controlled FUS hyperthermia.

MATERIALS AND METHODS

Cell Cultures

MSCs were obtained from the bone marrow of a syngeneic rat strain, Lewis 1A (RT1a) (Elevage Janvier, Le Genest St Isle, France), and were phenotypically and functionally characterized as described (8).

DNA Constructs and MSC Line Generation

Plasmid HSP-Luc expressing the luciferase gene under the control of a minimal HSP-70 promoter was a gift from Roy Smith (Boston University) (10). Plasmid pcDNA3.1 was from inVitrogen (CliniSciences, Montrouge, France). The MSC cell line expressing the luciferase gene under HSP-control (HSP-luc MSC) was cloned following cotransfection of MSCs with both plasmids using a commercial reagent (Effectene, Qiagen, Courtaboeuf, France). The phenotype and the differentiation properties of the HSP-luc MSC were assayed as described for unmodified MSCs (8). For in vitro studies of the heat induction of the luciferase reporter gene, cells were added with medium prewarmed at the induction temperature and placed on water bath prewarmed at the induction temperature. The duration of the heat shock was 20 minutes. At the end of the heating time, cells were added with fresh 37°C medium and placed back in incubator at 37°C and the expression of luciferase was measured at various time intervals.

MRI-CONTROLLED FUS HYPERTHERMIA

The experimental set up is illustrated in Figure 1A. Rats were installed in a plastic tube to reduce the amplitude of the kidney motion during the respiratory cycle. A circular window in front of the left flank allowed the ultrasound beam to reach the kidney, through a circular, 47 mm diameter, receiver-only surface coil. The MRI-controlled FUS system was set up as described (11). Briefly, during the heating procedure, magnetic resonance (MR) temperature mapping is used for feedback control of the deposited thermal energy. MR temperature mapping is based on the temperature dependence of the proton resonance frequency (PRF). Respiratory-gated, fat-suppressed, gradient-echo echo planar imaging (GE-EPI) sequences were used for fast PRF-based MR thermometry. One coronal slice [square 96 mm field of view (FOV), acquisition matrix 128×96, voxel size $0.75 \times 0.75 \times 5$ mm] was acquired at each respiratory cycle. The actual power applied to the transducer was automatically calculated and updated each time a new MR temperature map was available (Fig. 1B), according to the target temperature curve and based on the method described by Salomir et al. (12).

The heating curve consisted of two parts, as illustrated in Figure 1C. First, the temperature increased during two minutes from the physiological baseline (which was continuously monitored with an MR-compatible, endorectal thermocouple) to the targeted value. Second, a steady-state regimen at the focus point was maintained for five minutes. Standard deviation of the measured temperature in steady-state regimen ranged between 1.5°C and 2°C. Recorded fluctuations corresponded to experimental background whereas the mean value fitted the target temperature better than 1°C accuracy.

Animal Experiments and Experimental Protocol

The animal experiments reported in this study were performed in accordance with the local regulations for animal research. For all manipulations, rats were anesthetized with an intraperitoneal injection of 0.5 ml per 100 g bodyweight of 8% (w/w) chloral hydrate (Sigma, Saint Quentin Fallaviers, France). For MSC grafting in the kidney, four healthy 300 g Lewis RT 1A rats were injected in the left renal artery. The artery was accessed through a 2 cm lateral incision in the abdominal wall, and exposing the renal vascular pedicle by lifting the kidney out of the retroperitoneal cavity. Cells were injected using a 30-G needle under a magnifying binocular.

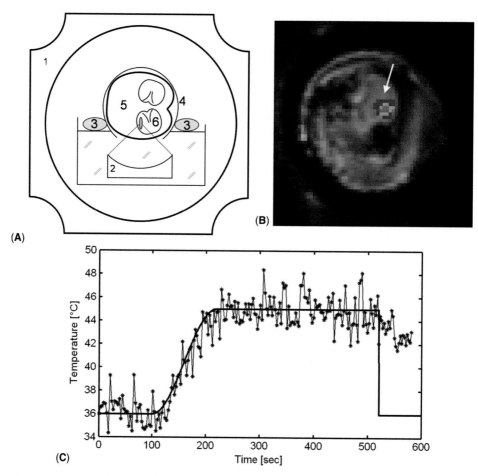

Figure 1 (*See color insert.*) Noninvasive local hyperthermia with MRI-controlled focused ultrasound in the kidney. (**A**) Schematic representation of the experimental setup (transversal section): (1) magnet, (2) focused ultrasound transducer showing the ultrasound beam and the focus spot, (3) MR receiver coil, (4) plastic tube, (5) rat, (6) kidney. (**B**) Example of MR temperature map (color levels: blue 39°C, green 42°C, and red 45°C). Field of view is 48 mm. *Arrow* indicates the kidney. (**C**) Example of temperature time course. A steady-state regime at the target temperature ($T = 45°C$) is maintained during five minutes. *Abbreviations*: MR, magnetic resonance; MRI, magnetic resonance imaging.

Luciferase Assay

Assay for luciferase was performed using a commercial kit following the manufacturer's recommendations (Promega, Charbonnières, France) on cells or tissue fragments that had been sonicated to homogeneity in the lysis buffer provided with the kit.

Histological Analysis

To assess MSC localization and luciferase expression, frozen serial microsections were performed. The expression of α-smooth muscle actin (SMA), an actin isoform expressed in vascular smooth muscle cells and which is expressed by MSCs, was assessed with a monoclonal antibody (clone 1A4, Sigma) and the antimouse horseradish peroxidase

Envision™+ system (Dakocytomation, Trappes, France), and the expression of luciferase was assessed with an antiluciferase peroxidase-conjugated polyclonal antibody (Abcam, Cambridge, U.K.). SMA expression was revealed with liquid diaminobenzidine (brown color) and luciferase expression with AEC (3 amino-9-ethylcarbazole) chromogen kit (Sigma) (red color).

RESULTS

By transfecting rat MSCs with two plasmids, one expressing the neomycin resistance gene and the other expressing the reporter gene luciferase downstream of an HSP-promoter, several HSP-luc MSC cell lines were obtained. These retained their MSC phenotype and their property to differentiate toward the adipocyte or osteogenic lineages (data not shown). We first examined the in vitro kinetics and temperature dependence of the expression of the luciferase transgene by HSP-luc MSC. Three cell lines were tested with similar results. The in vitro optimal temperature for the induction of the luciferase gene was found to be 45°C (Fig. 2A) for the given duration of the heat shock. This temperature falls within the reported optimal range of temperature for in vitro induction of HSP minimal promoter (13–15). Kinetic studies of luciferase expression at 45°C

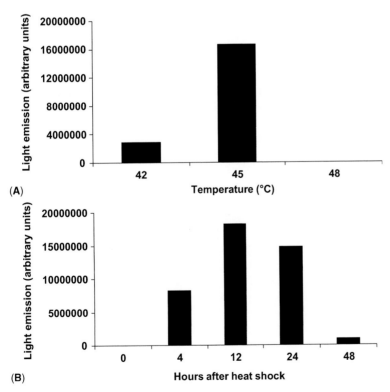

Figure 2   Induction of the expression of *luciferase* in HSP-luc MSC, in vitro study. (**A**) The HSP-luc MSC line was heated at different temperatures and the expression of luciferase quantified. Average of three experiments using three different cell lines. (**B**) The HSP-luc MSC line was heated at 45°C for different times and the expression of *luciferase* quantified. Average of two experiments using two different cell lines. *Abbreviations*: HSP, heat-shock promoter; MSC, mesenchymal stem cells.

showed a peak of expression 12 hours after heating (Fig. 2B). The expression of luciferase declined thereafter again in accordance with published data (10) with a return to background expression by 48 to 72 hours for the HSP-driven expression of marker proteins (10). Following these in vitro studies, a target temperature of 45°C and heat-shock duration of five minutes were chosen for the in vivo experiments. The left kidney of the rats was injected via one of the renal artery branches. In a volume of 300 μL of phosphate buffered saline, 300,000 cells were injected. Selective injection in one of the main branches of the renal artery was obtained and the corresponding injected territory could easily be visualized by the temporary bleaching upon injection. Either the upper or the lower pole of the kidney was injected following this approach. After surgical suture, the animals were then immediately subjected to MRI-controlled FUS hyperthermia. The injected pole was heated as described in the section entitled Methods. The heated area corresponded to an ellipsoid-shaped region of approximately $4 \times 4 \times 6$ mm, with a temperature gradient at the border of the heated region ranging from 2 to 4°C/mm. Animals (four animals) were then sacrificed 8 to 12 hours after the heating procedure. The kidney was removed and samples cut out within the heated area and control areas including injected-nonheated and noninjected-nonheated territories. Results showed expression of the luciferase in the kidney parenchyma that had been grafted and heated (Fig. 3A). Only background luciferase activity was observed in the noninjected territories (not shown). Histological analysis showed the presence of the grafted MSCs expressing SMA and luciferase in the heated area (Fig. 3B).

DISCUSSION

These results demonstrate for the first time the feasibility of the in vivo induction of a transgene that has been delivered in the kidney by modified MSCs and by noninvasive (MRI)-controlled FUS hyperthermia. Spatially and temporally controlled gene expression to a precise anatomic location is a general aim of gene therapy. Control of gene expression based on image-guided local heating has the potential to answer these questions as well as offer the advantage of being noninvasive (9). Recent reports demonstrated the feasibility of using ultrasonic heating to control transgene expression via HSP-induction (10,16,17). As MSCs are being increasingly used as cell therapy vectors, we try to answer the question whether it was feasible to induce a MSC-delivered transgene by image-guided local heating. Our study shows the feasibility of such an approach and allows to highlight the limitations that exist in this approach to date. The HSP-70 promoter is not uniquely temperature-driven. It is activated in cells exposed to environmental stress in general. Therefore, procedures used in cell culture and collection of MSCs could lead to activation of the HSP-70 promoter. Indeed, nonheated areas where MSCs were detected showed expression of luciferase presumably due to stress unrelated to the heat shock. This background level of expression was however less than the expression found in the heated regions and indicated specific heat-induced additional expression.

As we have shown previously (8), grafting of MSCs through the renal artery does not lead to a homogeneous distribution of MSCs throughout the renal cortex, presumably due to the anatomical variability of the renal arterial system. The MSCs were found to be located within the vessels of the interstitium and the glomerulus as previously reported (8). However this localization was assessed by histological analysis and may be heterogeneous. As a consequence, the number of MSCs in a given part of the kidney could not be quantified in this study. It has been shown that labeling stem cells with iron

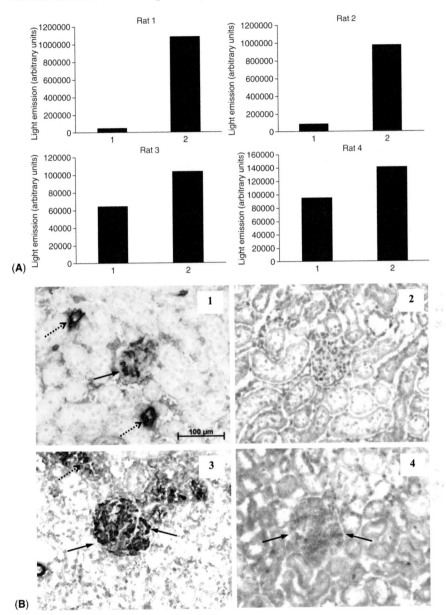

Figure 3 External beam of focused ultrasound induces luciferase activity in kidney at sites of HSP-luc MSC grafting. Ultrasound treatment was performed after grafting. (**A**) Luciferase activity as measured on tissue lysates from kidney, for four different rats; each measure is represented (1) injected/nonheated area; (2) injected/heated area. Results are expressed as arbitrary units. (**B**) Luciferase activity as detected on frozen tissue sections. (1 and 2) Control kidney sections that received MSCs but were not heated. (1) SMA-positive MSCs are seen in glomeruli showing grafted MSCs (*plain arrows*), and basal SMA staining is visualized in recipient vascular smooth muscle cells (*dashed arrows*), but there is no detectable luciferase in serial section stained with antiluciferase antibody (2). (3 and 4) Kidney sections that received MSCs and were heated show SMA-positive MSCs in glomeruli (3, *plain arrow*) and SMA expression in vascular smooth muscle cells (3, *dashed arrow*), but only MSCs in glomeruli are positive for luciferase (4, *plain arrow*). Magnification is identical in 1, 2, 3, and 4. *Abbreviations*: HSP, heat shock promoter; MSC, mesenchymal stem cells; SMA, α-smooth muscle actin.

particles may allow such quantification (8). However, temperature mapping with the PRF method in the presence of a high concentration of iron particles has not been firmly tested and was not used in this preliminary study.

The spatial definition of the heated area was obtained in a restricted $50\,mm^3$ area. Large volume heating techniques (11,18,19) have been described with mechanical displacement of the focused ultrasound transducer. However, they necessitate correction for temperature errors due to the magnetic field perturbation, which may be difficult to implement when dealing with the kidney. Ideally, covering of a larger volume should be done with electronic steering of the acoustic beam [phased-array technology (20)]. There are difficulties specific to the kidney, such as the quality of the temperature control that is easy to reach in the renal medullary due to the high blood flow and thus rapid heat exchange but more difficult in the cortex.

Finally, the temperature of 45°C was chosen following the in vitro experiments, for the single purpose of feasibility and is not a clinical applicable target, because of potential deleterious effect, as could be demonstrated for instance by some images of cell necrosis occurring within the heated area. Experiments are in progress with lower target temperatures.

In conclusion, our study demonstrates the feasibility to induce by a noninvasive heating method the expression of a transgene delivered in the kidney via genetically modified MSCs. MSCs are increasingly being used to direct the expression of a transgene in tissues. However the distribution of the grafted cells outside the target organ even after local injection is a concern and makes necessary the spatial and temporal monitoring of transgene expression. Study herein shows the potential interest of MRI-controlled FUS for that purpose.

ACKNOWLEDGMENTS

This work was supported by grants from the Association Française contre les Myopathies, the Institut National de la Santé et de la Recherche Médicale and by the EC-FP6-project DiMI, LSHB-CT-2005-512146. Support by the Conseil Régional d'Aquitaine, Ligue National Contre le Cancer, Imagerie du Petit Animal and Philips Medical Systems is gratefully acknowledged.

REFERENCES

1. Baksh D, Song L, Tuan RS. Adult mesenchymal stem cells: characterization, differentiation, and application in cell and gene therapy. J Cell Mol Med 2004; 8:301–316.
2. Deans RJ, Moseley AB. Mesenchymal stem cells: biology and potential clinical uses. Exp Hematol 2000; 28:875–884.
3. Pittenger MF, Martin BJ. Mesenchymal stem cells and their potential as cardiac therapeutics. Circ Res 2004; 95:9–20.
4. Fang B, Shi M, Liao L, Yang S, Liu Y, Zhao RC. Systemic infusion of FLK1(+) mesenchymal stem cells ameliorate carbon tetrachloride-induced liver fibrosis in mice. Transplantation 2004; 78:83–88.
5. Ortiz LA, Gambelli F, McBride C, et al. Mesenchymal stem cell engraftment in lung is enhanced in response to bleomycin exposure and ameliorates its fibrotic effects. Proc Natl Acad Sci U S A 2003; 100:8407–8411.
6. Bacigalupo A. Mesenchymal stem cells and haematopoietic stem cell transplantation. Best Pract Res Clin Haematol 2004; 17:387–399.

7. Bensidhoum M, Chapel A, Francois S, et al. Homing of in vitro expanded Stro-1- or Stro-1+ human mesenchymal stem cells into the NOD/SCID mouse and their role in supporting human CD34 cell engraftment. Blood 2004; 103:3313–3319.

8. Bos C, Delmas Y, Desmouliere A, et al. In vivo MR imaging of intravascularly injected magnetically labeled mesenchymal stem cells in rat kidney and liver. Radiology 2004; 233: 781–789.

9. Madio DP, van Gelderen P, DesPres D, et al. On the feasibility of MRI-guided focused ultrasound for local induction of gene expression. J Magn Reson Imaging 1998; 8:101–104.

10. Smith RC, Machluf M, Bromley P, Atala A, Walsh K. Spatial and temporal control of transgene expression through ultrasound-mediated induction of the heat shock protein 70B promoter in vivo. Hum Gene Ther 2002; 13:697–706.

11. Mougenot C, Salomir R, Palussiere J, Grenier N, Moonen CT. Automatic spatial and temporal temperature control for MR-guided focused ultrasound using fast 3D MR thermometry and multispiral trajectory of the focal point. Magn Reson Med 2004; 52:1005–1015.

12. Salomir R, Vimeux FC, de Zwart JA, Grenier N, Moonen CT. Hyperthermia by MR-guided focused ultrasound: accurate temperature control based on fast MRI and a physical model of local energy deposition and heat conduction. Magn Reson Med 2000; 43:342–347.

13. Vekris A, Maurange C, Moonen C, et al. Control of transgene expression using local hyperthermia in combination with a heat-sensitive promoter. J Gene Med 2000; 2:89–96.

14. Guilhon E, Voisin P, de Zwart JA, et al. Spatial and temporal control of transgene expression in vivo using a heat-sensitive promoter and MRI-guided focused ultrasound. J Gene Med 2003; 5:333–342.

15. Borrelli MJ, Schoenherr DM, Wong A, Bernock LJ, Corry PM. Heat-activated transgene expression from adenovirus vectors infected into human prostate cancer cells. Cancer Res 2001; 61:1113–1121.

16. Xu L, Zhao Y, Zhang Q, Li Y, Xu Y. Regulation of transgene expression in muscles by ultrasound-mediated hyperthermia. Gene Ther 2004; 11:894–900.

17. Silcox CE, Smith RC, King R, et al. MRI-guided ultrasonic heating allows spatial control of exogenous luciferase in canine prostate. Ultrasound Med Biol 2005; 31:965–970.

18. Palussiere J, Salomir R, Le Bail B, et al. Feasibility of MR-guided focused ultrasound with real-time temperature mapping and continuous sonication for ablation of VX2 carcinoma in rabbit thigh. Magn Reson Med 2003; 49:89–98.

19. Salomir R, Palussiere J, Vimeux FC, et al. Local hyperthermia with MR-guided focused ultrasound: spiral trajectory of the focal point optimized for temperature uniformity in the target region. J Magn Reson Imaging 2000; 12:571–583.

20. Hynynen K, McDannold N. MRI guided and monitored focused ultrasound thermal ablation methods: a review of progress. Int J Hyperthermia 2004; 20:725–737.

15
Ultrasound-Induced Apoptosis

Natalia Vykhodtseva and Manabu Kinoshita
Department of Radiology, Brigham and Women's Hospital and Harvard Medical School, Boston, Massachusetts, U.S.A.

APOPTOSIS AS A TARGET FOR SUCCESSFUL TUMOR TREATMENT

Lethal cell injury (cell death) has two main morphological expressions: necrosis and apoptosis. Necrosis is the succession of histological changes that occur when a cell has sustained irreversible damage. The main feature of necrotic change is the progressive deterioration of the functions of the cell cytoplasm. The cytoplasm contains the organelles, which are responsible for the metabolic, synthetic, energy-requiring, and energy-generating functions of the cell. Necrosis is always an accidental cell death that results from a severe irreversible cell injury, and it elicits a strong inflammation response. In contrast, apoptosis is a natural way for cell to die—an active, physiological process—by which an organism eliminates superfluous, damaged, mutated, or aged cells (1). It is one of the mechanisms of so-called "programmed cell death," in which a genetic program is activated that results in the death of an individual cell.

The main feature of apoptosis is the self-destruction of the cell nucleus, which contains the cell's genome. Apoptosis occurs through a well-organized sequence of events, whereby individual cells die without injuring neighboring cells and provoking no inflammation reaction (2–6). Cells destined to undergo apoptosis are earmarked via specific alterations in the cell surface phospholipid assembly that serve as signals for phagocytic cells to ingest the debris (7) as opposed to accidental death or necrosis, which produces a strong inflammatory response (8).

Enormous interest in cell death in the past several years has moved apoptosis to the forefront of scientific research. Apoptosis has been widely studied for many reasons. It is a mechanism by which tissue growth is regulated, balancing the effect of continued cell proliferation. It also plays a role in many pathological processes, including cancer and acquired immunodeficiency syndrome and is also implicated in neurodegenerative diseases. For the last two decades, a number of laboratories have studied apoptosis involved in cell death in cerebral ischemia (9–14). Apoptosis also occurs in cells subjected to cytotoxic drugs and ionizing radiation (15–20). It is widely accepted that hyperthermia at doses that fall within the therapeutic range triggers cell death by apoptosis (21–27), while severe hyperthermia produces necrosis (28,29).

Apoptosis can be differentiated from necrosis by means of morphological, biochemical, and molecular parameters. As observed by electron microscopy, the cells undergoing apoptotic cell death manifest morphologically distinct non-necrotic cellular destruction: cell shrinkage, chromatin margination, membrane blebbing, nuclear condensation, and then segmentation and division into apoptotic bodies (30). During apoptosis, DNA is cut by endonucleases at DNA-linked sites between nucleosomes, producing a number of multimers of nucleosomal DNA units in cell nuclei (31,32). DNA fragmentation in apoptotic cells is followed by cell death and removal from the tissue, usually within several hours (33).

Cancer is a disease characterized by an imbalance between cell division and cell death (34). Apoptosis is the best-defined cell death program counteracting tumor growth. It is characterized by the activation of a specific family of cysteine proteases, the caspases, followed by a series of caspase-mediated morphological changes such as the shrinkage of the cell, the condensation of the chromatin, and the disintegration of the cell into small fragments that can be engulfed by nearby cells without inciting inflammation (2,4–6). There is an overwhelming body of evidence suggesting the ability of tumor cells to avoid apoptosis is a major molecular force driving the progression of cancers (35). Apoptotic evasion represents one of the true hallmarks of cancer and appears to be a vital component in the immunogenic, chemotherapeutic, and radiotherapeutic resistance that characterizes the most aggressive of human cancers (34). In response to chemotherapeutic agents (e.g., DNA-damaging drugs), apoptotic-prone malignancies undergo apoptosis; however, patients develop progressive disease despite treatment because of defects in apoptotic pathway (36). Acquired defects in signaling pathways leading to programmed cell death or apoptosis are among the major characteristics of cancer (37). Thus, apoptosis is a goal of cancer therapy (38,39) that coincides with successful human malignancy treatment.

APOPTOSIS AND MOLECULAR TARGETS

Two Major Pathways for Apoptosis

Apoptotic signal pathways can be categorized into mainly two systems: one that involves the micro-organelle mitochondria and the other, the mitochondria-independent pathway (40,41). In a mitochondrial-independent apoptotic pathway, command and control centers for apoptosis can be sprung into action by signals transmitted through the cell surface receptors. In a mitochondrial-independent apoptotic pathway, death stimuli, such as the binding of Fas-L and tumor necrosis factor-α (TNF-α) to their target receptor (death receptors), will directly activate the downstream enzymes (caspases) for apoptotic induction (41). On the other hand, in a mitochondrial-dependent pathway, the intracellular signaling caused from the death stimuli will first be delivered to and concentrated at the mitochondria. Subsequently the mitochondria will "decide" whether the cell should live or die, and cytotoxic substances will be released from the mitochondria, triggering downstream caspase activation for apoptotic induction (40,42). In some type of cells (type II cells), mitochondrial-dependent apoptotic signal pathway is required for death signals caused by death receptors (43).

The Mitochondrial-Dependent Apoptotic Pathway

In the mitochondria-dependent apoptosis signal transduction, the signal transduction system can be separated into three stages. First, various intracellular molecules depending on the type of stimulus will be activated (step 1). Biological stress to any of the intracellular component, such as nuclear DNA damage, induction of defects in membrane permeability, disturbance of calcium homeostasis, endoplasmic reticulum (ER) stress, and so on can initiate the apoptotic signal cascade (44,45). After the signals are delivered to the mitochondria, a series of events will be triggered at the mitochondria, such as loss of the mitochondrial membrane potential ($\Delta\psi$m), and molecules necessary for downstream enzymatic activation will be released from the mitochondrial intermembrane space (step 2) (5,40,42). Finally, the released molecules will activate the downstream enzymes, e.g., caspases to complete the whole apoptotic signal transduction system (step 3) (46).

Among many factors, Bcl-2 family proteins are the key regulators of the mitochondrial-dependent apoptotic pathway. The *bcl-2* gene was first discovered as an oncogene for B cell lymphoma and constitutes a familial protein member. Four domains (BH1~4) have been identified as common domains that the Bcl-2 family proteins share (42). Bcl-2 family proteins can be categorized into two major groups depending on their functions: the antiapoptotic and proapoptotic groups. The antiapoptotic Bcl-2 proteins include Bcl-2 and Bcl-xL, which possess a strong antiapoptotic activity and share all of the four domains. On the other hand, the proapoptotic Bcl-2 family can be categorized into two groups according to their structures: the BH3-only group and the multidomain group. The BH3-only proteins, such as Bad, Bid, and Bmf, share only the BH3 domain, while the multidomain group, such as Bax and Bak, share from BH1 to BH3 domains. It has become clear that during the first step of apoptosis induction, BH3-only proteins, which are normally inactivated at the cytosole, translocate to the mitochondria to either activate multidomain Bcl-2 family proteins (Bax and Bak) or inactivate the antiapoptotic Bcl-2 proteins (Bcl-2 and Bcl-xL) (5,42). It has been confirmed from various experiments that multidomain Bcl-2 family proteins, such as Bax and Bak, undergo conformational changes during activation and form multimers (47,48). Bax and Bak multimers can form pores in artificial lipid membranes and are considered responsible for the release of molecules such as cytochrome c from the mitochondrial intermembrane space to the cytosole (49). There are also evidences that activated Bax and Bak can release cytochrome c through triggering a conformation change of the voltage-dependent anion channel (50), a component of the permeability transition pore at the outer mitochondrial membrane.

During the second phase, molecules that are being released from the mitochondrial intermembrane space include cytochrome c, second mitochondria-derived activator of caspase/direct inhibitor of apoptosis-binding protein with low isoelectric point (pI) (Smac/DIABLO) and apoptosis-inducing factor (AIF). Cytochrome c, which is a component of the electron transportation system for energy production [adenosine triphosphate (ATP) production] at the mitochondria, was the first mitochondrial protein shown to be released from mitochondria during apoptotic conditions (51). Release of cytochrome c into the cytosole sparks a caspase activation cascade to complete the apoptotic signal transduction system. Smac/DIABLO is another type of molecule that is released from the mitochondria during apoptosis and can trigger caspase activation by inhibiting caspase inhibitors (52). AIF, a 57 kDa protein localized at the mitochondria, is known to posses DNA degradation activity and is also again released to the cytosole during apoptosis stimulation (53). In the end of the second phase, with the activated caspases downstream of mitochondria, the mitochondria lose its $\Delta\psi$m, leading to its irreversible functional loss.

In the final stage, cytochrome c released to the cytosole, combined with apoptotic protease-activating factor-1 (54), activates caspase-9 composing a complex named apoptosome, which subsequently activates downstream caspase-3, and -7, which are the main executioners. Substrates of activated caspase-3 and -7 include a variety of targets such as inhibitor of caspase-activated DNase (55,56), lamin, and actin, the destruction of which is necessary for apoptotic cell death.

METHODS FOR APOPTOSIS DETECTION

Terminal Deoxynucleotidyl Transferase Biotin-dUTP Nick End Labeling

Fragmentation of the genomic DNA is one of the hallmarks of apoptosis. Strand break within the DNA occurs in apoptotic cell death by the activation of Ca/Mg-dependent endonucleases. By using terminal deoxynucleotidyl transferase to transfer 2′-deoxyuridine-5′-triphosphate (dUTP) to these strand breaks of cleaved DNA, the terminal deoxynucleotidyl transferase biotin-dUTP nick end labeling (TUNEL) method enables in situ detection of apoptotic cells. This method can be used both in vitro and in vivo. However, with the development of other apoptosis detection methods in vitro, now TUNEL is mostly used for in vivo apoptosis detection (57).

DNA Fragmentation Assay

As fragmentation of the genomic DNA is a hallmark for apoptosis, methods for observing or quantifying DNA fragmentation can be used for apoptosis detection especially in vitro. Fragmented DNA can be observed by electrophoresis of the genomic DNA, which will show a ladder formation. The amount of fragmented DNA can also be quantified by labeling the genomic DNA with [3H]-thymidine ([3H]-dT) isotope or the nucleotide analog 5-bromo-2′-deoxyuridine (58).

Annexin V/PI Staining Assay

Taking advantage of the fact that apoptotic cells externally expose phosphatidylserine (PS), a molecule that is located inside the cell, and that necrotic but not apoptotic cells import propidium iodide (PI), apoptotic and necrotic cells can be simultaneously quantified. Annexin V, a protein that has a strong affinity with PS, is usually labeled with FITC (Fluorescein, mistakenly abbreviated by its commonly used reactive isothiocyanate form, is currently the most commonly used fluorescent dye.) or other kinds of fluorescence to make PS exposure detectable. Cells that are simultaneously stained with fluorescent-conjugated Annexin V and PI can be analyzed by fluorescent microscope or by flow cytometry (59).

Caspase Activity Assay

By directly measuring specific caspase activity, apoptosis can be detected and quantified. As different caspases have different target substrates, not only the amount of apoptosis in the sample, but also the activity of each specific caspase can be measured. Different kinds of measurement methods such as measurement of the caspase activity in the whole sample or the caspase activity in each single cell are available (60).

Measurement of the $\Delta\psi$m

When the mitochondria are involved in apoptotic signal transduction, loss of $\Delta\psi$m accompanies the translocation of cytochrome c to the cytosole. By using fluorescent markers that accumulate only at mitochondrial membrane with viable potential, the loss of $\Delta\psi$m can be measured using flow cytometric analysis (61).

ULTRASOUND-INDUCED APOPTOSIS—EXPERIMENTAL DATA

Recently, it has been reported that ultrasound (US) can induce apoptosis both in vitro (62–69) and in vivo (70–74). In this section we will review and discuss the past accomplishments in this issue.

In Vitro Experimental Data

Most in vitro studies on US-induced apoptosis have been performed on leukemia and malignant lymphoid cell lines with or without the presence of gas-based US contrast agent in the culture medium. In these studies, US-induced apoptosis via mitochondria-caspase-dependent pathway (63–66).

The observation of US-induced apoptosis in cells in vitro was first reported by Ashush et al. (62). In their investigation, human leukemia cell lines, HL-60, K562, U937, and M1/2, were exposed to 750 KHz focused US. Apoptosis was morphologically confirmed by light and electron microscopic examination, and also evaluated biochemically by TUNEL and Annexin V/PI staining. This investigation was significant in that it has proven for the first time that US is capable to induce apoptotic cell death in vitro. At the same time, however, the question of "How" US is inducing apoptosis in these cells arose.

Mechanisms by which a cell commits suicide by apoptosis after mechanical stress induced by US are poorly known. US might induce apoptosis either by the activation of one type of molecular target or by multiple types of damage including those resulting from increased levels of free radicals within the cell, DNA double-strand breaks (DNA DSBs) produced by free radicals or shock waves, increased membrane permeability, disturbance of calcium homeostasis, etc.

Experiments performed by several groups confirmed the drop of $\Delta\psi$m (loss of $\Delta\psi$m) (63–66,68,69) and release of cytochrome c to the cytosole during apoptosis induction by US (65). Concurrently with these findings, caspase-3, a protease, which is usually activated downstream of mitochondria during apoptosis, was also found to be activated during apoptosis induction by US (63–66). Furthermore, downregulation of Bcl-2 and upregulation of Bax have been observed (63). These experimental evidences lead to the conclusion that the mitochondrial system is involved in the apoptosis signal transduction triggered by US.

Similar to ionizing radiation, US has been shown to cause both single and double-strand breaks in DNA (75–77). As DNA damage can trigger apoptosis, US-induced DNA damage was one candidate for the key trigger for US-induced apoptosis. DNA damage has been known to cause either cell cycle arrest or apoptosis through p53 activation. Under normal conditions, p53 is a short-lived protein. However, the status of p53 is drastically altered when cells are exposed to stress, including DNA damage (78). Activated p53 can downregulate Bcl-2 (79) and also has been suggested to directly activate Bax (80), both of which are favorable and necessary steps for apoptosis induction. Abdollahi et al. have attempted to evaluate the importance of DNA damage in US-induced apoptosis by investigating the role of p53. They showed that cells lacking p53 are resistant to US-induced apoptosis, concluding that the genomic DNA could be a possible target for US (67). Phosphorylation of histone H2AX, an indication for DNA DSB, has also been observed after US treatment of cells (69). However, according to the report from Ashush et al., although they observed DNA single-strand breaks after US treatment comparable with that induced by 10 Gy γ-irradiation, they found no evidence suggesting that US-induced apoptosis is related to cell cycle checkpoints or p53 status of the cell, as US-induced apoptosis in various cell lines regardless of p53 status (62). The possible role of DNA damage in US-induced apoptosis has not been settled and more research is required to answer this question.

US is known to possess the ability to produce free radicals through the occurrence of inertial cavitation (formation, growth, and collapse of gas microbubbles in liquids) (81). The violent collapse of the microbubbles can lead water homolysis and the creation of hydrogen atoms (˙H) and hydroxyl radicals (˙OH) (82–84). These primary radicals can recombine producing reactive oxygen species (ROS) such as superoxide and hydrogen peroxide. ROS may be also generated in cells by oxidative metabolic reactions and as a byproduct of mitochondrial respiration. These highly reactive species can interact with and damage proteins, lipids, and carbohydrates. Cells are able to defend themselves against ROS damage through the use of the enzymes, superoxide dismutase (SOD) and catalase. A defect or deficiency in the antioxidant defense system and/or the excessive intracellular generation of ROS render a cell oxidatively stressed (85). Involvement of ROS at different phases of the apoptotic pathway, such as induction of mitochondrial permeability transition and release of mitochondrial death factors, activation of intracellular caspases, and DNA damage, has been established (85). In this context, the role of free radicals in US-induced apoptosis was investigated. Several reports have confirmed the production of free radicals in the medium at a US exposure condition suitable for apoptosis induction (66,67,86). There are also evidences showing that cells are oxidatively stressed after US treatment (63,64). Furthermore, Honda et al. evaluated the role of free radicals, especially superoxide and hydrogen peroxide, in US-induced apoptosis by using antioxidant N-acetyl-cysteine (NAC) to inhibit ROS (64). They have shown that NAC can inhibit caspase-3 activation and DNA fragmentation but cannot stop the $\Delta\psi$m loss and concluded that intracellular ROS production (presumably from the mitochondria, which contain a large quantity of ROS) is one of the key elements for induction of apoptosis by US. Another group has observed downregulation of SOD, an enzyme, which scavenges ROS produced in the cell, after US treatment of cells. They suggested that US can cause apoptosis both by producing ROS and by inhibiting the ROS-scavenging mechanism at the same time (67).

Overall these data suggested that free radicals produced either directly by inertial cavitation or indirectly through mitochondria stimulated by US play an important role in US-induced apoptosis. This model seems to be convincing for the explanation of how US can cause apoptotic cell death. Feril et al., however, have reported that apoptosis can be induced under the condition where free radical is not produced (68). The role of free radicals in US-induced apoptosis has been questioned in this report and alternative mechanism such as cell mechanical destruction or disturbance of cell membranes has been proposed. A more careful and thorough investigations are necessary to solve this controversy.

Other factor such as loss of Ca^{2+} homeostasis after US treatment (64) has been investigated by Honda et al. They observed an increase in intracellular Ca^{2+} concentration after US exposure and confirmed that the source for the increased Ca^{2+} was the extracellular Ca^{2+} from the buffer medium. They also showed that inhibition of intracellular Ca^{2+} resulted in inhibition of DNA fragmentation and loss of $\Delta\psi$m but not of caspase-3 activity, concluding that increased Ca^{2+} was necessary for DNA fragmentation and loss of $\Delta\psi$m (64).

Although fragmented pieces of information on the mechanism(s) of US-induced apoptosis are accumulating, still the understanding of the exact mechanism(s) is far from complete. For example, while it seems that there is no question on the fact that US-induced apoptosis is using the mitochondrial pathway, the key molecules upstream of the mitochondrial event are not identified. Are the BH3-only Bcl-2 family proteins, which act as sensors for apoptotic stress in the cell, involved in the induction of apoptosis? Is the $\Delta\psi$m loss caused by direct physical disturbance of the mitochondria by US or is it caused by the activation of upstream molecules? What is the exact initiator for US-induced apoptosis and what are the links from the initiator to mitochondria? There are still so much more to be investigated and to be clarified.

In Vivo Experimental Data

Histological studies evaluating US effects on brain provided the evidence that US can induce apoptosis in the targeted tissue in vivo.

Apoptosis in US-Produced Thermal Lesions in Rabbit Brains

In the first study, the feasibility of focused ultrasound (FUS) to produce thermal ablation in the rabbit brain was investigated (70), and magnetic resonance imaging (MRI) thermometry (87) was used to correlate the temperature elevation with the degree of tissue damage. A short (10 seconds) FUS exposure (1.5 MHz) induced localized high temperature beyond 53°C to 60°C—threshold, which was found to be sufficient to produce localized lesions. Routine histological examination (hematoxylin and eosin, and cresyl violet staining) revealed both necrotic and apoptotic cells in the FUS-produced lesions. The apoptotic cells appeared as multiple rounded or oval bodies (apoptotic bodies) that were typically manifested as intensely dark purple-blue masses varying in size. To verify apoptotic cell death, in situ immunohistochemical staining based on labeling of DNA strand breaks that occur during apoptosis (57) was used. In TUNEL staining, apoptotic cells were identified by the presence of various types of chromatin condensation or apoptotic bodies (dark brown, round or oval in shape). Thus, the presence and location of apoptotic cells exhibiting DNA fragmentation indicate that apoptosis accompanies necrosis in cellular death induced by FUS.

From hyperthermia studies, it is known that tissue damage can occur at substantially lower temperatures, depending on the heating time and that low-temperature heating triggers cell death by apoptosis (27), while high-temperature heating produces necrosis (28,29). We continued to explore thermal effects of US and investigated threshold-level US heating to produce localized lesions (71). Using MRI thermometry and US phase array technology to induce threshold thermal exposures in the rabbit brains in vivo (88,89), we have demonstrated that US sonications close to the thermal threshold exposures induce apoptosis accompanying necrosis. At four hours after the sonications, the apoptotic cells constituted $9\% \pm 7\%$ of identifiable cells and the ratio of apoptotic cells to necrotic cells was about 1:3. By 48 hours, the number of apoptotic cells had increased up to $17\% \pm 9\%$ and was approximately equal to number of necrotic cells.

One of the possible mechanisms by which FUS-induced heating can activate apoptotic cell death pathway is the production of heat shock (stress) proteins. The stress protein response involves the immediate reprogramming of gene expression in cells exposed to insult leading to massive synthesis of heat shock proteins (HSP) (90). The HSPs are produced in abundant quantities in cells exposed to heat (91). These short-living proteins usually are degraded by the ubiquitin/proteasome system. Monney et al. (92) have demonstrated that blocking of the ubiquitin degradation pathway via a temperature-sensitive defect (at the nonpermissive temperature, 39°C) resulted in accumulation of a high amount of HSP and induction of apoptosis independent on the activation of caspases, the key enzymes involved in the apoptotic cascade events (93–95). These mechanisms leading to apoptosis may be relevant to the cells exposed to the relatively low-temperature heating induced by US. Both, US-induced shock proteins and temperature-sensitive defects in the ubiquitination pathway might result in accumulation of HSP to levels that were sufficient to trigger apoptosis. Ubiquitin-dependent degradation is known to be essential for numerous cellular processes such as a cell cycle control (96), gene transcription (97), chromatin maintenance (98), stress responses (99), etc. It mainly serves to rid the cell of abnormal or short-lived proteins (100). US-produced defects in this system might perturb cell homeostasis and promote cell death.

Inducing Apoptosis with Focused US and US Contrast Agent

In the third series of experiments, we explored the feasibility of FUS combined with US contrast agent (Optison®, Amersham Health AS, Norway) to produce localized lesions and investigated whether lesions were dominated by apoptosis rather than necrosis (72). This agent consists of preformed microbubbles, which can act as nucleation promotion agents for cavitation. Inducing apoptosis through nonthermal mechanisms would be advantageous, particularly in the brain where possible unwanted side effects such as inflammation and tissue edema, associated with thermal ablation, are undesirable.

It was found that US contrast agent combined with FUS reduced power requirements for lesion production more than a factor of 10 compared to what was needed to produce thermal lesions (without Optison) (72,101). The temperature threshold for damage was also lower than was found before without Optison, indicating that nonthermal mechanisms were involved in the lesion production. However, MRI-based thermometry correlated with the resulting lesions, offering a method to guide the procedure (101).

In histology, the lesions exhibited multiple red blood cell extravasations and destruction of blood vessels. At four hours after sonication, the lesions lost many cells and remaining cells exhibited both necrotic and apoptotic features. Overall, apoptosis dominated; the average ratio of TUNEL-positive cells to necrotic cells per microscopic field was more than 6:1 (32.3 ± 13.2 and 5.1 ± 3.4 cells, respectively). It was approximately 1:2 (5.8 ± 4.2 and 10.1 ± 5.8 cells) within the small areas without extravasations. In some areas, cells demonstrated a "messy" form of cell death; there were indistinguishable TUNEL positive-stained debris, possibly representing DNA fragments produced by inertial cavitation effects. At 48 hours, the tissue structure in the lesions was lost and the neurons and glial cells almost completely disappeared, and TUNEL-positive cell were observed only in the thin outer boundary zone.

In investigation of FUS combined with Optison with acoustic parameters suitable for noninvasive exposure through the skull (frequency: 690 kHz, the pulse duration: 10 msec, proton repetion frequency: 1 Hz), approximately 70% to 80% of the sonicated locations showed localized lesions in the rabbit brains associated with multiple apoptotic cells at a peak rare fractional pressure amplitude level of 2.3 MPa or higher (73).

These histological findings suggest that FUS combined with Optison might produce localized lesions mostly through cavitation-induced damage to blood vessels and blood flow disturbance. The cells then died mainly due to ischemia. Both necrotic and apoptotic cell death mechanisms are known to be activated after cerebral ischemia, and the dominant cell death phenotype is determined by the relative speed of each process (13).

Apoptosis is suggested to be the predominant form of cell death after brief ischemia caused by transient blood vessel occlusion or slowly developing blood flow disturbance, while rapid development of cell energy collapse resulted from severe or permanent ischemia leads to early membrane disruption and necrosis (102). It is possible that the cells with TUNEL-positive nuclei were in regions with transient or milder form of ischemia because these cells had a chance to activate the apoptotic mechanisms before the collapse of their energy metabolism and a loss of membrane integrity (13). The areas with few extravasations may have been regions with severe occluded blood vessels or even total cessation of the blood supply. The cells in such areas would undergo rapid development of energy collapse, leading to membrane disruption and necrosis. In contrast, apoptotic mechanisms would continue to dismantle the irreparably damaged cells with residual ATP levels (102).

US exposure can cause tissue ischemia especially if used with US contrast agent injected into the bloodstream. US produces radiation force, which has significant effects on microbubbles and provides a mechanism for manipulating them (103), including bubble displacement, trapping, and aggregation, which cause blood vessel occlusion and damage.

Even mild microcirculatory disturbances are known can trigger apoptosis (104). In our case, there were prominent effects on the blood vessels. An increased permeability of vessel walls, vascular stasis, moderate congestion, and extravasations as a result of the injury of the fine vasculature were observed in all lesions. The more severe damage resulted in thrombosis, occlusion, destruction of the vessel walls, and hemorrhages. Ischemia provokes perturbations to mitochondria consistent with the mitochondria death pathway, including permeability transition pore opening, loss of $\Delta\psi$m, and cytochrome c release (105).

Thus, FUS combined with Optison can produce lesions that are dominated by apoptosis, presumably induced mostly via ischemia after cavitation-produced damage to brain vasculature. These results are promising since apoptosis-dominant lesions will likely produce less inflammation, an important consideration especially for applications in the brain.

CONCLUSION

A treatment of cancer based on US induction of cell death via apoptosis through nonthermal mechanisms would offer a potentially effective therapeutic method. While work is needed to optimize the exposure parameters, these studies could lead to wider applications of focused US, especially in the brain, where skull heating could be reduced during transcranial sonication.

Future work should also investigate whether methods could be found to maximize the ratio of apoptotic to necrotic cells. The problem of how we can correlate the findings from in vitro experiments and in vivo experiments should also be solved. Finally, tests should be performed to determine whether apoptosis could be induced in tumors, since in vitro studies have found differences between normal and cancer cell sensitivity (63).

Previously, pulsed focused US combined with Optison was used to temporarily disrupt the blood-brain barrier for targeted delivery of therapeutic agents (drugs, genes, etc.) to the brain (106). It was demonstrated that using the same technique but different parameters, local lesions in the brain can be produced. Combined, these approaches could result in a possible strategy to use FUS in conjunction with contrast agent for the treatment of brain tumors: first, destroy any visible tumor using the approach described here, and second, disrupt the blood-brain barrier in the surrounding tissue to deliver therapeutic agents to kill the proliferating tumor cells and to stop the angiogenesis.

REFERENCES

1. Afford S, Randhawa S. Apoptosis. Mol Pathol 2000; 53(2):55–63.
2. Kerr JF, Wyllie AH, Currie AR. Apoptosis: a basic biological phenomenon with wide-ranging implications in tissue kinetics. Br J Cancer 1972; 26(4):239–257.
3. Kerr JF, Winterford CM, Harmon BV. Apoptosis. Its significance in cancer and cancer therapy. Cancer 1994; 73(8):2013–2026.
4. Strasser A, O'Connor L, Dixit VM. Apoptosis signaling. Annu Rev Biochem 2000; 69:217–245.
5. Ferri KF, Kroemer G. Organelle-specific initiation of cell death pathways. Nat Cell Biol 2001; 3(11):E255–E263.

6. Kaufmann SH, Hengartner MO. Programmed cell death: alive and well in the new millennium. Trends Cell Biol 2001; 11(12):526–534.

7. Pervaiz S, Clement MV. A permissive apoptotic environment: function of a decrease in intracellular superoxide anion and cytosolic acidification. Biochem Biophys Res Commun 2002; 290(4):1145–1150.

8. Majno G, Joris I. Apoptosis, oncosis, and necrosis. An overview of cell death. Am J Pathol 1995; 146(1):3–15.

9. Linnik MD, Zobrist RH, Hatfield MD. Evidence supporting a role for programmed cell death in focal cerebral ischemia in rats. Stroke 1993; 24(12):2002–2008; discussion 2008–2009.

10. Li Y, Powers C, Jiang N, et al. Intact, injured, necrotic and apoptotic cells after focal cerebral ischemia in the rat. J Neurol Sci 1998; 156(2):119–132.

11. Lo EH, Dalkara T, Moskowitz MA. Mechanisms, challenges and opportunities in stroke. Nat Rev Neurosci 2003; 4(5):399–415.

12. Lo EH, Moskowitz MA, Jacobs TP. Exciting, radical, suicidal: how brain cells die after stroke. Stroke 2005; 36(2):189–192.

13. Unal-Cevik I, Kilinc M, Can A, et al. Apoptotic and necrotic death mechanisms are concomitantly activated in the same cell after cerebral ischemia. Stroke 2004; 35(9): 2189–2194.

14. Charriaut-Marlangue C. Apoptosis: a target for neuroprotection. Therapie 2004; 59(2): 185–190.

15. Di Pietro R, Falcieri E, Centurione L, et al. Ultrastructural patterns of cell damage and death following gamma radiation exposure of murine erythroleukemia cells. Scanning Microsc 1994; 8(3):667–673.

16. Di Pietro C, Piro S, Tabbi G, et al. Cellular and molecular effects of protons: apoptosis induction and potential implications for cancer therapy. Apoptosis 2006; 11(1):57–66.

17. Harms-Ringdahl M, Nicotera P, Radford IR. Radiation induced apoptosis. Mutat Res 1996; 366(2):171–179.

18. Meijer AE, Ekedahl J, Joseph B, et al. High-LET radiation induces apoptosis in lymphoblastoid cell lines derived from atazia-telangiectasia patients. Int J Radiat Biol 2001; 77(3):309–317.

19. Belyaev IY, Czene S, Harms-Ringdahl M. Changes in chromatin conformation during radiation-induced apoptosis in human lymphocytes. Radiat Res 2001; 156(4):355–364.

20. Belloni P, Meschini R, Czene S, et al. Studies on radiation-induced apoptosis in G0 human lymphocytes. Int J Radiat Biol 2005; 81(8):587–599.

21. Sakaguchi Y, Stephens LC, Makino M, et al. Apoptosis in tumors and normal tissues induced by whole body hyperthermia in rats. Cancer Res 1995; 55(22):5459–5464.

22. Moroi J, Kashiwagi S, Kim S, et al. Regional differences in apoptosis in murine gliosarcoma (T9) induced by mild hyperthermia. Int J Hyperthermia 1996; 12(3):345–354.

23. Nakano H, Kurihara K, Okamoto M, et al. Heat-induced apoptosis and p53 in cultured mammalian cells. Int J Radiat Biol 1997; 71(5):519–529.

24. Fuse T, Yoon KW, Kato T, et al. Heat-induced apoptosis in human glioblastoma cell line A172. Neurosurgery 1998; 42(4):843–849.

25. Ohnishi K, Ohnishi T. Heat-induced p53-dependent signal transduction and its role in hyperthermic cancer therapy. Int J Hyperthermia 2001; 17(5):415–427.

26. Hildebrandt B, Wust P, Ahlers O, et al. The cellular and molecular basis of hyperthermia. Crit Rev Oncol Hematol 2002; 43(1):33–56.

27. Dewhirst MW, Vujaskovic Z, Jones E, et al. Re-setting the biologic rationale for thermal therapy. Int J Hyperthermia 2005; 21(8):779–790.

28. Harmon BV, Corder AM, Collins RJ, et al. Cell death induced in a murine mastocytoma by 42–47 degrees C heating in vitro: evidence that the form of death changes from apoptosis to necrosis above a critical heat load. Int J Radiat Biol 1990; 58(5):845–858.

29. Fairbairn DW, Walburger DK, Fairbairn JJ, et al. Key morphologic changes and DNA strand breaks in human lymphoid cells: discriminating apoptosis from necrosis. Scanning 1996; 18(6): 407–416.

30. Darzynkiewicz Z, Juan G, Li X, et al. Cytometry in cell necrobiology: analysis of apoptosis and accidental cell death (necrosis). Cytometry 1997; 27(1):1–20.

31. Thiry M. Highly sensitive immunodetection of DNA on sections with exogenous terminal deoxynucleotidyl transferase and non-isotopic nucleotide analogues. J Histochem Cytochem 1992; 40(3):411–419.

32. Migheli A, Attanasio A, Schiffer D. Ultrastructural detection of DNA strand breaks in apoptotic neural cells by in situ end-labelling techniques. J Pathol 1995; 176(1):27–35.

33. Bursch W, Paffe S, Putz B, et al. Determination of the length of the histological stages of apoptosis in normal liver and in altered hepatic foci of rats. Carcinogenesis 1990; 11(5): 847–853.

34. Hanahan D, Weinberg RA. The hallmarks of cancer. Cell 2000; 100(1):57–70.

35. McKenzie S, Kyprianou N. Apoptosis evasion: the role of survival pathways in prostate cancer progression and therapeutic resistance. J Cell Biochem 2006; 97(1):18–32.

36. Mueller T, Voigt W, Simon H, et al. Failure of activation of caspase-9 induces a higher threshold for apoptosis and cisplatin resistance in testicular cancer. Cancer Res 2003; 63(2): 513–521.

37. Jaattela M. Multiple cell death pathways as regulators of tumour initiation and progression. Oncogene 2004; 23(16):2746–2756.

38. Spierings DC, de Vries EG, Vellenga E, et al. Loss of drug-induced activation of the CD95 apoptotic pathway in a cisplatin-resistant testicular germ cell tumor cell line. Cell Death Differ 2003; 10(7):808–822.

39. Blagosklonny MV. Prospective strategies to enforce selectively cell death in cancer cells. Oncogene 2004; 23(16):2967–2975.

40. Green DR, Kroemer G. The pathophysiology of mitochondrial cell death. Science 2004; 305 (5684):626–629.

41. Nagata S. Apoptosis by death factor. Cell 1997; 88(3):355–365.

42. Tsujimoto Y. Cell death regulation by the Bcl-2 protein family in the mitochondria. J Cell Physiol 2003; 195(2):158–167.

43. Wei MC, Lindsten T, Mootha VK, et al. tBID, a membrane-targeted death ligand, oligomerizes BAK to release cytochrome c. Genes Dev 2000; 14(16):2060–2071.

44. Szegezdi E, Fitzgerald U, Samali A. Caspase-12 and ER-stress-mediated apoptosis: the story so far. Ann N Y Acad Sci 2003; 1010:186–194.

45. Norbury CJ, Zhivotovsky B. DNA damage-induced apoptosis. Oncogene 2004; 23(16): 2797–2808.

46. Riedl SJ, Shi Y. Molecular mechanisms of caspase regulation during apoptosis. Nat Rev Mol Cell Biol 2004; 5(11):897–907.

47. Desagher S, Osen-Sand A, Nichols A, et al. Bid-induced conformational change of Bax is responsible for mitochondrial cytochrome c release during apoptosis. J Cell Biol 1999; 144(5): 891–901.

48. Eskes R, Desagher S, Antonsson B, et al. Bid induces the oligomerization and insertion of Bax into the outer mitochondrial membrane. Mol Cell Biol 2000; 20(3):929–935.

49. Saito M, Korsmeyer SJ, Schlesinger PH. BAX-dependent transport of cytochrome c reconstituted in pure liposomes. Nat Cell Biol 2000; 2(8):553–555.

50. Shimizu S, Narita M, Tsujimoto Y. Bcl-2 family proteins regulate the release of apoptogenic cytochrome c by the mitochondrial channel VDAC. Nature 1999; 399(6735):483–487.

51. Liu X, Kim CN, Yang J, et al. Induction of apoptotic program in cell-free extracts: requirement for dATP and cytochrome c. Cell 1996; 86(1):147–157.

52. Du C, Fang M, Li Y, et al. Smac, a mitochondrial protein that promotes cytochrome c-dependent caspase activation by eliminating IAP inhibition. Cell 2000; 102(1):33–42.

53. Susin SA, Zamzami N, Castedo M, et al. Bcl-2 inhibits the mitochondrial release of an apoptogenic protease. J Exp Med 1996; 184(4):1331–1341.

54. Zou H, Henzel WJ, Liu X, et al. Apaf-1, a human protein homologous to *C. elegans* CED-4, participates in cytochrome c-dependent activation of caspase-3. Cell 1997; 90(3): 405–413.

55. Sakahira H, Enari M, Nagata S. Cleavage of CAD inhibitor in CAD activation and DNA degradation during apoptosis. Nature 1998; 391(6662):96–99.
56. Enari M, Sakahira H, Yokoyama H, et al. A caspase-activated DNase that degrades DNA during apoptosis, and its inhibitor ICAD. Nature 1998; 391(6662):43–50.
57. Gavrieli Y, Sherman Y, Ben-Sasson SA. Identification of programmed cell death in situ via specific labeling of nuclear DNA fragmentation. J Cell Biol 1992; 119(3):493–501.
58. Kaufmann SH, Mesner PW Jr, Samejima K, et al. Detection of DNA cleavage in apoptotic cells. Methods Enzymol 2000; 322:3–15.
59. Darzynkiewicz Z, Bedner E. Analysis of apoptotic cells by flow and laser scanning cytometry. Methods Enzymol 2000; 322:18–39.
60. Stennicke HR, Salvesen GS. Caspase assays. Methods Enzymol 2000; 322:91–100.
61. Reers M, Smiley ST, Mottola-Hartshorn C, et al. Mitochondrial membrane potential monitored by JC-1 dye. Methods Enzymol 1995; 260:406–417.
62. Ashush H, Rozenszajn LA, Blass M, et al. Apoptosis induction of human myeloid leukemic cells by ultrasound exposure. Cancer Res 2000; 60(4):1014–1020.
63. Lagneaux L, de Meulenaer EC, Delforge A, et al. Ultrasonic low-energy treatment: a novel approach to induce apoptosis in human leukemic cells. Exp Hematol 2002; 30(11):1293–1301.
64. Honda H, Kondo T, Zhao QL, et al. Role of intracellular calcium ions and reactive oxygen species in apoptosis induced by ultrasound. Ultrasound Med Biol 2004; 30(5):683–692.
65. Firestein F, Rozenszajn LA, Shemesh-Darvish L, et al. Induction of apoptosis by ultrasound application in human malignant lymphoid cells: role of mitochondria-caspase pathway activation. Ann N Y Acad Sci 2003; 1010:163–166.
66. Honda H, Zhao QL, Kondo T. Effects of dissolved gases and an echo contrast agent on apoptosis induced by ultrasound and its mechanism via the mitochondria-caspase pathway. Ultrasound Med Biol 2002; 28(5):673–682.
67. Abdollahi A, Domhan S, Jenne JW, et al. Apoptosis signals in lymphoblasts induced by focused ultrasound. Faseb J 2004; 18(12):1413–1414.
68. Feril LB Jr, Kondo T, Cui ZG, et al. Apoptosis induced by the sonomechanical effects of low intensity pulsed ultrasound in a human leukemia cell line. Cancer Lett 2005; 221(2): 145–152.
69. Ando H, Feril LB Jr, Kondo T, et al. An echo-contrast agent, Levovist, lowers the ultrasound intensity required to induce apoptosis of human leukemia cells. Cancer Lett 2006; 242(1): 37–45.
70. Vykhodtseva N, Sorrentino V, Jolesz FA, et al. MRI detection of the thermal effects of focused ultrasound on the brain. Ultrasound Med Biol 2000; 26(5):871–880.
71. Vykhodtseva N, McDannold N, Martin H, et al. Apoptosis in ultrasound-produced threshold lesions in the rabbit brain. Ultrasound Med Biol 2001; 27(1):111–117.
72. Vykhodtseva N, McDannold N, Hynynen K. Induction of apoptosis in vivo in the rabbit brain with focused ultrasound. Proceedings of the 5th International Symposium on Therapeutic Ultrasound, Boston, USA, 2006.
73. Hynynen K, McDannold N, Sheikov NA, et al. Local and reversible blood-brain barrier disruption by noninvasive focused ultrasound at frequencies suitable for trans-skull sonications. Neuroimage 2005; 24(1):12–20.
74. McDannold N, Vykhodtseva N, Jolesz FA, et al. MRI investigation of the threshold for thermally induced blood-brain barrier disruption and brain tissue damage in the rabbit brain. Magn Reson Med 2004; 51(5):913–923.
75. Kondo T, Kano E. Effect of free radicals induced by ultrasonic cavitation on cell killing. Int J Radiat Biol 1988; 54(3):475–486.
76. Miller DL, Thomas RM, Frazier ME. Ultrasonic cavitation indirectly induces single strand breaks in DNA of viable cells in vitro by the action of residual hydrogen peroxide. Ultrasound Med Biol 1991; 17(7):729–735.
77. Miller DL, Thomas RM. The role of cavitation in the induction of cellular DNA damage by ultrasound and lithotripter shock waves in vitro. Ultrasound Med Biol 1996; 22(5): 681–687.

78. Giaccia AJ, Kastan MB. The complexity of p53 modulation: emerging patterns from divergent signals. Genes Dev 1998; 12(19):2973–2983.

79. Haldar S, Negrini M, Monne M, et al. Down-regulation of bcl-2 by p53 in breast cancer cells. Cancer Res 1994; 54(8):2095–2097.

80. Chipuk JE, Kuwana T, Bouchier-Hayes L, et al. Direct activation of Bax by p53 mediates mitochondrial membrane permeabilization and apoptosis. Science 2004; 303(5660): 1010–1014.

81. Kondo T, Murali Krishna C, Riesz P. Sonolysis, radiolysis, and hydrogen peroxide photolysis of pyrimidine derivatives in aqueous solutions: a spin-trapping study. Radiat Res 1988; 116(1):56–73.

82. Miyoshi N, Sostaric JZ, Riesz P. Correlation between sonochemistry of surfactant solutions and human leukemia cell killing by ultrasound and porphyrins. Free Radic Biol Med 2003; 34(6):710–719.

83. Makino K, Mossoba MM, Riesz P. Formation of .OH and .H in aqueous solutions by ultrasound using clinical equipment. Radiat Res 1983; 96(2):416–421.

84. Riesz P, Christman CL. Sonochemical free radical formation in aqueous solutions. Fed Proc 1986; 45(10):2485–2492.

85. Le Bras M, Clement MV, Pervaiz S, et al. Reactive oxygen species and the mitochondrial signaling pathway of cell death. Histol Histopathol 2005; 20(1):205–219.

86. Feril LB Jr, Kondo T, Zhao QL, et al. Enhancement of ultrasound-induced apoptosis and cell lysis by echo-contrast agents. Ultrasound Med Biol 2003; 29(2):331–337.

87. Hynynen K, Vykhodtseva NI, Chung AH, et al. Thermal effects of focused ultrasound on the brain: determination with MR imaging. Radiology 1997; 204(1):247–253.

88. Cain CA, Umemura S. Concentric-ring and sector-vortex phased-array applicators for ultrasound hyperthermia. IEEE Trans Microwav Theory Tech 1986; 34(5):542–551.

89. Fjield T, Hynynen K. The combined concentric-ring and sector-vortex phased array for MRI guided ultrasound surgery. IEEE Trans Ultrason Ferroelectr Freq Control 1997; 44(5): 1157–1167.

90. Calderwood SK. Regulatory interfaces between the stress protein response and other gene expression programs in the cell. Methods 2005; 35(2):139–148.

91. Calderwood SK, Theriault JR, Gong J. How is the immune response affected by hyperthermia and heat shock proteins? Int J Hyperthermia 2005; 21(8):713–716.

92. Monney L, Otter I, Olivier R, et al. Defects in the ubiquitin pathway induce caspase-independent apoptosis blocked by Bcl-2. J Biol Chem 1998; 273(11):6121–6131.

93. Alnemri ES, Livingston DJ, Nicholson DW, et al. Human ICE/CED-3 protease nomenclature. Cell 1996; 87(2):171.

94. Yuan J. Molecular control of life and death. Curr Opin Cell Biol 1995; 7(2):211–214.

95. Yuan J. Genetic control of cellular suicide. Reprod Toxicol 1997; 11(2-3):377–384.

96. Glotzer M. The mechanism and control of cytokinesis. Curr Opin Cell Biol 1997; 9(6): 815–823.

97. Scheffner M, Werness BA, Huibregtse JM, et al. The E6 oncoprotein encoded by human papillomavirus types 16 and 18 promotes the degradation of p53. Cell 1990; 63(6): 1129–1136.

98. Hunt LT, Dayhoff MO. Amino-terminal sequence identity of ubiquitin and the nonhistone component of nuclear protein A24. Biochem Biophys Res Commun 1977; 74(2):650–655.

99. Lowe J, Landon M, Fergusson J, et al. Ubiquitin response to cell stress. J Neuropathol Exp Neurol 1995; 54 S6–S7.

100. Jennissen HP. Ubiquitin and the enigma of intracellular protein degradation. Eur J Biochem 1995; 231(1):1–30.

101. McDannold N, Vykhodtseva N, Hynynen K. Microbubble contrast agent with focused ultrasound to create brain lesions at low power levels: MR imaging and histologic study in rabbits. Radiology 2006; 241(1):95–106.

102. Nicotera P, Leist M, Fava E, et al. Energy requirement for caspase activation and neuronal cell death. Brain Pathol 2000; 10(2):276–282.

103. Dayton P, Klibanov A, Brandenburger G, et al. Acoustic radiation force in vivo: a mechanism to assist targeting of microbubbles. Ultrasound Med Biol 1999; 25(8): 1195–1201.

104. Vexler ZS, Roberts TP, Bollen AW, et al. Transient cerebral ischemia. Association of apoptosis induction with hypoperfusion. J Clin Invest 1997; 99(6):1453–1459.

105. Gurevich RM, Regula KM, Kirshenbaum LA. Serpin protein CrmA suppresses hypoxia-mediated apoptosis of ventricular myocytes. Circulation 2001; 103(15):1984–1991.

106. Hynynen K, McDannold N, Vykhodtseva N, et al. Noninvasive MR imaging-guided focal opening of the blood-brain barrier in rabbits. Radiology 2001; 220(3):640–646.

Index

Aberration correction, 75–77
Abnormal bleeding, 112
Absorption, US, 12–13
Acoustic cavitation, 17–18
Acoustic characterization, MRIgFUS for, 48–50
Acoustic hemostasis, 91
Acoustic impedance, tissue, 13
Acoustic streaming, 17
Acute pain, 112
α-Smooth muscle actin (SMA), 174
5-Aminolevulinic acid (5-ALA), 154
Angioplasty, 151
Animals models
    drug/gene therapy in
        using sonoporation, 150–152
Annexin V/PI staining assay, 184
Apoptosis, ultrasound-induced, 181–189
    apoptosis detection, methods for, 184
        Δψm, measurement, 184
        Annexin V/PI staining assay, 184
        caspase activity assay, 184
        DNA fragmentation assay, 184
        terminal deoxynucleotidyl transferase
            biotin-dUTP nick end labeling, 184
    experimental data, 184–189
    with focused US and US-contrast agent, 188–189
    and molecular targets, 181. *See also* Molecular targets
    necrosis versus, 181
    for tumor treatment, 181–182
    in US-produced thermal lesions in
        rabbit brains, 187
    in vitro experimental data, 185–186
    in vivo experimental data, 187–189
Apoptosis-inducing factor (AIF), 183
Arterial venous malformations (AVMs), 91
Arterio venous malformation (AVM), 145
Arthritic joints, MRIgFUS treatment for, 90–91
Attenuation, US, 12–13
ATX-70, 153
ATX-S10, 153
Automated feedback control, in MRIgFUS, 45–46
Axillary lymph node sampling, 108

Bcl-2 family proteins, 183, 185
Biological effects of US, 14–18
    blood perfusion effects, 15
    cavitation, 17–18
    mechanical effects, 16–17
    thermal effects, 15–16
Blood perfusion effects, by US, 15
Blood–brain barrier (BBB) opening, 91, 131,
        161–167
    BBB opening, 92–93
    BBBD via heat, 162–163
    BBBD via ultrasound alone, 162
    via ultrasound combined with an ultrasound
            contrast agent, 163–166
        mechanism, 164
Bones
    bone tumors, MRIgFUS treatment for, 89
    MR-guided focused ultrasound of bone, 141–143
        percutaneous radiofrequency ablation
            techniques, 143
        radiofrequency electrodes, 143
Brain, 129–133. *See also* Skull
    brain tumor, MRIgFUS treatment for, 89–90
    clinical MRI-guided focused ultrasound system,
            131–132
    clinical potential, 132–133
    large gain therapeutic ultrasound arrays,
            development, 131
Breast cancer
    ablation, disadvantages of, 108–109
    MRIgFUS treatment for, 87
Breast fibroadenoma, MRIgFUS treatment for, 85
Breast MRIgFUS, 101–110
    advantages, 108–109
    clinical applications, 104–106
    effectiveness, 105
    histopathology, 106–108
    patient selection criteria, 101–102
    Phase I clinical trial, 105
    Phase II clinical trial, 106
    prerequisites, 103
    techniques, 102–104

Breast-conservation treatment (BCT), 101
Bubble oscillations, 17
Bubble-enhanced heating, 63

Calcein (fluorescein-methylene-iminodiacetic
      acid), 149
Cancer treatment, MRIgFUS treatment for, 86–90
   bone tumors, 89
   brain tumor, 89–90
   breast cancer, 87. *See also separate entry*
   ExAblate® 3000, 90
   liver cancer, 87–88
   prostate cancer, 88
   renal tumors, 88–89
Caspase activity assay, 184
Cavitation, 17–18
   cavitation-based clinical applications, of
      MRIgFUS, 91–92
   cell cultures, 172
   detection, in phased array surgery, 56–58
   inertial cavitation in vivo, 18
   threshold pressure for, 17
Closed-loop feedback control, in MRIgFUS, 44–47
Closed-loop image-guided FUS system, 83
Computed axial tomography (CAT), 114
Computed tomography (CT) scan, 114
Craniotomy, 129
Cytochrome c, 183

Decoy oligonucleotides, 151, 152
Δψm, measurement, 184
Deoxynucleotidyl transferase to transfer 2'-
      deoxyuridine-5'-triphosphate (dUTP), 184
Diffusion MRI, 47
Diffusion weighting, 27
DNA double-strand breaks (DNA DSBs), 185
DNA fragmentation assay, 184
Drug delivery
   by ultrasound in vitro, 147–149
   by ultrasound in vivo, 149–152
Drug/gene therapy in animals models using
      sonoporation, 150–152

Elastography, 47
Electroporation, 150
Endometrial destruction techniques, 118
EPI techniques, 27
ExAblate 2000 system, 85, 116, 121, 124
ExAblate® 3000 system, 90

External US-guided devices, 2
Extracorporeal focused ultrasound, 33

Fast gradient-echo (FSE) acquisition strategy,
      28, 30, 32
Fibroadenoma, 102–105
   FUS treatment of, 102
Fibroids
   fibroids, uterine. *See* Uterine fibroids
   imaging, advantages for, 114
   large fibroids treatment
      MRIgFUS in, 137–138
   MR appearance of, 116–117
Field modeling, in radiation therapy, 70–74
   finite difference (FD) method in, 71
   finite element modeling (FEM) method in, 71–73
   k-space method, 73
   modeling propagation methods in, 71
   temporal or spatial planar projection (spectral)
      method in, 71
Fields, ultrasound, 8–11
   electrical focusing, 10–11
   focused ultrasonic fields, 9–11
   from a planar transducer, 8–9
   reflectors, 10
   ultrasonic lenses, 10
Finite difference (FD) method, 71
Finite element modeling (FEM) method, 71–73
Finite difference time-domain (FDTD) method, 73
Flow cytometers, 149
Fluorescence, 149
Focused ultrasound surgery (FUS) system, 1, 9–11,
      55–65. *See also* Phased array surgery
      system
   for brain tumors, 132–133
   spherically curved transducers, 9–10
   and US-contrast agent
      inducing apoptosis with, 188–189
Free radicals, sonodynamic effect via, 153–154
FUS. *See* Focused ultrasound

Gadolinium imaging, 116, 122
Gene therapy 92
Gonadotrophin-releasing hormone (GNRH)
      agonists, 138
Green fluorescent protein (GFP), 149

Heat shock promoter-driven transgene in kidney,
      US-induced expression

[Heat shock promoter-driven transgene in kidney, US-induced expression]
by genetically modified MSCs, 171–178
animal experiments and experimental protocol, 173–174
histological analysis, 174–175
luciferase assay, 174
materials and methods, 172–173
cell cultures, 172
DNA constructs, 173
MSC line generation, 173
MRI-controlled FUS hyperthermia, 173–175
results, 175–176
Heat shock proteins (HSP), 187
Herceptin®, 93
High-intensity focused ultrasound (HIFU)
procedures, 88
for prostate cancer, 88
for renal tumors, 88–89
Hypercellular white fibroid, 116
Hyperthermia, 187
MRI-guided, 83
Hysterectomy, 118

Ideal tumor surgery, 1, 82–84
Image-guided therapy, for uterine fibroids, 119
Inertial cavitation, 18, 154, 164
Integrated therapy delivery systems, 55–64
MRI-guided ultrasound phased array surgery system, 55–62. See also Phased array surgery system
Interstitial laser therapy (ILT), 132
Interstitial ultrasound probes, MRI-compatible, 44
Intracellular drug/gene delivery in vivo by sonoporation, 150
Intravenous conscious sedation (IVCS), 121

k-space method, 73

Laparoscopic hysterectomy, 118
Leiomyomata uteri, 111. See also Uterine fibroids
Lethal cell injury (cell death), 181 necrosis, 181
apoptosis, 181. See also separate entry
Liver cancer, MRIgFUS treatment for, 87–88
Liver MR-guided focused ultrasound, 138–141
difficulties, 140
overcoming, 140
respiratory movement, 140
Luciferase assay, 174, 177

Magnetic resonance imaging (MRI)
MRI-controlled FUS hyperthermia, 173–175
temperature sensitivity of, 25–29. See also Temperature sensitivity
Magnetic resonance imaging guided breast focused ultrasound surgery. See Breast MRIgFUS
Magnetic resonance imaging–guided focused ultrasound (MRIgFUS) surgery
for breast fibroadenoma, 85
cancer treatment, 86–90. See also separate entry
clinical applications, 85–86
clinical MRI-guided focused ultrasound system, 131–132
closed-loop feedback control, 44–47
development of technology, 81–84
experimental MRIgFUS devices, 43–44
experimental uses of, 43–50
MRI-compatible interstitial ultrasound probes, 44
MRI-compatible transesophageal probes, 44
MRI-compatible transrectal probes, 44
new clinical applications of, 137–145
for bones, 141–143. See also Bones
kidney, 141
in large fibroids treatment, 137–138
liver MR-guided focused ultrasound, 138–141.
See also individual entry
renal tumors, 141
new potential areas of treatment, 143–145
for non-neoplastic diseases, 90–93. See also separate entry
for slow-flow arterial venous malformations, 145
for soft-tissue abnormalities, 144
for tissue and acoustic characterization, 48–50
therapy delivery system for, 84–85
tissue damage induced by, detection, 47–48
for uterine fibroid, 86
uterine fibroids and, 111–125.
See also Uterine fibroids
Magnetic resonance temperature imaging (MRTI)
advanced MRTI and future directions, 37–38
fundamental principles of, 25–38. See also Proton resonance frequency; Temperature sensitivity
MRTI acquisition strategies for ultrasound ablation, 33–36
Mechanical effects, by US, 16–17
Medical therapy, for uterine fibroids, 119–120
Mesenchymal stem cells (MSCs), 171–178.
See also under Heat shock promoter-driven transgene
Metastatic bone tumors,
MRIgFUS treatment for, 89
Mitochondrial-dependent apoptotic pathway, 182–183
Molecular diffusion coefficient of water (D), 25
Molecular targets
apoptosis and, 182–183

[Molecular targets
  apoptosis and]
    mitochondrial-dependent apoptotic pathway,
      182–183
    pathways for apoptosis, 182
Molecular water mobility, 25
MR elastography (MRE) methods, 47
MRTI. *See* Magnetic resonance temperature
    imaging
Myolysis, 119
Myomectomy, 118

N-acetyl-cysteine (NAC), 186
Necrosis, 181
Noninvasive local hyperthermia, 176–178
  with MRI-controlled FUS in kidney, 174
Noninvasive real-time closed loop ablation
    methodology, 84
Noninvasive surgical procedures, 1
Nonlinear propagation, 14
Non-neoplastic diseases, MRIgFUS application of,
    90–93
  arthritic joints, 90–91
  BBB opening, 92–93
  cavitation-based clinical applications, 91–92
  gene therapy 92
  vascular occlusion, 91
Nonsurgical ablation, 108
Nuclear factor-kappa B (NFκB), 151

Oligodeoxynucleotide (ODN), 152
Optison, 148

p53 Activation, 151, 185
Pelvic imaging, MRI in, 114
Pelvic pressure, 112
Pennes bioheat transfer equation, 74
Percutaneous radiofrequency ablation
    techniques, 143
Phased array surgery system, MRI-guided, 55–62
  cavitation detection, 56–58
  description, 55–62
  future directions, 63–64
  MR imaging, 59–60
  safety monitoring, 56
  sonications, 59
  temperature monitoring, 60–62
  transducer array, 56
  treatment effect verification, 62

[Phased array surgery system, MRI-guided]
  treatment execution, 62
  treatment planning, 58–59
  treatment table, 56
  ultrasound reflection detection, 56–58
  US surgery using, 11
Phase-difference techniques, 32
Phosphatidylserine (PS), 184
Phosphorylation, 185
Photodynamic diagnosis (PDD), 153
Photodynamic therapy (PDT), 153
Piezoelectric effect, 6
Polarized polycrystalline ferroelectrics, 6
Porphyrins, 153–155
Propidium iodide (PI), 184
Prostate cancer, MRIgFUS treatment for, 88
Proton resonance frequency (PRF), 25–35, 173
  temperature sensitivity of water PRF, 29–33
Protoporphyrin IX (PPIX), 154

Quality of life (QOL)
  uterine fibroid–specific QOL instrument, 117,
    120, 123

Reactive oxygen species (ROS), 186
Renal tumors
  MRIgFUS treatment for, 88–89, 141
Repetition time (TR) baseline image, 28

Safety monitoring, in phased array surgery, 56
Second generation MRI-guided focused ultrasound
    system, 63
Sentinel lymph node (SLN) surgery, 108
Shear wave properties, 13–14
Singlet oxygen, sonodynamic effect via, 153
Skull
  focusing through human skull, 130–131
  ultrasound propagation through, 130
Slow-flow arterial venous malformations,
    MRIgFUS for, 145
Soft-tissue abnormalities, MRIgFUS for, 144
Sonications, 45
  in phased array surgery, 59
Sonodynamic therapy, 152–155
  in vitro versus in vivo sonodynamic effect,
    154–155
  sonodynamic effect
    via free radicals, 153–154
    via singlet oxygen, 153

[Sonodynamic therapy]
  using tumor-accumulating porphyrins, 153
Sonoporation
  evaluation methods, 149
  in vitro, 147–148
  in vivo, 150–152
    drug/gene therapy in animals models, 150–152
    intracellular drug/gene delivery, 150
  limitations, 148
  microbubbles in, 148
Spatio-temporal resolution, 33
Spectral planar projection techniques, 71–72
Spherically curved transducers, 9–10
Spin-lattice relaxation time (T_1), temperature
        sensitivity of, 28–29
    fast gradient-recalled echo (FSE) acquisition
        strategy, 28, 30, 32
    repetition time (TR) baseline image, 28
Stokes–Einstein relationship, 25–26
Superoxide dismutase (SOD), 186
Symptom severity scale (SSS), 123
Systemic agents, target delivery of, 152

Targeted drug delivery, 147–155
  drug delivery by ultrasound in vitro, 147–149
  drug delivery by ultrasound in vivo, 149–152
  sonoporation in vitro, 147–148. *See also*
        Sonoporation
  target delivery of systemic agents, 152
  ultrasound-induced cell lysis, 152–155. *See also*
        Sonodynamic therapy
Temperature monitoring, with MRI, 60–62, 63
Temperature sensitivity
  of molecular diffusion coefficient of
        water (D), 25
  of MRI, 25–29
  of spin-lattice relaxation time (T_1), 28–29
  temperature-sensitive MRI methods, 82
  of water PRF, 29–33
Temporal or spatial planar projection (spectral)
        method, 71
Terminal deoxynucleotidyl transferase biotin-dUTP
        nick end labeling (TUNEL) method, 184
Therapeutic ultrasound, fundamental principles,
        5–18
Therapy delivery system for MRIgFUS treatment,
        84–85
Thermal ablations, MRI role during, 83, 132
Thermal coagulation, 2
Thermal dose, in radiation therapy, 74–75
  Pennes bioheat transfer equation, 74
Thermal effects, by US, 15–16
Thermal lesions in rabbit brains, apoptosis in, 187
Thermometry, MRI-based, 49, 55

Tissue
  acoustic impedance, 13
  nonlinear propagation, 14
  shear wave properties, 13–14
  tissue characterization, MRIgFUS for, 48–50
  tissue damage induced by MRIgFUS
    MRI detection methods for, 47–48
  US propagation through, 12–14
    absorption and attenuation, 12–13
    speed of sound, 12
Trackless brain surgery, 85
Transducers, ultrasound, 6–7
  planar, 8–9
  spherically curved, 9–10
  transducer array, in phased array surgery, 56
Transesophageal probes, MRI-compatible, 44
Transrectal probes, MRI-compatible, 44
Transrectal US surgery devices, 2
Transvaginal ultrasonography (TVUS), 113
Treatment effect verification, in phased array
        surgery, 62
Treatment execution, in phased array surgery, 62
Treatment planning
  in phased array surgery, 58–59
  in radiation therapy, 69–78
    aberration correction, 75–77
    field modeling, 70–74. *See also* Field
        modeling
    thermal dose, 74–75
Treatment table, in phased array surgery, 56
Tumor necrosis factor-α (TNF-α), 182
Tumor treatment, apoptosis as target for, 181–182
Tumor-accumulating porphyrins
  sonodynamic therapy using, 153. *See also*
        Sonodynamic therapy

Ultrasound (US). *See also* Therapeutic
        ultrasound
  ablation, MRTI acquisition strategies for, 33–36
  biological effects of, 14–18. *See also* Biological
        effects
  delivery and MRI thermometry, 63
  generation of, 6–8
  propagation through skull, 130
  propagation through tissue, 12–14. *See also*
        Tissue
  ultrasound fields, 8–11. *See also* Fields
  ultrasound transducers, 6–7
  US driving system, 7–8
  US hyperthermia
    2-D MR thermometry-based control of, 46
  US reflection detection, in phased array surgery,
        56–58
  US surgery using phased arrays, 11

[Ultrasound (US)]
US-induced apoptosis, 181–189.
See also Apoptosis
US-induced cell lysis enhancement
by tumor-accumulating sonosensitizers,
152–155
US-induced expression
of heat shock promoter-driven transgene,
171–178. *See also* Heat shock
promoter-driven transgene
US-induced sonoporation, 150
Uterine fibroids
classification, 112
definition, 111
diagnosis, 113–117
imaging examination, 113–116
physical examination, 113
etiology and pathogenesis, 112
image-guided therapy, 119
incidence, 111–112
medical therapy, 119–120
MR appearance of, 114–115
MRIgFUS for, 120–125
clinical outcome study, 123–125
clinical trials and results, 122–123
ExAblate 2000 table, 121, 124
feasibility study, 123
patient selection, 120–121
procedure day, 121

[Uterine fibroids
MRIgFUS for]
skin injuries, 121
skin preparation, 121
MRIgFUS treatment for, 86
surgical therapy, 118–119
endometrial destruction techniques, 118
hysterectomy, 118
laparoscopic hysterectomy, 118
myolysis, 119
myomectomy, 118
symptoms, 112
abnormal bleeding, 112
acute pain, 112
pelvic pressure, 112
treatment, 117–118
outcome, assessing, 117–118
uterine fibroid embolization (UFE), 119
uterine fibroid symptoms quality of life
(UFS-QOL), 117
Uterine myomas, 118

Vascular occlusion, MRIgFUS treatment for, 91

Xenopus oocyte, 147